Effect of Processing on Sensory Quality and Bioactive Components in Food Products

Effect of Processing on Sensory Quality and Bioactive Components in Food Products

Guest Editors

Antonio José Pérez-López
Luis Noguera-Artiaga

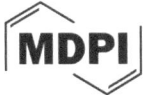

Basel • Beijing • Wuhan • Barcelona • Belgrade • Novi Sad • Cluj • Manchester

Guest Editors

Antonio José Pérez-López
San Antonio Catholic University
Murcia
Spain

Luis Noguera-Artiaga
Universidad Miguel Hernández de Elche
Orihuela
Spain

Editorial Office
MDPI AG
Grosspeteranlage 5
4052 Basel, Switzerland

This is a reprint of the Special Issue, published open access by the journal *Foods* (ISSN 2304-8158), freely accessible at: https://www.mdpi.com/journal/foods/special_issues/Sensory_Quality_Bioactive_Components.

For citation purposes, cite each article independently as indicated on the article page online and as indicated below:

Lastname, A.A.; Lastname, B.B. Article Title. *Journal Name* **Year**, *Volume Number*, Page Range.

ISBN 978-3-7258-2955-2 (Hbk)
ISBN 978-3-7258-2956-9 (PDF)
https://doi.org/10.3390/books978-3-7258-2956-9

© 2025 by the authors. Articles in this book are Open Access and distributed under the Creative Commons Attribution (CC BY) license. The book as a whole is distributed by MDPI under the terms and conditions of the Creative Commons Attribution-NonCommercial-NoDerivs (CC BY-NC-ND) license (https://creativecommons.org/licenses/by-nc-nd/4.0/).

Contents

About the Editors vii

Paula Torán-Pereg, Shuyana Deba-Rementeria, Olaia Estrada, Guillermo Pardo and Laura Vázquez-Araújo
Physicochemical and Sensory Evaluation Data to Drive the Development of a Green Chili Pepper Hot Sauce from Unexploited Raw Materials
Reprinted from: *Foods* **2023**, *12*, 3536, https://doi.org/10.3390/foods12193536 1

Ramiro Alonso-Salinas, Santiago López-Miranda, Ana González-Báidez, Antonio José Pérez-López, Luis Noguera-Artiaga, Estrella Núñez-Delicado, et al.
Effect of Potassium Permanganate, Ultraviolet Radiation and Titanium Oxide as Ethylene Scavengers on Preservation of Postharvest Quality and Sensory Attributes of Broccoli Stored with Tomatoes
Reprinted from: *Foods* **2023**, *12*, 2418, https://doi.org/10.3390/foods12122418 15

Helena Núñez, Aldonza Jaques, Karyn Belmonte, Andrés Córdova, German Lafuente and Cristian Ramírez
Effect of CO_2 Laser Microperforation Pretreatment on the Dehydration of Apple Slices during Refractive Window Drying
Reprinted from: *Foods* **2023**, *12*, 2187, https://doi.org/10.3390/foods12112187 32

Noluthando Noxolo Aruwajoye, Nana Millicent Duduzile Buthelezi, Asanda Mditshwa, Samson Zeray Tesfay and Lembe Samukelo Magwaza
Assessing the Impact of Roasting Temperatures on Biochemical and Sensory Quality of Macadamia Nuts (*Macadamia integrifolia*)
Reprinted from: *Foods* **2023**, *12*, 2116, https://doi.org/10.3390/foods12112116 46

Baoyuan Zang, Zhichang Qiu, Zhenjia Zheng, Bin Zhang and Xuguang Qiao
Quality Improvement of Garlic Paste by Whey Protein Isolate Combined with High Hydrostatic Pressure Treatment
Reprinted from: *Foods* **2023**, *12*, 1500, https://doi.org/10.3390/foods12071500 62

Tiantian Tang, Min Zhang and Bhesh Bhandari
Effects of Novel Preparation Technology on Flavor of Vegetable-Soy Sauce Compound Condiment
Reprinted from: *Foods* **2023**, *12*, 1263, https://doi.org/10.3390/foods12061263 75

Pan Gao, Yunpeng Ding, Zhe Chen, Zhangtao Zhou, Wu Zhong, Chuanrong Hu, et al.
Characteristics and Antioxidant Activity of Walnut Oil Using Various Pretreatment and Processing Technologies
Reprinted from: *Foods* **2022**, *11*, 1698, https://doi.org/10.3390/foods11121698 92

Vicente Manuel Gómez-López, Luis Noguera-Artiaga, Fernando Figueroa-Morales, Francisco Girón, Ángel Antonio Carbonell-Barrachina, José Antonio Gabaldón and Antonio Jose Pérez-López
Effect of Pulsed Light on Quality of Shelled Walnuts
Reprinted from: *Foods* **2022**, *11*, 1186, https://doi.org/10.3390/foods11091186 103

Beatriz Muñoz-Rosique, Eva Salazar, Julio Tapiador, Begoña Peinado and Luis Tejada
Effect of Salt Reduction on the Quality of Boneless Dry-Cured Ham from Iberian and White Commercially Crossed Pigs
Reprinted from: *Foods* **2022**, *11*, 812, https://doi.org/10.3390/foods11060812 115

Lijia Zhang, Xiaobo Dong, Xi Feng, Salam A. Ibrahim, Wen Huang and Ying Liu
Effects of Drying Process on the Volatile and Non-Volatile Flavor Compounds of *Lentinula edodes*
Reprinted from: *Foods* **2022**, *11*, 2836, https://doi.org/10.3390/foods10112836 . . . . **129**

Monika Janowicz, Agnieszka Ciurzyńska and Andrzej Lenart
Effect of Osmotic Pretreatment Combined with Vacuum Impregnation or High Pressure on the Water Diffusion Coefficients of Convection Drying: Case Study on Apples
Reprinted from: *Foods* **2021**, *10*, 2605, https://doi.org/10.3390/foods10112605 . . . . **142**

Yu-Jung Tsai, Li-Yun Lin, Kai-Min Yang, Yi-Chan Chiang, Min-Hung Chen and Po-Yuan Chiang
Effects of Roasting Sweet Potato (*Ipomoea batatas* L. Lam.): Quality, Volatile Compound Composition, and Sensory Evaluation
Reprinted from: *Foods* **2021**, *10*, 2602, https://doi.org/10.3390/foods10112602 . . . . **158**

Angela Mariela González-Montemayor, José Fernando Solanilla-Duque, Adriana C. Flores-Gallegos, Claudia Magdalena López-Badillo, Juan Alberto Ascacio-Valdés and Raúl Rodríguez-Herrera
Green Bean, Pea and Mesquite Whole Pod Flours Nutritional and Functional Properties and Their Effect on Sourdough Bread
Reprinted from: *Foods* **2021**, *10*, 2227, https://doi.org/10.3390/foods10092227 . . . . **171**

Paola Sánchez-Bravo, Luis Noguera-Artiaga, Vicente M. Gómez-López, Ángel A. Carbonell-Barrachina, José A. Gabaldón and Antonio J. Pérez-López
Impact of Non-Thermal Technologies on the Quality of Nuts: A Review
Reprinted from: *Foods* **2022**, *11*, 3891, https://doi.org/10.3390/foods11233891 . . . . **186**

Ana Belén Díaz, Enrique Durán-Guerrero, Cristina Lasanta and Remedios Castro
From the Raw Materials to the Bottled Product: Influence of the Entire Production Process on the Organoleptic Profile of Industrial Beers
Reprinted from: *Foods* **2022**, *11*, 3215, https://doi.org/10.3390/foods11203215 . . . . **200**

About the Editors

Antonio J. Pérez-López

Prof. Dr. Antonio Jose Perez-Lopez is a food engineer (1996) and graduate in Food Science and Technology (1999). He received his master's degree in Biotechnology and Tropical Fruits (2001) from Miguel Hernández University of Elche. Then, he received his PhD from the Miguel Hernández University of Elche (Spain) in 2004. Antonio Jose is an Associate Professor at the Catholic University of San Antonio of Murcia. He is also a researcher in three research groups, namely Food Processing, Molecular Encapsulation and Recognition, and Fruit and Vegetable Preservation. His research is based on the study of sensory analysis in food and the impact that agricultural practices have on the quality of these characteristics. He has published various works comparing organic foods with traditional ones, performing sensory analysis in the development of new foods, and examining the influence and characterization of aromatic profiles in different foods, as well as quality improvement through the use of non-thermal treatments. He has also written multiple publications on conservation in post-collection technology, among other studies. Currently, as a professor and researcher, he teaches on modules as part of the degrees of Human Nutrition and Dietetics as well as Food Science and Technology. He is also a professor in different master's degrees such as Nutrition and Food Safety, Teacher Training, and Bibliographic Search and Analysis for Future Science Doctors.

Luis Noguera-Artiaga

Luis Noguera Artiaga is a graduate in Food Science and Technology (2014) and received his master's degree in Advanced Research Techniques in Fruit Growing (2015) from the Miguel Hernández University of Elche. Then, he received his first PhD from the University of Sonora (Mexico) in 2019, and he received his second PhD from the Miguel Hernández University of Elche in 2020. Luis is an Assistant Professor at the Institute of Agro-Food and Agro-Environmental Research and Innovation at the Miguel Hernández University of Elche. His research is based on the study of sensory analysis in food and the impact that agricultural practices have on the quality of these characteristics. Among other factors, he studies the influence that different types of irrigation have on the quality of agri-food products by studying their physical, chemical, functional, bio-functional and sensory properties. In addition, he studies the impact that aroma has on the flavor and quality of food by analyzing its volatile organic compounds. Luis has participated in the training of sensory analysis panels at wine, vegetable, paprika, beer, ice cream, and chocolate companies. He has conducted more than 100 consumer studies (national and international) and he has accumulated more than 5000 hours of experience in sensory analysis as a panelist in descriptive and discriminative tests on all types of foods.

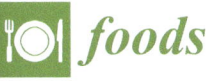

Article

Physicochemical and Sensory Evaluation Data to Drive the Development of a Green Chili Pepper Hot Sauce from Unexploited Raw Materials

Paula Torán-Pereg [1,2], Shuyana Deba-Rementeria [1,2], Olaia Estrada [1], Guillermo Pardo [3] and Laura Vázquez-Araújo [1,2,*]

[1] BCC Innovation, Technology Center in Gastronomy, Basque Culinary Center, 20009 Donostia-San Sebastián, Spain
[2] Basque Culinary Center, Faculty of Gastronomic Sciences, Mondragon Unibertsitatea, 20009 Donostia-San Sebastián, Spain
[3] Basque Centre for Climate Change (BC3), 48940 Leioa, Spain
* Correspondence: lvazquez@bculinary.com

Abstract: The present study shows the set of analyses conducted during the development of a hot chili pepper sauce to valorize green peppers usually discarded in the Espelette region (France). A traditional production process was used as the inspiration for product development, and two different fermentation processes were assessed and characterized by measuring pH, sugar content, instrumental color, volatile composition, and conducting sensory (discriminant test) and microbiological analyses (total plate count). Significant differences were observed among pepper mash samples with respect to their physicochemical characteristics, but the products were considered similar from a sensory standpoint. Both sensory and physicochemical tests suggested that the ingredients added to make the sauces were determinant and had a higher impact on the organoleptic profile of the final product than the fermentation process. Finally, a Napping® test was conducted to determine the attributes that could differentiate the product from the hot sauces found in the current market. The results of the present research allowed the optimization of the elaboration process of the new product, saving time and ingredient costs. The procedures shown in the study could be used as an example of a new product development process in which physicochemical and sensory data are collected and used for decision making.

Keywords: Espelette; new product development; food waste; fermentation; Napping®

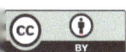

1. Introduction

The geographical origin of peppers (*Capsicum* spp.) has been reported to be tropical America [1] but, thanks to its adaptability to different environments, this plant has spread across different parts of the world, mainly warm-temperature regions [2,3]. Over 20 to 30 species of pepper have been identified, including five domesticated species: *C. annuum*, *C. chinese*, *C. pubescens*, *C. frutescens*, and *C. baccatum* [4,5]. This huge biodiversity has given rise to a great variety of fruits with unique morphologic (e.g., shape and size) and organoleptic characteristics (e.g., color, flavor, pungency), and different gastronomic cultures have developed diverse products and applications from peppers (e.g., fresh, dried, processed as spices, pickled, pastes, sauces, or roasted).

Espelette peppers (*C. annuum* var. Gorria) are one of the most renowned peppers in the Basque Country. Their growth in specific natural conditions (e.g., landscape, weather, soil, plant varieties, etc.), together with localized human factors (e.g., habits, culture, specific know-how, etc.), allowed the registration of Espelette peppers as having Protected Designation of Origin (PDO *Piment d'Espelette—Ezpeletako Biperra*, in the French and Basque languages, respectively) status in the European Union in 2012 [6]. The specifications of this regulation indicate that at least 80% of the surface of the pepper must be red when harvested to belong to the "Espelette pepper" PDO [7], among other requirements. At the end of the harvesting season (before 1 December), when the sun is less intense and the plant is at the end of its vegetative cycle, some fruits are not completely ripened (still being green) and are characterized by their intense spiciness. Because of the lack of commercial outlets, tons of green fruits remain on the plant and end up being discarded.

Gastronomy has been proven useful for identifying and up-cycling discarded foods, transforming them into new ingredients with higher values and acceptance [8–11]. Different Asian, African, and American food cultures are characterized by chili peppers, demonstrating that spicy food is particularly popular in some gastronomies [1,12–14]. Although traditional Basque cuisine is not recognized as being spicy, hot sauces are spreading to food cultures in which this flavor characteristic is not typical. These sauces are market-oriented products of which consumption is globally increasing, probably due to factors such as increases in trade, migration, travelling, and the current trend of consuming ethnic foods in the western regions [13,15–17].

The production processes of some of these sauces (e.g., tabasco, sriracha) include a fermentation process of the peppers, which can last from two weeks to three years [18,19]. In this fermentation, peppers are mashed together with salt, generating a selective environment in which the growth of lactic-acid bacteria (LAB) is favored [20]. The selected microorganisms metabolize the different components of the food matrix and produce organic acids, volatile compounds, etc., which bring the distinctive organoleptic properties and contribute to the nutritional profile of the resulting product, increasing its value and driving consumers' acceptance [21]. Fermentation processes can be classified in two main categories: spontaneous fermentations and driven fermentations. The first one, which has been widely used in homemade and culinary fields [22,23], results from the competition between the autochthonous microorganisms (yeasts, fungi, aerobic and anaerobic bacteria) present in the product, but these spontaneous fermentations may easily fail due to contamination [24]. Driven fermentations require the addition of a specific starter (e.g., a lactic acid bacteria strain), ensuring a more standardized product. Previous research has reported that the use of autochthonous isolated bacteria is a preferable process to drive a specific fermentation, because these bacteria may be better adapted to the raw material [25,26]. To finish the hot pepper sauce making process, after the fermentation, the pepper mash is generally mixed with other ingredients such as vinegar, garlic, sugar, water, vegetables, etc., to obtain a specific final product [18]. Considering all the ingredients, and the complexity of flavor of this product category, the role of fermentation could be linked to the preservation of the raw materials more than bringing specific sensory notes to the final product.

The aim of this study was to develop a green chili pepper hot sauce to valorize the unexploited green peppers of the Espelette region, using sensory and physicochemical data to propose an optimized process and successful product. Different methods, that allowed characterization of the process, prototypes, and products, were used in the present research, including sugars determination, instrumental color, volatile composition, discriminant sensory tests, and Napping®.

2. Materials and Methods

2.1. Reagents

Ultrapure water (Type I, 18.2 mΩ-cm) was from an Elga Purelab Flex 3 (ELGA LabWater, High Wycombe, UK). Sodium chloride (99.9%) was supplied by VWR (VWR Inc., Darmstadt, Germany). Analytical quality grade standards of glucose (1000 mg L^{-1}), fructose, and sucrose were supplied by Sigma-Aldrich (Merck KGaA, Darmstadt, Germany). Sodium hydroxide solution (1 mol L^{-1}) and sodium acetate anhydrous (>99%) (HPLC mobile phase) were supplied by Panreac AppliChem (Panreac AppliChem, Barcelona, Spain) and Sigma-Aldrich (Merck KgaA, Darmstadt, Germany), respectively. Peptone saline solution, Man, Rogosa and Sharpe (MRS) agar and nutrient agar were from VWR (VWR Inc., Darmstadt, Germany). The alkane standard mixture for gas chromatography–

mass spectrometry compound identification was purchased from Sigma-Aldrich (Merck KgaA, Darmstadt, Germany).

2.2. Pepper Samples and Sauce Making Samples

Green peppers (*C. annuum* var. Gorria) were obtained from a local producer from Espelette (France). The samples were harvested during the last week of November 2021, washed in tap water, and stored in a freezer ($-20\ °C$) until processing. The list of ingredients and summary of the processes used to make and analyze the 3 prototypes is shown in Figure 1; the main differences among them were linked to the fermentation process, to assess the impact of this stage in the final product.

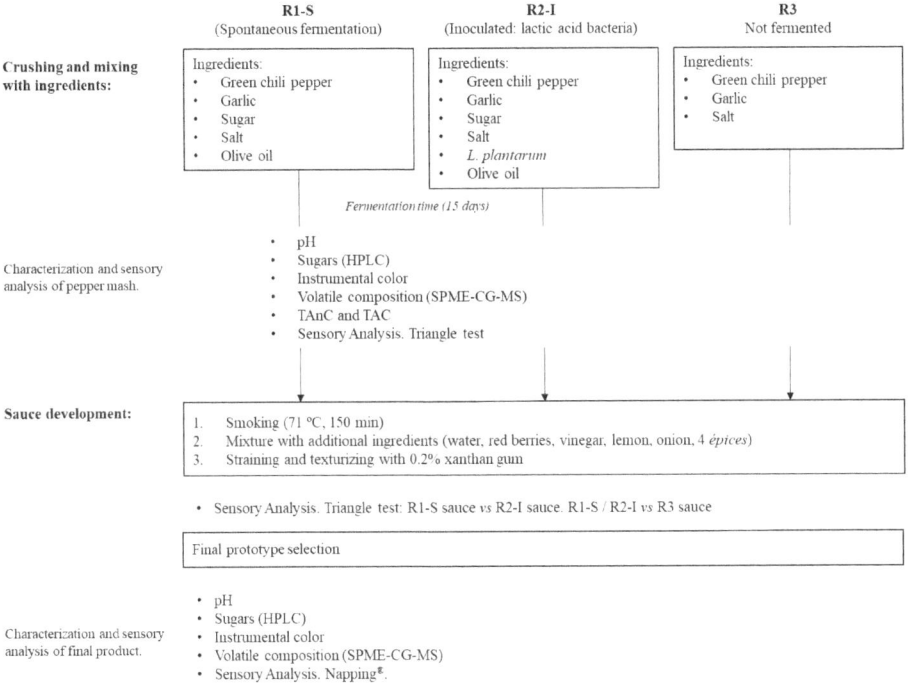

Figure 1. Scheme of the processes studied during the present research.

The peduncles of the fruits were removed, and the rest of the peppers were mashed in a blender with different ingredients (Thermomix TM6, Wuppertal, Germany). The samples to be fermented (R1 and R2) were transferred to sterilized glass jars (500 g/jar); one batch was left to ferment using the autochthonous microorganisms (spontaneous fermentation, R1-S), and the other one was inoculated with *Lactobacillus plantarum* Harvest LB-1 (0.08% as suggested by the producer of the starter; Chr Hansen, Hvidovre, Denmark) (R2-I). *L. plantarum* was chosen due to being one of the multiple lactic-acid bacteria found in peppers, which has been previously studied in pepper fermentation [25,27,28]. The samples were covered with 20 mL extra virgin olive oil (Urzante, Tudela, Spain) to avoid the surface coming into contact with the oxygen of the head space, sealed tightly, and stored at room temperature (21–24 °C) for 15 days. One of the samples (R3) was directly processed without fermentation into the final product; therefore, sugar was not added to this sample, and it was considered an example of the "original mash" at time 0 days. The three mash samples (R1-S, R2-I, and R3) were smoked (at 72 °C for 150 min) and mixed with other ingredients to finish the formula of the sauce (Figure 1). Then, samples were strained and thickened with xanthan gum (0.2%), obtaining 3 different prototypes of sauce.

2.3. Characterization of the Fermentation Process and Products: Green Chili Pepper Mashes and Sauces

The original mix, the fermented mash, and the final products were analyzed using different physicochemical analyses. Microbiological analyses were performed to verify that the fermentation procedures used in R1-S and R2-I were driven by different microorganisms and, therefore, that using the starter added in R2-I could result in a different product. All analyses were run in triplicate. In addition, sensory tests were performed to determine the differences among samples.

2.3.1. Determination of pH

The pH was determined at 20 ± 0.5 °C using a digital pH meter (Crison Basic 20, Crison instruments, Barcelona, Spain) calibrated with standard buffer solutions.

2.3.2. Microbiological Analysis

The mash samples were diluted in tenfold series in saline peptone solution (0.85% NaCl and 1% peptone) and plated onto different culture media to quantify the presence of different microorganisms using a traditional Plate Count Agar (PCA) method (ISO 4833-1:2013) [29]: nutrient agar for total viable colonies in aerobic conditions (30 °C for 48 h) and MRS agar for lactic acid bacteria (37 °C for 72 h, in anaerobic conditions).

2.3.3. Determination of Sugars

Sugars determinations were conducted as reported by Razola-Díaz et al. [30] with some modifications. Freeze-dried mash samples were diluted 1:100 (v/v) with ultrapure water at 60 °C, then shaken for 30 min, and centrifugated at $2367 \times g$ for 10 min. The supernatant was filtered using a 25 mm, 0.45 μm nylon VWR® Syrenge Filter (VWR Inc., Darmstadt, Germany), and 50 μL were injected in the same equipment as Deba-Rementeria et al. [8], using the same column and conditions indicated by these authors. Calibration curves for glucose, fructose, and sucrose, were used to quantify the presence of these compounds, identified by retention time.

2.3.4. Instrumental Color

The color of the samples was measured with a Chroma Meter CR 400 (Konica Minolta, Inc., Osaka, Japan). CIE $L^*a^*b^*$ color space, an illuminant D65, and a 10° observer were used as references. Data were expressed with the L^*, a^*, and b^* values and then, chroma $[C^* = (a^{*2} + b^{*2})^{1/2}]$, hue angle $[H = \tan^{-1}(b^*/a^*)]$, and total color change $[\Delta E^* = [(L^* - L_0^*)^2 + (a^* - a_0^*)^2 + (b^* - b_0^*)^2]^{1/2}]$ were calculated. Ten measurements were made for each of the samples' replicates.

2.3.5. Analysis of Volatile Composition

The volatile compositions of the samples were determined by headspace solid phase micro-extraction (HS-SPME) using the same conditions, fiber, column, and equipment reported by Deba-Rementeria et al. [31]. A total of 0.5 g of freeze-dried sample was weighted and ultrapure water (10 mL) and NaCl (1.0 g) were added into the 40 mL vial with polypropylene caps and PTFE/silicone septa for the extraction and processing as reported by these authors. Retention indexes of a commercial alkane standard mixture (Sigma-Aldrich, Steinheim, Germany) were used to identify the compounds, as well as the NIST 17 Mass Spectral and Retention Index Libraries [32]. The identification was considered tentative when only based on mass spectral data; a linear retention similarity filter was set at ± 10 units. The relative abundance of each compound was expressed as the percentage (%) of the total arbitrary area units.

2.3.6. Sensory Analysis of the Samples

The protocol for the consumer study was approved by the ethics committee of Mondragon Unibertsitatea (IEB-20221115). All articles from the Declaration of Helsinki and the 2016/679 EU Regulation on the protection of natural persons regarding the processing of personal data and on the free movement of such data were met. The experimental procedure was explained to and a written consent indicating voluntary participation was obtained from each participant prior to beginning the study. The tasting sessions were conducted in a sensory lab with individual booths and controlled temperature and relative humidity (21 ± 2 °C; 55 ± 5% RH); the illumination was a combination of natural and non-natural light (fluorescent). To determine if sensory differences could be perceptive between products, a triangle test was performed following the UNE-EN ISO 4120:2022 procedure, considering a = 0.05 and the recommended randomization design (ABB, AAB, ABA, BAA, BBA, BAB) [33]. A panel of 25 assessors trained for discriminant tests participated in the study and conducted a series of triangle tests in different sessions: (1) R1-S mash sample vs. R2-I mash sample; (2) R1-S sauce vs. R2-I sauce; and (3) R1-S and R2-I sauces vs. R3 sauce. Cream and breadsticks were provided for palate cleansing between samples.

After observing that the prototypes were considered similar from a sensory standpoint, a Napping® test [34] was conducted with the R3 sample to identify similitudes and differences between the developed sauce and similar products found in the local supermarkets (13 samples; shown in Table 1). A total of 21 professional chefs/gastronomes participated in the session to ensure familiarity with the product category. Approximately 10 mL of each sample were served in 20 mL disposable cups coded with 3-digit random numbers. Participants were asked to smell and taste the sauces and place them in an A3 paper (297 × 420 mm), close together or further apart, depending on their similarities/differences. In addition, assessors were instructed to include descriptors for each sauce/group of sauces. Cream and breadsticks were provided for palate cleansing between samples.

Table 1. Sauce samples tested in the Napping® test.

Code	Hot Sauce Type	Origin
200	Tabasco	USA
383	Tabasco chipotle	USA
274	Green tabasco	USA
958	Mexican green sauce	Mexico
394	Mexican red sauce	Mexico
664	Valentina	Mexico
060	Thai sriracha	Thailand
765	Spanish sriracha	Spain
491	Pasilla sauce	Denmark
587	Soya-based chilli sauce	Japan
332	Gochujang	South Korea
605	Kimchi	Japan
986	R3—sample	Spain

2.4. Data Analysis

Physicochemical and microbiological determinations were analyzed using one-way Analysis of Variance (ANOVA) using "recipe" as factor, followed by post-hoc Tukey's HSD test (α = 0.05). The results of the triangular test were analyzed as suggested by the UNE-EN ISO 4120:2008 procedure [33]; the significance was determined by considering the minimum number of correct responses. A multiple-factor analysis was carried out with the Napping® test [35]. The results were analyzed using XLSTAT (Version, 2021.5, Addinsoft, Denver, CO, USA) [36].

3. Results and Discussion

3.1. Mash Characterizations: Role of the Fermentation Process

Table 2 shows the initial pH of the original green chili pepper mash without fermentation, corresponding to sample R3 (5.2), and both R1-S and R2-I mash samples after 15 days of fermentation, which had a significantly lower pH value ($p \leq 0.05$). The inoculated sample (R2-I) reached a lower pH (3.7) than the spontaneously fermented sample (4.8).

Similar results have been reported by other authors; Di Cagno et al. [25] showed that spontaneously fermented red and yellow peppers (C. annuum L.) had higher pH values (pH above 4.8) than those inoculated with autochthonous bacteria (L. plantarum PE21, L. curvatus PE4, and W. confuse PE36) (approximately 3.6). Aryee et al. [17] reported a decrease of pH from 5.24 to 4.87 after 14 days of fermentation in habanero peppers (C. chinese) fermented spontaneously in a brine with a 5% salt concentration. The pH of Tabasco pepper mash (C. fructescens grinded with 8% salt), changed from 4.7 to 3.9–3.7, depending on the material of the container (plastic and wood, respectively), after the first month of a spontaneous fermentation [37]. The results of the present study suggested that using a low salt concentration, together with the inoculation of a commercial L. plantarum strain, favored the pH decrease. These results support the use of microorganisms well-adapted to the medium to promote the fermentation process. Reaching low pH values is recommended to ensure food safety while avoiding refrigeration of the product, because shelf stable hot sauces must have a pH below 4.6 [38].

Table 2. Physicochemical and microbiological characteristics of the three green chili pepper mash samples.

Mash Samples (Time in Days)	pH	Sugars (mg g^{-1})			Log CFU/mL	
		Sucrose	Glucose	Fructose	TAC	TanC
R1-S (T15)	4.83 b	1.53 c	28.85 c	29.11 b	3.5 b	5.2 ab
R2-I (T15)	3.66 c	1.70 b	24.41 b	28.43 b	3.8 b	8.8 a
R3 (T0)	5.22 a	25.25 a	17.13 a	18.04 a	5.6 a	4.6 b
p-value	0.0001	<0.0001	0.001	<0.001	0.001	0.024

Note: Different letters within the column indicate different post hoc groupings by Tukey's HSD ($p \leq 0.05$).

Significant differences were found in total aerobic counts (TAC) and total anaerobic counts (TanC) among the samples (Table 2). TAC significantly decreased during fermentation in both the R1-S and R2-I samples, probably due to the lack of a proper environment for aerobic microorganism development. TanC increased in both samples during fermentation, starting from 4.6 log CFU ml^{-1} and reaching a significantly different amount in R2-I T15 (8.8 log CFU mL^{-1}), the sample inoculated with L. plantarum. No significant differences were found between the pepper mashes T0 and R1-S at T15, although a slight increase was observed after 15 days of fermentation. Di Cagno et al. [25] showed an increment in lactic acid bacteria counts (L. plantarum, L. curvatus, and W. confusa) in peppers fermented at 35 °C during 15 days in a brine (1% NaCl), passing from approximately 4 log CFU/g to 9 log CFU/g; these authors reported higher increments in the samples in which starters were used. An increase in LAB count was also reported by Janiszewska-Turak et al. [27], who studied the differences between a spontaneous fermentation of green peppers (C. anuumm L.) vs. a fermentation driven by an inoculated starter of Levilactobacillus brevis, Limoslactobacillus fermentum, and L. plantarum. Fermentation time was different between the present study and the one reported by Janiszewska-Turak et al. [27] (15 days and 7 days, respectively), which may have led to a different result than the one obtained in the present study.

All color parameters varied significantly ($p \leq 0.05$) during the fermentation process (Table 3). Lightness (L^*), the blue-yellow coordinate (b^*), chroma, and hue increments were significantly higher in the R2-I mash sample. On the contrary, the red-green coordinate (a^*) and the total color transformation, represented by ΔE^*, were higher in the mash sample of the spontaneous fermentation (R1-S). The fermented samples' colors were significantly different from the original mash, ΔE^* being over 5 in both the R1-S (T15) and R2-I (T15) samples; ΔE^* has been reported to show differences between treated and untreated samples when being over 0.5 in citrus products [31,39]. Janiszewska-Turak et al. [27] reported that, in general, the L^*, a^*, and b^* coordinates increased during the fermentation of green peppers driven by different microorganisms, with a higher increase of L^* in the samples fermented by *L. plantarum*, and a higher increase of a^* in the spontaneously fermented samples.

Table 3. Instrumental color characteristics of the three different green chili pepper mash samples.

Mash Samples (Time in Days)	L^*	a^*	b^*	Chroma	Hue (Rad.)	ΔE^*
R1-S (T15)	43.45 b	2.45 a	35.67 b	35.75 b	1.50 b	11.92 a
R2-I (T15)	46.12 a	1.97 b	38.62 a	38.67 a	1.52 a	5.66 b
R3 (T0)	42.12 c	−7.87 c	33.02 c	33.95 c	1.34 c	-
p-value	<0.0001	<0.0001	<0.0001	<0.0001	<0.0001	<0.0001

Note: Different letters within the column indicate different post hoc groupings by Tukey's HSD ($p \leq 0.05$).

The volatile compositions of the mash samples are shown in Table 4. In general, the volatile compositions of the mash samples were mainly represented by compounds found in garlic such as diallyl disulfide or allyl methyl trisulfide [40,41], and other compounds previously found in chili peppers (e.g., 2-Isobutyl-3-methoxypyrazine, several aldehydes and alcohols [42]). Significant differences were found among samples, suggesting that the fermentation process influenced the aromatic profile of the samples.

To assess if the differences found in the physicochemical compositions of the mashes were perceived by the human senses, triangle tests were conducted with a trained panel of 25 assessors. Results showed that no significant differences were perceived between fermented mashes (correct answers = 10; at least 13 correct answers were needed to consider samples to be significantly different considering a = 0.05), suggesting that the different processes led to products that could be considered different from a sensory standpoint. The pungency of the mash samples could have influenced the perception of the differences identified in their volatile compositions or sugars profiles. Therefore, because other ingredients would be later incorporated to finish the product, and these could have a significant effect on their perception, additional triangle tests were conducted to determine if the three samples of sauce prototypes were perceived as different. No significant differences were detected among sauce samples, suggesting that, in general, the ingredients had a higher effect on the flavor of the sauces than the production process. The results of the sensory tests leads to the conclusion that the fermentation stage, although typically conducted in other products of the same category [18,19], was unnecessary to develop the proposed new product of the present research, probably because the contribution of the fermentation to the organoleptic properties of the sauce was limited in this product.

Table 4. Volatile composition of the mash samples expressed in relative abundance (% of total area).

Compound	RI (Exp)	RI (Lit)	R1-S (T15)	R2-1 (T15)	R3 (T0)	p-Value	Descriptor *
Hexanal	808	810	1.68	3.07	2.23	0.337	Fresh green, fatty, grass, leafy.
Disulfide, methyl 2-propenyl	922	920	4.59	5.02	5.03	0.862	Alliaceous, garlic, green, onion.
2-Heptenal	953	954	8.42	17.76	8.75	0.082	Pungent, green, vegetable.
Dimethyl trisulfide	963	976	0.83 b	0.52 b	2.10 a	**0.004**	Sulfureous, alliaceous, cooked.
1-Octen-3-ol	978	978	1.99	5.41	4.18	0.217	Sweet, mushroom, fungal, earthy.
Limonene	1034	1026	19.65 a	7.21 b	1.03 b	**0.007**	Citrus, range, fresh, sweet.
3-Octen-2-one	1044	1040	0.21	0.39	0.15	0.132	Earthy, spicy, herbal, sweet, mushroom.
Benzene acetaldehyde	1048	1045	0.55	0.27	0.31	0.516	Green, sweet, floral.
2-Octenal	1055	1056	1.58 b	4.17 a	1.20 b	**0.014**	Fatty, green, herbal.
2-Octen-1-ol	1065	n.d.	0.95	1.84	1.66	0.297	Green, vegetable.
1-Octanol	1069	n.d.	5.07	0.63	0.08	0.414	Waxy, green, orange.
Diallyl disulphide	1075	1087	12.70	16.45	14.25	0.714	Alliaceous, onion, garlic, metallic.
Allyl disulfide	1090	1087	3.94	1.97	1.81	0.248	Alliaceous, onion, garlic, metallic.
Allyl (E)-1-Propenyl disulfide	1096	n.d.	2.14	4.39	5.97	0.144	Sulfurous, alliaceous.
Linalool	1098	1095	3.07	1.37	n.d.	0.408	Citrus, floral, sweet.
Nonanal	1104	1102	4.47	0.31	0.62	0.442	Waxy, aldehydic, rose.
Allyl methyl trisulfide	1135	1135	8.42	9.51	16.04	0.171	Alliaceous, creamy, garlic, onion.
2,6-Nonadienal	1149	1154	n.d. b	n.d. b	0.19 a	**<0.0001**	Green, fatty, dry, cucumber.
2-Nonenal	1157	1162	1.04 b	0.67 b	1.67 a	**0.002**	Fatty, green, waxy, cucumber.
2-Isobutyl-3-methoxypyrazine	1173	1183	n.d. b	n.d. b	0.28 a	**<0.0001**	Green pea, green bell pepper.
3-Vinyl-1,2-dithi-4-ene	1181	1180	2.82 b	1.99 b	10.96 a	**<0.001**	n.d.
Methyl salicylate	1186	1190	0.19 b	0.23 b	0.57 a	**0.001**	Wintergreen mint.
UNK.	1188	n.d.	2.11 ab	1.69 b	3.41 a	**0.017**	n.d.
UNK.	1206	1214	1.75 b	1.55 b	6.85 a	**0.001**	n.d.
2,4-Nonadienal	1212	1215	n.d. b	0.71 a	0.26 b	**<0.0001**	Fatty, melon, waxy.
2-Decenal	1261	1264	1.74 ab	3.55 a	0.15 b	**0.004**	Waxy, fatty, earthy, coriander.
Allyl trisulfide	1294	1300	7.97	7.28	7.55	0.869	Sulfurous, green, onion, garlic, metallic.
2,4-Decadienal	1312	1312	0.97	1.00	0.79	0.263	Fatty, oily, green.
Allyl trisulfide	1317	1300	0.40	0.19	0.54	0.383	Alliaceous, creamy, garlic, onion.
Eugenol	1340	1352	0.24	0.14	0.33	0.563	Sweet, spicy, clove, woody.
b-Phenylethyl butyrate	1398	1447	0.18	0.45	0.58	0.070	Musty, sweet, floral.
Tetradecane	1400	1400	0.32 a	0.25 ab	0.15 b	**0.029**	Mild, waxy.
b-Chamigrene	1473	1475	n.d. b	n.d. b	0.30 a	**<0.001**	n.d.

Legend: Retention indexes (RI), experimental (Exp) and found in literature (Lit). Bold letter to highlight the compounds significantly different among samples. Different letters within the row indicate different post hoc groupings by Tukey's HSD ($p \leq 0.05$). UNK: unknown compounds. * TGSC Information System [43].

The use of different sensory tests, such as discriminant tests, combined with physicochemical data has proven to be useful in the decision-making process of different product developments such as ice cream recipe reformulations [44], testing the application of degreening treatments in citrus [45], or estimating the shelf lives of fish broth products [46]. The present study supports the need to use at least simple sensory tests, as well as physicochemical data, in the design process of a product.

3.2. Final Product Characterization

Tables 5 and 6 show the physicochemical characteristics and volatile composition of the final sauce sample. The mixture of the mashes with the additional ingredients significantly modified their characteristics, resulting in what could be considered a kind of product with homogeneous sensory characteristics. The pH of the final product was significantly lower ($p < 0.05$) than the pH of the mashes, probably due to the addition of lemon juice, comprising 8%. The pH reached after adding this ingredient (pH = 3.3) ensured the absence of pathogen bacteria growth because it is under 4 [47], and supported the results of the sensory tests, confirming that the fermentation stage was not useful to differentiate the flavor of the product, nor was it necessary from a technical standpoint.

Table 5. Main physicochemical characteristics of the sauce prototype.

	Mean	SD
pH	3.3	0.17
Sucrose (mg g^{-1})	0.85	0.18
Glucose (mg g^{-1})	16.96	3.51
Fructose (mg g^{-1})	17.50	3.51
L^*	23.67	0.86
a^*	19.37	1.63
b^*	7.16	0.71
Chroma	20.65	1.76
Hue (rad.)	0.35	0.01

Table 6. Volatile composition of the final sauce sample (% of total area).

Compound	RI (Exp)	RI (Lit)	Mean (%)	SD	Descriptor *
Hexanal	802	810	0.21	0.01	Fresh green, fatty, grass, leafy.
3,4-Dimethylthiophene	903	888	0.23	0.13	Savory roasted onion.
Disulfide, methyl 2-propenyl	913	922	0.83	0.22	Alliaceous, garlic, green, onion.
a-Pinene	932	930	0.19	0.09	Dry, woody, resinous-piney.
2-Heptenal	952	954	2.69	0.51	Pungent, green, vegetable.
b-Myrcene	988	989	0.45	0.13	Woody, vegetative, citrus, fruity, tropical.
p-Cymene	1022	1031	0.49	0.16	Fresh, citrus, terpene, woody, spice.
Limonene	1027	1026	15.76	1.19	Citrus, range, fresh, sweet.
Benzene acetaldehyde	1038	1048	0.09	0.02	Green, sweet, floral.
1-Octanol	1069	1071	0.30	0.16	Waxy, green, orange.
Diallyl disulfide	1075	1087	6.69	1.72	Alliaceous, onion, garlic, metallic.
o-Guaiacol	1080	1088	0.38	0.11	Phenolic, smoky, spicy, medicinal.
Allyl (Z)-1-Propenyl disulfide	1089	1104	0.51	0.34	Sulfurous, alliaceous.
Allyl (E)-1-Propenyl disulfide	1096	n.d.	1.86	0.75	Sulfurous, alliaceous.
Linalool	1098	1098	2.41	1.53	Citrus, floral, sweet.
Nonanal	1103	1102	0.31	0.07	Waxy, aldehydic, rose.
Phenylethyl alcohol	1107	n.d.	0.14	0.01	Floral, rose, dried rose.
Fenchol	1114	1117	0.04	0.02	Camphor, pine, woody.
Allyl methyl trisulfide	1131	1135	2.76	1.51	Alliaceous, creamy, garlic, onion.
2-Nonenal	1157	1162	0.25	0.05	Fatty, green, waxy, cucumber.
Isoborneol	1165	1156	0.15	0.01	Balsam, camphor, herbal, woody.

Table 6. *Cont.*

Compound	RI (Exp)	RI (Lit)	Mean (%)	SD	Descriptor *
Terpinen-4-ol	1176	1177	3.47	0.41	Musty, dusty.
3-Vinyl-1,2-dithiacyclohex-4-ene	1180	1180	1.26	1.16	n.d.
Methyl salicylate	1186	1190	0.31	0.15	Wintergreen mint.
a-Terpineol	1190	1197	1.04	0.25	Pine, terpene, lilac, citrus, woody.
Estragole	1193	1200	0.06	0.02	Sweet sassafras, anise, spice, green.
p-Cumic aldehyde	1238	1240	0.49	0.11	Spicy, cumin, green, herbal.
2-Decenal	1261	1264	0.64	0.25	Waxy, fatty, earthy, coriander.
E-Cinnamaldehyde	1267	1260	0.54	0.07	Sweet, spice, candy, cinnamon.
Ethyl guaiacol	1269	1280	0.43	0.12	Spicy, clove-like, medicinal.
Anethole	1281	1283	0.23	0.07	Sweet, anise, licorice, mimosa.
Isosafrole	1284	n.d.	0.78	0.09	Sweet, sassafras, spicy.
Allyl trisulfide	1293	1300	3.06	1.53	Sulfurous, green, onion, garlic, metallic.
a-Terpinyl acetate	1344	1347	0.48	0.09	Herbal, bergamot, lavender, lime, citrus.
Eugenol	1353	1353	35.33	3.26	Sweet, spicy, clove, woody.
Neryl acetate	1358	1366	0.62	0.11	Floral, rose, soapy, citrus, dewy pear.
Copaene	1372	1376	1.27	0.29	n.d.
Nerol acetate	1376	1365	0.14	0.08	Floral, rose, soapy, citrus, dewy pear.
Methyl eugenol	1396	1403	1.27	0.07	Sweet, spicy, clove, carnation, cinnamon.
Caryophyllene	1399	n.d.	0.59	0.19	Sweet, woody, spice, clove.
E-b-Caryophyllene	1415	1416	7.54	0.63	Spicy, clove, woody, nut skin.
Humulene	1450	1452	0.85	0.24	Woody, oceanic-watery, spicy-clove.
a-Muurolene	1493	1500	0.14	0.01	Herbal, woody, spicy.
b-Bisabolene	1504	1509	0.42	0.11	Balsamic, citrus, myrrh, spicy.
Myristicine	1513	1516	1.85	0.13	Spicy, warm, balsamic, woody.
Elemicin	1542	1547	0.45	0.03	Spice, flower.

Legend: Retention indexes (RI), experimental (Exp) and found in literature (Lit). * TGSC Information System [43].

Sugars and color parameters were also heavily influenced by the additional ingredients. Although green chili peppers were the main ingredient of the sauce, the presence of other ingredients such as lemon juice and red fruits completely modified the sugar content and color of the final product, having higher a^* coordinate values (redder than the mash samples) and lower b^* coordinate values (bluer than the mash samples).

Finally, the volatile composition of the sauce was significantly affected by the presence of the additional ingredients (Table 6). Approximately 18 volatile compounds of the mash samples were also present in the sauce samples, but limonene and eugenol represented over 50% of the total area of the volatile profile of the sauce samples, suggesting the importance of the additional ingredients (lemon juice and 4 *épices*) in the aromatic profile of the product. The final sauce had over 45 different volatile compounds from different chemical groups (terpenes, benzene derivatives, sulfide derivatives, etc.) showing the complexity of the product and confirming the difficulty of perceiving the flavors coming from the potential fermentation stage.

With the aim of mapping the new product in the food market, and understanding the similarities and differences among competitors, a Napping® test was also developed by food experts (chefs and gastronomes) who could aid in positioning and describing the new product. Figure 2 shows the symmetric plot of all the sauces listed in Table 1, explaining the 39% variability of the samples.

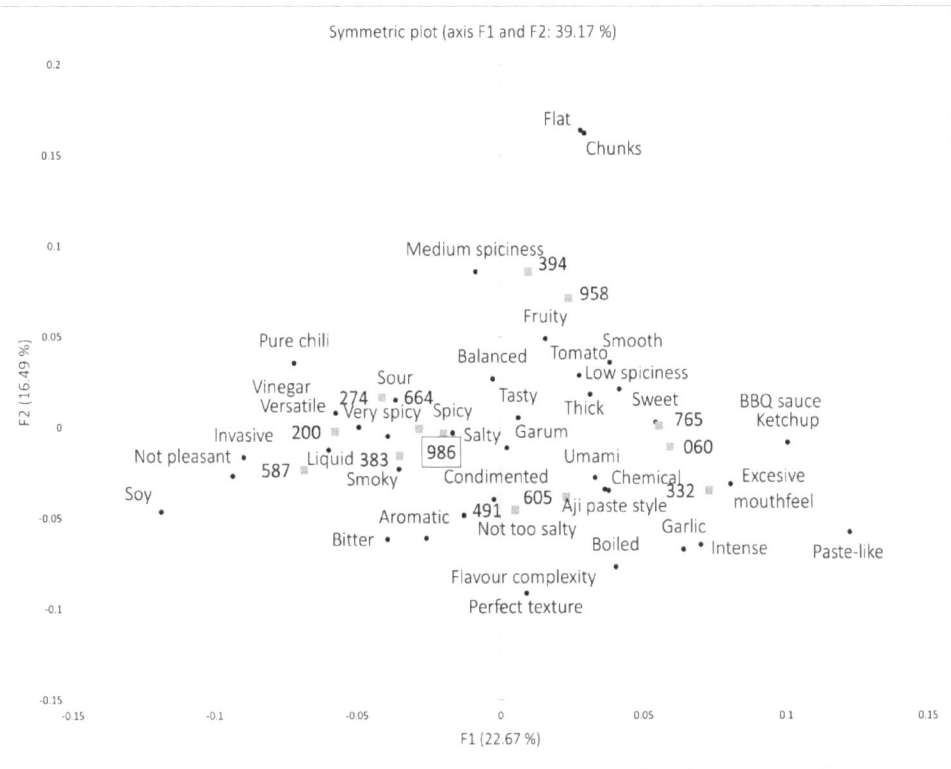

Figure 2. Results of the Napping® test conducted with the samples listed in Table 1. Note: cubes refer to sauce samples and dots to the descriptors for each sauce/group of sauces.

The sample developed during the present research was described as "sour", "spicy", "smoky", or "balanced", features shared with commercial sauces such as Valentina (664) and Tabasco chipotle (383), and that could be used to communicate its profile and encourage the selection of the developed product by consumers who prefer these attributes over other ones such as "sweet", "dense", or "bitter", which were used to describe other products such as Spanish sriracha (765), Gochujang (332) and Soya-based chili sauce (587). Different studies have shown that the intensive consumption of spicy foods could favor the ability to discriminate flavors in this type of product [12,48]; therefore, it is possible that heavy consumers or sensory experts in the corresponding food category (hot sauces) could detect subtle differences among the products. Further studies should be conducted to determine if consumers from different food cultures (e.g., gastronomies with high vs. low use of spicy ingredients) have different discriminatory abilities for these hot sauces.

4. Conclusions

Results of the present research suggest that the fermentation stage of the production process of some hot chili pepper sauces could be avoided depending on the additional ingredients used to finish the product. Physicochemical characteristics should always be analyzed and considered for food product development, but sensory tests are also key to avoid investing time and resources when a new product is developed (e.g., imitating traditional methods). Considering the gastronomy culture for which the product was developed in the present study, the fermentation stage of the process could be avoided, reducing the number of unit operations and ingredients (starter), and optimizing the processing time (from 15 days to 1 day).

Author Contributions: Conceptualization, P.T.-P. and L.V.-A.; methodology, P.T.-P. and L.V.-A. formal analysis, P.T.-P., S.D.-R., O.E., G.P. and L.V.-A.; investigation, P.T.-P., S.D.-R., O.E., G.P. and L.V.-A.; writing—original draft preparation, P.T.-P. and L.V.-A.; writing—review and editing, P.T.-P., S.D.-R., O.E., G.P. and L.V.-A.; supervision, L.V.-A.; funding acquisition, L.V.-A. All authors have read and agreed to the published version of the manuscript.

Funding: This research was funded by BASQUE GOVERNMENT (Departamento de Desarrollo Económico e Infraestructuras de la Viceconsejería de Agricultura, Pesca e Industria Alimentaria del Gobierno Vasco).

Data Availability Statement: The data used to support the findings of this study can be made available by the corresponding author upon request.

Conflicts of Interest: The authors declare no conflict of interest.

References

1. Pickersgill, B. Genetic resources and breeding of *Capsicum* spp. *Euphytica* **1997**, *96*, 129–133. [CrossRef]
2. Fári, M. Pepper (*Capsicum annuum* L.). In *Biotechnology in Agriculture and Forestry*; Bajaj, Y.P.S., Ed.; Springer: Berlin, Germany, 1986; Volume 2, pp. 345–362. [CrossRef]
3. Eshbaugh, W.H. The taxonomy of the genus capsicum. In *Peppers: Botany, Production and Uses*; Russo, V., Ed.; CAB International: Wallingford, UK, 2012; pp. 14–28.
4. Long, J. *El Chile. Fruto Ancestral*, 1st ed.; Catálogo Artes de México: Mexico City, Mexico, 2017; ISBN 6074612404.
5. Pathirana, R. Peppers: Vegetable and Spice Capsicums. *N. Z. J. Crop Hortic. Sci.* **2013**, *41*, 102–103. [CrossRef]
6. Durand, C. An Introduction to Geographical Indications and the Transformative Effect of Successful GI Products. In Promoting Intellectual Property Rights in the ASEAN Region. Available online: https://internationalipcooperation.eu/sites/default/files/arise-docs/2022/ARISEplusIPR_jan2022_Claire-Durand_An-Introduction-to-Geographical-Indications-and-the-Transformative-Effect-of-Successful-GI-Products.pdf (accessed on 12 September 2023).
7. Official Journal of the European Communities. Available online: https://eur-lex.europa.eu/LexUriServ/LexUriServ.do?uri=OJ.C:2001:354:0009:0011:EN:PDF (accessed on 25 July 2023).
8. Deba-Rementeria, S.; Zugazua-Ganado, M.; Estrada, O.; Regefalk, J.; Vázquez-Araújo, L. Characterization of salt-preserved orange peel using physico-chemical, microbiological, and sensory analyses. *LWT* **2021**, *148*, 111769. [CrossRef]
9. Rodríguez Valerón, N.; Prado Vásquez, D.; Rodgers, R.; Rugset, O.; Munk, R. From waste to a new sustainable ingredient in the kitchen: Red king crab abdominal flap (*Paralithodes camtschaticus*). *Int. J. Gastron. Food Sci.* **2021**, *27*, 100455. [CrossRef]
10. Torán-Pereg, P.; Del Noval, B.; Valenzuela, S.; Martínez, J.; Prado, D.; Perisé, R.; Arboleya, J.C. Microbiological and sensory characterization of kombucha SCOBY for culinary applications. *Int. J. Gastron. Food Sci.* **2021**, *23*, 100314. [CrossRef]
11. Boronat, Ò.; Sintes, P.; Celis, F.; Díez, M.; Ortiz, J.; Aguiló-Aguayo, I.; Martin-Gómez, H. Development of added-value culinary ingredients from fish waste: Fish bones and fish scales. *Int. J. Gastron. Food Sci.* **2023**, *31*, 100657. [CrossRef]
12. Rozin, P.; Schiller, D. The nature and acquisition of a preference for chili pepper by humans. *Motiv. Emot.* **1980**, *4*, 77–101. [CrossRef]
13. Kim, H.J.; Chung, S.J.; Kim, K.O.; Nielsen, B.; Ishii, R.; O'Mahony, M. A cross-cultural study of acceptability and food pairing for hot sauces. *Appetite* **2018**, *123*, 306–316. [CrossRef]
14. Trachootham, D.; Satoh-Kuriwada, S.; Lam-ubol, A.; Promkam, C.; Chotechuang, N.; Sasano, T.; Shoji, N. Differences in Taste Perception and Spicy Preference: A Thai–Japanese Cross-cultural Study. *Chem. Senses* **2018**, *43*, 65–74. [CrossRef]
15. Josiam, B.M.; Monteiro, P.A. Tandoori tastes: Perceptions of Indian restaurants in America. *Int. J. Contemp. Hosp. Manag.* **2004**, *16*, 18–26. [CrossRef]
16. Spence, C. Why is piquant/spicy food so popular? *Int. J. Gastron. Food Sci.* **2018**, *12*, 16–21. [CrossRef]
17. Aryee, N.A.; Owusu-Kwarteng, J.; Senwo, Z.; Alvarez, M.N. Characterizing fermented habanero pepper (*Capsicum chinense* L.). *Food Chem. Adv.* **2022**, *1*, 100137. [CrossRef]
18. Watts, E.G.; Janes, M.E.; Prinyawiwatkul, W.; Shen, Y.; Xu, Z.; Johnson, D. Microbiological changes and their impact on quality characteristics of red hot chilli pepper mash during natural fermentation. *Int. J. Food Sci. Technol.* **2018**, *53*, 1816–1823. [CrossRef]
19. Sinsawasdi, V.K.; Rattanapanone, N.; Toschka, H.Y. *The Science of Thai Cuisine: Chemical Properties and Sensory Attributes*, 1st ed.; CRC Press: Boca Raton, FL, USA, 2022; p. 272. [CrossRef]
20. Vatansever, S.; Vegi, A.; Garden-Robinson, J.; Hall, C.A., III. The effect of fermentation on the physicochemical characteristics of dry-salted vegetables. *J. Food Res.* **2017**, *6*, 32–40. [CrossRef]
21. Ruiz Rodríguez, L.; Zamora Gasga, V.M.; Pescuma, M.; Van Nieuwenhove, C.; Mozzi, F.; Sánchez Burgos, J.A. Fruits and fruit by-products as sources of bioactive compounds. Benefits and trends of lactic acid fermentation in the development of novel fruit-based functional beverages. *Food Res. Int.* **2021**, *140*, 109854. [CrossRef] [PubMed]

22. Katz, S.E. *The Art of Fermentation: An In-Depth Exploration of Essential Concepts and Processes from around the World*, 1st ed.; Chelsea Green Publishing: Chelsea, VT, USA, 2012; ISBN 9781603582865.
23. Redzepi, R.; Zilber, D. *The Noma Guide to Fermentation: Including Koji, Kombuchas, Shoyus, Misos, Vinegars, Garums, Lacto-Ferments, and Black Fruits and Vegetables*, 1st ed.; Artisian: New York, NY, USA, 2018; ISBN 9781579657185.
24. Di Cagno, R.; Filannino, P.; Gobbetti, M. vegetable and fruit fermentation by lactic acid bacteria. In *Biotechnology of Lactic Acid Bacteria: Novel Applications*, 2nd ed.; Mozzi, F., Raya, R.R., Vignolo, G.M., Eds.; John Wiley & Sons, Ltd.: Chichester, UK, 2015; pp. 216–230.
25. Di Cagno, R.; Surico, R.F.; Minervini, G.; De Angelis, M.; Rizzello, C.G.; Gobbetti, M. Use of autochthonous starters to ferment red and yellow peppers (*Capsicum annum* L.) to be stored at room temperature. *Int. J. Food. Microbiol.* **2009**, *130*, 108–116. [CrossRef]
26. Torres, S.; Verón, H.; Contreras, L.; Isla, M.I. An overview of plant-autochthonous microorganisms and fermented vegetable foods. *Food Sci. Hum. Wellness* **2020**, *9*, 112–123. [CrossRef]
27. Janiszewska-Turak, E.; Witrowa-Rajchert, D.; Rybak, K.; Rolof, J.; Pobiega, K.; Wózniak, Ł.; Gramza-Michałowska, A. The influence of lactic acid fermentation on selected properties of pickled red, yellow, and green bell peppers. *Molecules* **2022**, *27*, 8637. [CrossRef]
28. López-Salas, D.; Oney-Montalvo, J.E.; Ramírez-Rivera, E.; Ramírez-Sucre, M.O.; Rodríguez-Buenfil, I.M. Fermentation of habanero pepper by two lactic acid bacteria and its effect on the production of volatile compounds. *Fermentation* **2022**, *8*, 219. [CrossRef]
29. AENOR (Asociación Española de Normalización y Certificación). Método horizontal para el recuento de microorganismos. In *Microbiología de la Cadena Alimentaria*; Part I; AENOR: Madrid, Spain, 2014.
30. Razola-Díaz, M.d.C.; Verardo, V.; Martín-García, B.; Díaz-de-Cerio, E.; García-Villanova, B.; Guerra-Hernández, E.J. Establishment of acid hydrolysis by box-behnken methodology as pretreatment to obtain reducing sugars from tiger nut byproducts. *Agronomy* **2020**, *10*, 477. [CrossRef]
31. Deba-Rementeria, S.; Estrada, O.; Issa-Issa, H.; Vázquez-Araújo, L. Orange peel fermentation using *Lactiplantibacillus plantarum*: Microbiological analysis and physico-chemical characterisation. *Int. J. Food Sci. Technol.* **2022**, *57*, 5542–5552. [CrossRef]
32. National Institute of Standards and Technology (NIST). Search for Species Data by Chemical Name. Available online: https://webbook.nist.gov/chemistry/name-ser/ (accessed on 25 July 2023).
33. AENOR (Asociación Española de Normalización y Certificación). Metodología: Prueba triangular. In *Análisis Sensorial*; AENOR: Madrid, Spain, 2022.
34. Pagès, J. Collection and analysis of perceived product inter-distance using multiple factor analysis: Application to the study of 10 white wines from the Loire Valley. *Food Qual. Pref.* **2003**, *16*, 642–649. [CrossRef]
35. Romeo-Arroyo, E.; Mora, M.; Noguera-Artiaga, L.; Vázquez-Araújo, L. Tea pairings: Impact of aromatic congruence on acceptance and sweetness perception. *Curr. Res. Nutr. Food Sci.* **2023**, *6*, 100432. [CrossRef]
36. Addinsoft. XLSTAT Statistical and Data Analysis Solution. New York, NY, USA. 2023. Available online: https://www.xlstat.com/es (accessed on 26 July 2023).
37. Foong Ming, K. Physicochemical Properties of Pepper Mash Fermented in Wood and Plastic. Master's Thesis, Louisiana State University and Agricultural and Mechanical College, Baton Rouge, LA, USA, 2005.
38. Food and Drug Administration, Department of Health and Human Services. 21 CFR Part 114. Code of Federal Regulations. Available online: https://www.ecfr.gov/current/title-21/chapter-I/subchapter-B/part-114?toc=1 (accessed on 12 September 2023).
39. Cserhalmi, Z.; Sass-Kiss, Á.; Tóth-Markus, M.; Lechner, N. Study of pulsed electric field treated citrus juices. *Innov. Food Sci. Emerg. Technol.* **2006**, *7*, 49–54. [CrossRef]
40. Abe, K.; Hori, Y.; Myoda, T. Volatile compounds of fresh and processed garlic. *Exp. Ther. Med.* **2020**, *19*, 1585–1593. [CrossRef] [PubMed]
41. Keleş, D.; Taşkın, H.; Baktemur, G.; Kafkas, E.; Büyükalac, S. Comparitive study on volatile aroma compounds of two different garlic types (Kastamonu and Chinese) using Gas Chromatography Mass Spectrometry (Hs-Gc/Ms) Technique. *Afr. J. Tradit. Complement. Altern. Med.* **2014**, *11*, 217–220. [CrossRef]
42. Forero, M.D.; Quijano, C.E.; Pino, J.A. Volatile compounds of chile pepper (*Capsicum annuum* L. var. glabriusculum) at two ripening stages. *Flavour Fragr. J.* **2009**, *24*, 25–30. [CrossRef]
43. TGSC Information System. Available online: http://www.thegoodscentscompany.com/ (accessed on 5 May 2023).
44. Balthazar, C.; Silva, H.; Celeguini, R.M.S.; Santos, R.; Pastore, G.M.; Conte Junior, C.A.; Freitas, M.; Nogueira, L.; Silva, M.; Cruz, A.G. Effect of galactooligosaccharide addition on the physical, optical, and sensory acceptance of vanilla ice cream. *J. Dairy Sci.* **2015**, *98*, 4266–4272. [CrossRef]
45. Morales, J.; Tárrega, A.; Salvador, A.; Navarro, P.; Besada, C. Impact of ethylene degreening treatment on sensory properties and consumer response to citrus fruits. *Food Res. Int.* **2020**, *127*, 108641. [CrossRef] [PubMed]
46. Moisés, S.G.; Guamis, B.; Roig-Sagués, A.X.; Codina-Torrella, I.; Hernández-Herrero, M.M. Effect of Ultra-High-Pressure Homogenization processing on the microbiological, physicochemical, and sensory characteristics of fish broth. *Foods* **2022**, *11*, 3969. [CrossRef]

47. Rahman, M.S. pH in food preservation. In *Handbook of Food Preservation*, 2nd ed.; Rahman, M.S., Ed.; CRC Press: Boca Raton, FL, USA, 2007; pp. 287–298.
48. Ludy, M.J.; Mattes, R.D. Comparison of sensory, physiological, personality, and cultural attributes in regular spicy food users and non-users. *Appetite* **2012**, *58*, 19–27. [CrossRef] [PubMed]

Disclaimer/Publisher's Note: The statements, opinions and data contained in all publications are solely those of the individual author(s) and contributor(s) and not of MDPI and/or the editor(s). MDPI and/or the editor(s) disclaim responsibility for any injury to people or property resulting from any ideas, methods, instructions or products referred to in the content.

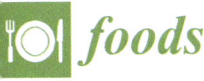

Article

Effect of Potassium Permanganate, Ultraviolet Radiation and Titanium Oxide as Ethylene Scavengers on Preservation of Postharvest Quality and Sensory Attributes of Broccoli Stored with Tomatoes

Ramiro Alonso-Salinas [1,2], Santiago López-Miranda [1,2,*], Ana González-Báidez [1,2], Antonio José Pérez-López [1,2], Luis Noguera-Artiaga [3], Estrella Núñez-Delicado [4], Ángel Carbonell-Barrachina [3] and José Ramón Acosta-Motos [1,2]

1. Plant Biotechnology for Food and Agriculture Group (BioVegA2), Universidad Católica San Antonio de Murcia, Avenida de los Jerónimos 135, Guadalupe, 30107 Murcia, Spain; ralonso@ucam.edu (R.A.-S.); agonzalez@ucam.edu (A.G.-B.); ajperez@ucam.edu (A.J.P.-L.); jracosta@ucam.edu (J.R.A.-M.)
2. Plant Biotechnology, Agriculture and Climate Resilience Group, UCAM-CEBAS-CSIC, Associated Unit to CSIC by CEBAS-CSIC, DP, 30100 Murcia, Spain
3. Research Group "Food Quality and Safety", Centro de Investigación e Innovación Agroalimentaria y Agroambiental (CIAGRO-UMH), Miguel Hernández University, Carretera de Beniel, Km 3.2, 03312 Orihuela, Spain; lnoguera@umh.es (L.N.-A.); angel.carbonell@umh.es (Á.C.-B.)
4. Molecular Recognition and Encapsulation Group (REM), UCAM Universidad Católica de Murcia, Avenida de los Jerónimos 135, Guadalupe, 30107 Murcia, Spain; enunez@ucam.edu
* Correspondence: slmiranda@ucam.edu

Abstract: This study introduces an effective solution to enhance the postharvest preservation of broccoli, a vegetable highly sensitive to ethylene, a hormone produced by climacteric fruits such as tomatoes. The proposed method involves a triple combination of ethylene elimination techniques: potassium permanganate ($KMnO_4$) filters combined with ultraviolet radiation (UV-C) and titanium oxide (TiO_2), along with a continuous airflow to facilitate contact between ethylene and these oxidizing agents. The effectiveness of this approach was evaluated using various analytical techniques, including measurements of weight, soluble solids content, total acidity, maturity index, color, chlorophyll, total phenolic compounds, and sensory analysis conducted by experts. The results demonstrated a significant improvement in the physicochemical quality of postharvest broccoli when treated with the complete system. Notably, broccoli subjected to this innovative method exhibited enhanced organoleptic quality, with heightened flavors and aromas associated with fresh green produce. The implementation of this novel technique holds great potential for the food industry as it reduces postharvest losses, extends the shelf life of broccoli, and ultimately enhances product quality while minimizing waste. The successful development and implementation of this new technique can significantly improve the sustainability of the food industry while ensuring the provision of high-quality food to consumers.

Keywords: *Brassica oleracea* var. *italica*; climacteric fruit; ethylene scavengers; *Solanum lycopersicum* L.; susceptible vegetable

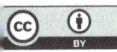

1. Introduction

Reducing food waste is a crucial task nowadays due to its economic, social, and environmental impact. It is estimated that worldwide, one-third of all food produced is lost or wasted, which is equivalent to approximately 1.3 billion tons annually [1]. This issue not only poses a problem in terms of wasted resources and loss of profits for farmers and the food industry but also has a negative impact on the environment due to the emission of greenhouse gases and the degradation of ecosystems [2]. One effective way to reduce food waste is through postharvest activities, which occur after harvesting but before distribution and retail sale. Simultaneous storage of crops can be an effective strategy to minimize food waste during the postharvest period.

The simultaneous conservation of broccoli and tomatoes at the same temperatures can have different effects on the agri-food industry due to their distinct optimal storage requirements [3–6]. Firstly, it is important to consider that broccoli is sensitive to ethylene, while tomatoes are ethylene producers [5,7,8]. When stored together, tomatoes can expedite the ripening process of broccoli due to ethylene release, leading to a reduction in broccoli's shelf life. Generally, broccoli should be stored at lower temperatures than tomatoes to preserve its freshness and quality for a longer period. At the same temperature, ethylene can cause the broccoli to soften and wilt more rapidly than normal, compromising its shelf life and overall quality. Additionally, direct contact between tomatoes and broccoli can result in surface damage to the broccoli, further impacting its quality. However, the joint conservation of broccoli and tomatoes can yield beneficial effects for the agri-food industry if managed appropriately, such as efficiency in transport, cost reduction, and product availability. For instance, controlled storage techniques can be employed to prolong the freshness of broccoli and minimize the impact of tomato ethylene on its ripening process. Moreover, since tomato and broccoli are two widely consumed crops [9], their combined storage can enhance the efficiency and profitability of distribution and wholesale processes.

Broccoli is an important crop worldwide due to its high nutritional value and growing demand in international markets. According to FAO data [9], over 27 million tons of broccoli were produced worldwide in 2020, with China being the main producer, followed by India, the United States, and Spain. Broccoli is a nutrient-rich cruciferous vegetable that has been associated with a range of health benefits. It is a good source of fiber, vitamin C, vitamin K, folate, iron, and potassium. Additionally, it contains antioxidant and anti-inflammatory compounds such as glucosinolates and carotenoids [10]. Regular consumption of broccoli and other cruciferous vegetables has been shown to be associated with a decreased risk of certain types of cancer, including lung, colon, prostate, and breast cancer. It may also help improve cardiovascular health, reduce inflammation, and enhance cognitive function [11,12]. Furthermore, broccoli is a low-calorie food and can be a healthy option for those looking to lose weight or maintain a healthy weight. Overall, broccoli is highly nutritious and beneficial for health, and its inclusion in a balanced diet is recommended. Tomatoes, on the other hand, are natural producers of ethylene, a plant hormone that is released in a gaseous form and regulates various physiological processes in plants, including ripening and senescence [13,14]. Ethylene production in tomatoes increases during ripening and aging, making them highly ethylene-sensitive fruits [15,16]. Moreover, tomatoes can also impact the ripening and aging of other fruits and vegetables in close proximity, due to ethylene release. For this reason, it is necessary to avoid storing tomatoes together with other fruits and vegetables, especially if they are highly sensitive to ethylene.

There are natural actions that can mitigate the effects of ethylene. Firstly, the amount of ethylene produced by tomatoes can vary depending on their degree of ripeness [5]. Ripe tomatoes produce more ethylene than less ripe ones, so the impact of ethylene on broccoli may be reduced if stored with less ripe tomatoes. Additionally, fresh high-quality broccoli is better able to withstand the effects of tomato ethylene and maintain its quality for a longer period, while lower-quality and less fresh broccoli may be more susceptible to ethylene's effects. On the other hand, there are several ethylene-removal technologies that can prevent the negative effects of this hormone on sensitive foods such as broccoli [17]. Potassium permanganate [18,19], ultraviolet radiation [20,21], and titanium oxide [22,23] are three different technologies that can be used to eliminate ethylene from the storage environment of fruits and vegetables. Each of these technologies has its own advantages, differences, and mode of action. Potassium permanganate acts by oxidizing ethylene into carbon dioxide and water, while ultraviolet radiation and titanium oxide eliminate ethylene by producing hydroxyl radicals, which react with ethylene to form carbon dioxide and water. Although all three methods aim to remove ethylene, potassium permanganate is more effective in high humidity environments, while ultraviolet radiation and titanium oxide are more effective in low humidity environments. In terms of similarities, the three methods do not require direct contact with the fruits, making them non-invasive and allowing for longer storage periods. Furthermore, all three methods can help delay fruit ripening and extend the shelf life of produce, which is a crucial factor in the food industry.

The aim of this work is to investigate the effect of potassium permanganate, ultraviolet radiation, and titanium oxide on the postharvest conservation of broccoli when it is grown together with tomatoes at the same temperature for a period of 21 days.

2. Materials and Methods

2.1. Plant Material

A total of 25 kg of broccoli *Brassica oleracea* var *Italica* were procured from "Hoyamar S.Coop" in Murcia, Spain. The broccoli was harvested using conventional techniques and immediately stored at a temperature of $1 \pm 1\ °C$ for 24 h prior to laboratory transportation for subsequent analysis. The classification of the harvested produce based on caliper measurements was conducted by the supplier on the same day of harvest, which took place on 18 May 2022. Furthermore, to ensure homogeneity, a harvest index analysis was performed on a representative sample of 10 randomly selected broccoli florets from the supplied batch, employing the same methodology as the subsequent investigations. The resultant harvest indexes are presented in Table 1. Then, the broccoli was cooled and transported the following day (19 May 2022) to the laboratory. In addition, 25 kg of tomatoes were supplied by "ExpoÁguilas S.Coop" (Murcia, Spain) and were stored alongside the broccoli, except for the control treatment broccoli, to analyse the ethylene produced by this climacteric fruit on a vegetable that is sensitive to this gas, such as broccoli. The choice of tomato for combined storage with broccoli in this study was based on its status as a well-studied climacteric fruit. Additionally, in the production region where the study was conducted (Region of Murcia, Spain), both vegetables share a harvest season for a significant part of the year, and it is common for producing companies to cultivate them together due to the local climatic conditions and production techniques.

Table 1. Harvest indexes of broccoli and tomato. The means ± standard error of the means (SEM) are shown. $n = 10$.

Parameters	Weight (g)	SSC (%)	TA (%)	Colour
Broccoli	468.71 ± 10	7.64 ± 0.7	1.01 ± 0.05	a^*: −4.3 ± 0.5 b^*: 6.1 ± 0.8 L^*: 24.3 ± 1.9
Tomato	184.22 ± 4.11	5.06 ± 0.12	3.83 ± 0.10	a^*: 34.8 ± 3.1 b^*: 24.2 ± 2.8 L^*: 40.7 ± 4.0
Method	Navigator balance, Ohaus Europe Gmbh (Nänikon, Switzerland).	Pocket Brix–acidity meter, Atago (Tokyo, Japan).	Pocket Brix–acidity meter, Atago (Tokyo, Japan).	Colourpin II, Natural Color System (Stockholm, Sweden).

2.2. Experimental Design

A total of 45 florets of broccoli (25 kg) were randomly distributed into five 150 L (volume) conservation chambers (CCs) (Eurofred Cool Head RCG200, Eurofred S.A., Barcelona, Catalonia, Spain) for the different treatments analyzed. In addition, a total of 85 tomatoes (25 kg) were randomly distributed into 4 (except for the control treatment) 150 L (volume) conservation chambers (CCs) (Eurofred Cool Head RCG200, Eurofred S.A., Barcelona, Catalonia, Spain).

Following Alonso-Salinas [24], the filters utilized in this study consisted of $KMnO_4$ immobilized onto the active centers of zeolite, promoting enhanced interaction between this oxidizing agent and ethylene. The patented filter composition in terms of granulometry and additional adsorbent substances was developed by the Spanish company "Nuevas Tecnologías Agroalimentarias KEEPCOOL" (Molina de Segura, Spain) under patent number 2548787 (2016). To facilitate ethylene removal while preventing the ingress of water or interfering particles, the adsorbing material was enveloped with a semi-permeable paper. This paper allowed the entry of ethylene-rich air while facilitating the egress of purified air free from this phytohormone.

Ethylene filters served as the sole technology for ethylene removal and were installed within an M-CAM 50 device (KEEPCCOL, Molina de Segura, Spain), which functioned as an air-flow-forcing apparatus. This configuration ensured that all air circulating within the conservation chambers (CCs) passed through the ethylene filter. The airflow volume inside the system was 750 L min^{-1}, indicating that all the air was recirculated within 12 s, as the chamber had a capacity of 150 L.

Furthermore, this system integrated a photocatalytic ultraviolet light system UV-C (TUV 254 nm, Philips, Amsterdam, The Netherlands) and titanium dioxide TiO_2 (in mesh format) to support the $KMnO_4$ filters in effectively eliminating ethylene. Titanium dioxide is a semiconductor material widely utilized as a photocatalyst for ethylene degradation. Its effectiveness in this role is primarily attributed to its exceptional photochemical reactivity and physical properties, such as high brightness (resulting from its high refractive index) and resistance to discoloration [25]. The mechanism of ethylene elimination through UV light radiation on titanium dioxide is described by Pathak and colleagues [26]. In summary, the reaction is based on the fact that, following irradiation with UV wavelengths (hv) (around 240–380 nm), titanium dioxide generates electrons (e-) that, upon acting on the ambient water, produce highly reactive hydroxyl radicals ($\cdot$OH). These radicals, in turn, react with organic compounds such as ethylene, resulting in the production of CO_2 and water [27,28]. To mitigate any potential adverse effects, the application of ultraviolet (UV) light and titanium oxide was targeted specifically at the air exiting the filters rather than the fruit itself. This precautionary measure was taken due to the enclosed nature of the device, which featured only two air inlet and outlet openings. The light beam was directed towards the ethylene component, ensuring that the fruit remained unaffected by the UV light treatment. Figure 1 provides a comprehensive diagram of the system, offering clarity regarding the operational process.

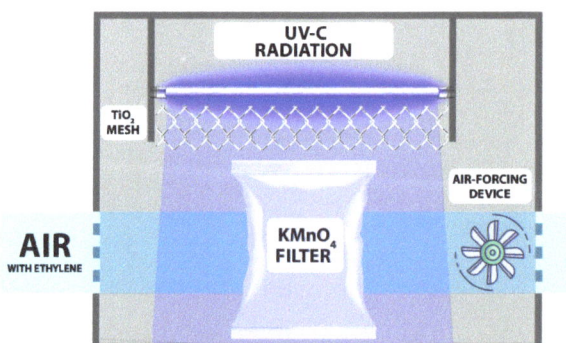

Figure 1. Ethylene scavenger diagram.

The selection of $KMnO_4$, UV-C radiation, and TiO_2 was based on several factors. Firstly, according to sources in the literature [5,18,25,29], $KMnO_4$ was found to be more effective than 1-MCP for ethylene removal. Additionally, $KMnO_4$ is more practical for implementation in the food industry due to its affordability compared with palladium. Furthermore, the inclusion of UV light and TiO_2 was chosen due to their ease of application and their ability to enhance the performance of $KMnO_4$.

The treatments were categorized based on ethylene removal, preservation temperature, and relative humidity, as outlined in Table 2.

Table 2. Treatment classification according to storage temperature (°C), relative humidity (%) and presence of ethylene scavengers.

Treatments	Broc-Control	Broc-Tomato	Broc-Tom + KMnO$_4$	Broc-Tom + KMnO$_4$ + UV-C	Broc-Tom + KMnO$_4$ + UV-C + TiO$_2$
Temperature	1 °C	1 °C	1 °C	1 °C	1 °C
Relative humidity	90%	90%	90%	90%	90%
Ethylene scavenger	None	None	Filter	Filter + UV-C	Filter + UV-C + TiO$_2$

2.3. Physicochemical Variables

All physicochemical analyses were conducted in quintuplicate ($n = 5$) at regular intervals during the entire storage period, specifically on the following days: 0, 7, 15, and 21 (spanning from 19 May 2022 to 8 June 2022). The shelf life of the broccoli was determined to be 21 days, according to the recommended commercial lifetime provided by the supplying company. This time was selected to align with the optimal quality and freshness of the broccoli, ensuring its suitability for commercial purposes. Similar storage durations have also been reported in previous studies [30,31].

The concentration of ethylene (C_2H_4) was quantified using a gas analyser (Felix Three F-950, Felix Instruments, Camas, WA, USA) and reported in nmol kg^{-1} h^{-1}. The gas analyser operated at a measuring flow rate of 1 mL s^{-1}, and five measurements were conducted for each analysis and treatment day. To avoid disruption to the internal atmosphere of the chambers, a sealed access point was opened to insert a sonde for ethylene concentration measurements.

The gas analyser had a resolution of 0.1 ppm, and its lower limit of detection was 0.15 ppm. In order to assess potential variations, ethylene measurements were taken 6 h after the beginning of the study on day 0, since the initial ethylene concentration inside the chambers was 0 when the broccoli and tomatoes arrived at the laboratory. This allowed for the observation of any discernible differences in ethylene levels.

The weight measurements were conducted using a precision balance (Navigator balance, Ohaus Europe Gmbh Nänikon, Greifensee, Switzerland), and the results reported in grams. The determination of soluble solid content (SSC), pH, and total acidity (TA) in the fruit samples followed the method adapted from Zhang et al. [32].

To obtain the measurements, 20 g of broccoli was taken and combined with 20 mL of distilled water. The mixture was homogenized for 30 s using an Ultra turrax T25 mixer (LabWare Wilmington, DE, USA). Subsequently, the homogenate was subjected to centrifugation at 3600× g for 10 min at 4 °C, employing an Eppendorf centrifuge 5810 (Hamburg, Germany). The resulting supernatant, referred to as "broccoli extract" in the manuscript, was utilized for the determination of SSC, pH, TA, and total phenolic content (TPC).

The soluble solid content (SSC) of the broccoli extract was analyzed using a digital refractometer (Pocket Brix–acidity meter, Atago Tokyo, Japan) at a temperature of 20 °C. The results were expressed as a percentage of sugar equivalent in grams per 100 g (g 100 g^{-1}). The pH of the broccoli extract was measured using a pH meter (Testo 206-pH2, Testo, Barcelona, Spain). The determination of total acidity (TA) in the broccoli extract followed the method described by Zang et al. [32] and utilized a Pocket Brix–acidity meter (Atago, Tokyo, Japan). The results of TA were reported as grams per liter (g L^{-1}). To assess the maturity index (MI) of the broccoli, the SSC (%) was divided by the TA (%). The MI is a dimensionless parameter that provides insight into the maturity and quality of the broccoli sample.

The total phenolic content (TPC) of the broccoli was determined using a colorimetric method at a wavelength of 765 nm. Folin–Ciocalteu reagent was employed following a modified protocol of Kidron et al. [33]. The Folin–Ciocalteu reaction involved mixing 100 µL of the broccoli extract with 150 µL of Folin–Ciocalteu reagent, 450 µL of 20% Na$_2$CO$_3$, and 2300 µL of distilled water. After a 2 h dark reaction, the absorbance of the sample was measured against a blank using a spectrophotometer (Shimadzu model UV-1603, Japan). A calibration curve (y = 0.5206x + 0.0899; R^2 = 0.998) was created using gallic acid as the standard within a range of 25–250 µg mL^{-1}. The TPC was expressed as grams of gallic acid equivalent per kilogram of fresh broccoli (g kg^{-1}).

The method proposed by Gou et al. [30] was adapted for the analysis of chlorophyll a, chlorophyll b, and total chlorophyll in broccoli samples. A sample weighing 20 g was homogenized using an Ultra Turrax T25 mixer (LabWare, Wilmington, DE, USA) with the addition of 20 g of an acetone–water mixture (80/20 w/w). The resulting homogenate was centrifuged at 3600× g for 5 min. The supernatant was collected after filtration and the absorbance measured at 645 nm and 663 nm using a Shimadzu UV-1603 spectrophotometer (Shimadzu, Japan). Concentrations of chlorophyll a, chlorophyll b, and total chlorophyll were calculated using the following formulas and expressed as mL g^{-1}:

$$\text{Chlorophyll a} = \frac{(20.2 \times \text{Absorbance}645 - 8.02 \times \text{Absorbance}663) \times V(mL)}{m(g)} \quad (1)$$

$$\text{Chlorophyll b} = \frac{(34.7 \times \text{Absorbance}663 - 7.12 \times \text{Absorbance}645) \times V(mL)}{m(g)} \quad (2)$$

$$\text{Total chlorophyll} = \frac{(20.2 \times \text{Absorbance}645 + 34.7 \times \text{Absorbance}663) \times V(mL)}{m(g)} \quad (3)$$

m = broccoli sample mass expressed in grams.
V = the volume of the extraction solution in millilitres.

The color was determined according to the CIELAB system using a colorimeter (Hunterlab Colorflex EZ, Hunterlab Reston, VA, USA) to measure the color of the florets of five broccolis per treatment and conservation period (0, 7, 15 and 21 days), taking a measurement of CIELAB parameters in two different positions of each fruit and calculating the average. The parameters determined were the coordinates a* (red-green coordinate, red component when positive, green when negative), b* (yellow-blue coordinate, yellow component when positive, blue when negative), and the L parameter, which is a measure of color brightness or lightness referring to the grayscale scale of 0 to 100, where 0 represents absolute black and 100 represents absolute white.

2.4. Descriptive Sensory Analysis

The descriptive sensory analysis was carried out by a trained panel comprising 8 highly skilled panellists. The panelists, consisting of 5 females aged between 35 and 56 years, were members of the Food Quality and Safety research group at the Universidad Miguel Hernández de Elche (UMH), Orihuela, Spain. Each panelist possessed extensive experience with fruits and vegetables, with more than 1000 h of training. The methodology employed for the descriptive sensory analysis was previously outlined by Noguera-Artiaga et al. [34]. The scale used ranged from 10 (extremely high intensity) to 0 (no intensity) with 0.5 increments. Prior to the analysis of the samples, 3 training sessions were held in which the lexicon to be used was defined. In these sessions, the panel worked with different broccoli cultivars at day 0 and day 21. From more than 70 descriptors analysed, the final selection was limited to 30, distributed in the visual (green color, yellow color, homogeneity of color, general ID, opening of inflorescences), olfactory (broccoli ID, green vegetable, ripe vegetable, earthy, fermented, sulfurous), gustatory (broccoli ID, green vegetable, ripe vegetable, earthy, fermented, sulfurous, woody, sweet, sour, bitter, astringency, aftertaste), and textural (spicy, hardness, crunchiness, chewiness, juiciness, fibrousness, and residual particles) phases. The samples were presented to the panelists on odor-free disposable plates at room temperature of approximately 22 °C. Each sample was assigned a unique 3-digit code to ensure blind testing. To cleanse their palates between samples, the panelists were provided with mineral water and unsalted crackers. The analyses were conducted in triplicate, with each sample being evaluated three times ($n = 3$).

2.5. Statistical Analysis

The descriptive statistics, including the mean and standard error of the mean (SEM), were calculated using StatGraphics Centurion XV software from StatPoint Technologies (Warrenton, VA, USA). The normality of the data was assessed using the Shapiro–Wilk test, and the homogeneity of variance was examined using Bartlett's test. For the comparison of the 5 treatments across 12 variables on days 7, 15, and 21 of the experiment, a 1-way analysis of variance (ANOVA) was performed. A principal component analysis (PCA) was conducted to identify principal components with eigenvalues greater than or equal to 1.0. Subsequently, a partial least square discriminant analysis was carried out. These analyses explained 82.97% of the variation within the dataset at the end of the 21-day experiment. The sensory analysis data were subjected to an analysis of variance (1-way ANOVA), comparing day 0 with day 21 of the experiment. Tukey's multiple range test was utilized to compare means and detect significant differences between the treatments (p-value < 0.05).

3. Results and Discussion

3.1. Ethylene

Regarding ethylene accumulation throughout the assay, the control treatment with only broccoli (Broc-Control) showed little change due to its low ethylene production. The maximum accumulation was observed in the treatment where broccoli and tomato were grown together without any ethylene eliminators (Broc-Tom), indicating that the tomato was responsible for this increase, as a climacteric fruit capable of producing this gas during postharvest after the fruit is separated from the plant. Ethylene decrease was progressive as the number of ethylene eliminators increased (Broc-Tom + $KMnO_4$ > Broc-Tom + $KMnO_4$ + UV-C > Broc-Tom + $KMnO_4$ + UV-C + TiO_2), with the triple combination treatment accumulating less gas (Broc-Tom + $KMnO_4$ + UV-C + TiO_2) even at levels very close to the control treatment (Broc-Control) (Figure 2).

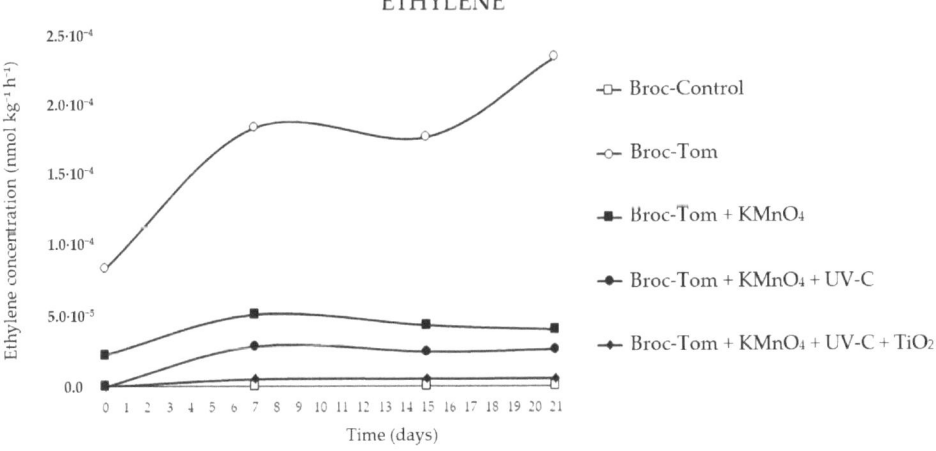

Figure 2. Ethylene concentration (nmol kg^{-1} h^{-1}) over the storage period for treatments (Broc-Control, Broc-Tom, Broc-Tom + $KMnO_4$, Broc-Tom + $KMnO_4$ + UV-C, Broc-Tom + $KMnO_4$ + UV-C + TiO_2).

Minimizing ethylene concentration during the storage of broccoli is highly desirable to reduce the occurrence of floret damage and internal breakdown. Alonso-Salinas et al. [19] demonstrated a 52% reduction in ethylene concentration in peaches stored at 1 ± 1 °C using an ethylene elimination system incorporating $KMnO_4$ + UV-C. Previous studies have examined the individual effectiveness of $KMnO_4$ and UV-C as ethylene scavengers [35–37] However, the combination of $KMnO_4$ + UV-C employed in this study showed even greater efficacy. Moreover, the present study introduces a novel finding, demonstrating that the triple combination of $KMnO_4$ + UV-C + TiO_2 exhibited an even more significant effect.

In a study by Álvarez-Hernández et al. [38], the application of ethylene scavengers based on $KMnO_4$ onto apricots stored at 2 °C led to a reduction close to 100% in ethylene concentration; these results are similar to those obtained in our study when applying the triple combination of $KMnO_4$ + UV-C + TiO_2 to broccoli, but in our study this effect was observed from the beginning of the trial. In recent years, studies on the effect of titanium dioxide–UV on ethylene have focused on its application as a component of films or packaging for fruits. Among them, Fonseca et al. [39] in 2021 evaluated the effectiveness of polyethylene foam nets coated with a photocatalytic nanocomposite composed of gelatine and titanium dioxide to degrade ethylene produced by papayas (*Carica papaya* L.) of the 'Golden' variety. The fruits treated with gelatine of titanium dioxide and irradiated with UV light showed a 60% lower ethylene accumulation than the fruit in the control group after four days of storage. De Chiara et al. [40] applied a powder composed of titanium dioxide and silicon dioxide in different proportions for the preservation of tomatoes of the 'Camone' variety. In the tomatoes treated with the 80–20 (TiO_2-SiO_2) ratio and exposed to UV light, ethylene was completely degraded after 14 days of study. Again, the triple combination of $KMnO_4$ + UV-C + TiO_2 used in our study reduced ethylene concentration in broccoli from the beginning of the trial.

3.2. Physicochemical Variables

Table 3 illustrates the changes in physicochemical variables of broccoli throughout the entire storage period for each treatment. At the end of the experiment (day 21), the treatments Broc-Control and Broc-Tom + $KMnO_4$ + UV-C + TiO_2 demonstrated superior preservation performance and/or longer shelf life compared with the other treatments, and, on the other hand, the Broc-Tomato treatment showed the worst performance. The raw data for weight, pH, SSC, TA, and MI and raw data for color parameters a*, b*, and L are presented in the Supplementary Materials (Supplementary Tables S1 and S2), including the results of the parameters indicated on all days studied (0, 7, 15, and 21).

After 21 days of study, weight loss was observed in all tested treatments, with the Broc-Tomato treatment experiencing the greatest weight loss, decreasing by up to 39.38% of the initial weight. Among the other treatments, there were no significant differences, but weight loss was lower in the Broc-Control treatment with 43.99% and Broc-Tom + $KMnO_4$ + UV-C + TiO_2 treatment with 35.02% (Table 3). Analysis of how time affected each of the treatments (Supplementary Figure S1) revealed that the pattern of weight loss was the same, with significant differences between day 0 and 7, between day 7 and the other analyzed days, and no differences between day 14 and 21. However, weight loss was faster with the Broc-Tomato treatment. Previous studies on ethylene scavengers also reported a reduction in loss of weight of stored broccoli [41].

After 21 days of testing, a pH increase was observed in all analyzed treatments compared with 0 days but was significantly higher in the Broc-Tomato treatment with 11.42%, compared with the others. Among the other treatments, there were significant differences between Broc-Tom + $KMnO_4$ = Broc-Tom + $KMnO_4$ + UV-C, with an increase in pH of 8.14% on average, and Broc-Control = Broc-Tom + $KMnO_4$ + UV-C + TiO_2, with an increase in pH of 6.37 on average (Table 3). Analysis of how time affected each of the treatments (Supplementary Figure S1) revealed that the pattern of pH increase was the same, except for the Broc-Tomato treatment which showed significant differences on all days analyzed.

Table 3. Evolution from day 0 to day 21 of the weight expressed in grams, maturity variables as pH, solid soluble content (SSC) expressed as percentage, total acidity (TA) expressed as g L^{-1}, and mature index (MI) as the SSC (%)/TA (%). Total phenol contents (TPC) expressed as mg g^{-1}, chlorophyll variables chlorophyll a, chlorophyll b, and total chlorophyll expressed as mL g^{-1}, and color parameters a*, b*, and L in broccoli subjected to the different treatments (Broc-Control, Broc-Tom, Broc-Tom + KMnO$_4$, Broc-Tom + KMnO$_4$ + UV-C, Broc-Tom + KMnO$_4$ + UV-C + TiO$_2$).

Treatments	Weight (%)		pH		SSC (%)	
	Day 0	Day 21	Day 0	Day 21	Day 0	Day 21
Broc-Control		56.01 ± 3.08 a		6.78 ± 0.04 c		9.58 ± 0.07 c
Broc-Tomato		39.38 ± 1.41 c		7.12 ± 0.04 a		11.66 ± 0.10 a
Broc-Tom + KMnO$_4$	100	45.56 ± 1.49 b	6.39 ± 0.03	6.95 ± 0.03 b	7.83 ± 0.33	10.33 ± 0.07 b
Broc-Tom + KMnO$_4$ + UV-C		51.20 ± 2.38 a		6.87 ± 0.01 b		9.99 ± 0.09 b
Broc-Tom + KMnO$_4$ + UV-C + TiO$_2$		64.98 ± 3.50 a		6.82 ± 0.02 c		10.01 ± 0.10 b
		F = 6.21 **		F = 17.96 ***		F = 86.33 **

Treatments	TA		MI		TPC	
	Day 0	Day 21	Day 0	Day 21	Day 0	Day 21
Broc-Control		0.75 ± 0.02 a		2.58 ± 0.06 c		27.10 ± 0.29 a
Broc-Tomato		0.54 ± 0.01 b		4.37 ± 0.08 a		11.63 ± 1.02 c
Broc-Tom + KMnO$_4$	0.93 ± 0.05	0.69 ± 0.02 a	1.70 ± 0.09	3.01 ± 0.10 b	36.41 ± 1.24	20.11 ± 1.57 b
Broc-Tom + KMnO$_4$ + UV-C		0.71 ± 0.03 a		2.86 ± 0.14 bc		24.47 ± 0.78 ab
Broc-Tom + KMnO$_4$ + UV-C + TiO$_2$		0.70 ± 0.02 a		2.90 ± 0.10 bc		27.25 ± 0.60 a
		F = 12.84 ***		F = 49.31 ***		F = 46.96 ***

Treatments	Chlorophyll a		Chlorophyll b		Total Chlorophyll	
	Day 0	Day 21	Day 0	Day 21	Day 0	Day 21
Broc-Control		1.81 ± 0.24 a		11.37 ± 0.52 a		18.23 ± 0.38 a
Broc-Tomato		1.33 ± 0.21 b		5.49 ± 0.68 d		9.87 ± 0.62 d
Broc-Tom + KMnO$_4$	2.19 ± 0.26	1.60 ± 0.13 ab	10.41 ± 1.13	7.22 ± 0.23 c	18.62 ± 1.26	12.68 ± 0.31 c
Broc-Tom + KMnO$_4$ + UV-C		1.62 ± 0.09 ab		8.13 ± 0.28 bc		13.91 ± 0.36 bc
Broc-Tom + KMnO$_4$ + UV-C + TiO$_2$		1.80 ± 0.12 a		9.08 ± 0.29 b		15.41 ± 0.22 b
		F = 4.84 *		F = 35.65 ***		F = 60.06 ***

Treatments	Colour a*		Colour b*		Colour L	
	Day 0	Day 21	Day 0	Day 21	Day 0	Day 21
Broc-Control		−8.17 ± 0.39 a		14.45 ± 0.52 b		25.63 ± 1.41 b
Broc-Tomato		−15.26 ± 1.56 c		24.86 ± 1.36 a		49.63 ± 2.96 a
Broc-Tom + KMnO$_4$	−4.52 ± 0.23	−12.69 ± 1.02 bc	6.26 ± 0.30	17.18 ± 0.69 b	25.69 ± 0.68	30.33 ± 1.22 b
Broc-Tom + KMnO$_4$ + UV-C		−10.80 ± 0.47 ab		15.04 ± 0.94 b		28.95 ± 0.86 b
Broc-Tom + KMnO$_4$ + UV-C + TiO$_2$		−8.48 ± 0.27 a		14.61 ± 1.19 b		26.11 ± 0.92 b
		F = 11.28 ***		F = 19.83 ***		F = 36.08 ***

The means ± standard error of the means (SEM) are shown. Different letters for each treatment represent statistically significant differences according to Tukey's test, n = 5 per treatment and day. *, **, ***, significant at $p < 0.05$, 0.01, and 0.001, respectively.

After 21 days was, for both variables in this study, increases and decreases in SSC and AT, respectively, were observed for all treatments studied compared with 0 days of trial. The highest increase in SSC was observed in the Broc-Tomato treatment, with 48.91% compared with day 0. The lowest increase was observed in the Broc-Control treatment, with 22.35%. The treatments with some type of mechanism to eliminate ethylene had intermediate results with average increases of 29.12% (Table 3). In the case of TA, significant decreases were observed only in the Broc-Tomato treatment, with a decrease of 41.94%. The rest of the treatments showed similar responses with average decreases of 23.39% (Table 3). Therefore, an increase in the maturity index, which is calculated as the ratio between total soluble solids and total acidity, is an important indicator of postharvest quality in broccoli, indicating accelerated product ripening that affects its quality and shelf life. The MI also increased over time in this study, with the main differences observed in the Broc-Control (51.76%) and Broc-Tomato (2.57-fold) treatments. Treatments with two (Broc-Tom + KMnO$_4$ + UV-C) or three types of mechanisms (Broc-Tom + KMnO$_4$ + UV-C + TiO$_2$) for ethylene removal responded similarly to the control treatment, with slightly higher average increases of 69.71% (Table 3). Analysis of how time affected each of the treatments (Supplementary Figure S1) revealed that the pattern of SSC increase was the same, except for the Broc-Tomato treatment which showed significant differences on all days analyzed. Regarding decreases in TA, it is noteworthy that there were no differences in any of the treatments studied between day 0 and 7, and that the decreases were not very pronounced on day 14 (Supplementary Figure S1). The increase in the MI showed very similar trends, except in the Broc-Tomato treatment where no significant differences were observed on days 7 and 14 (Supplementary Figure S1).

Phenolic compounds are a class of chemical compounds widely distributed in nature and found in numerous plants, including broccoli. These compounds are important in nutrition due to their antioxidant, anti-inflammatory, antimicrobial, and anticancer properties. In broccoli, phenolic compounds, particularly glucosinolates and flavonoids, are responsible for its health benefits. Glucosinolates are compounds that convert into isothiocyanates when vegetables are cut or chewed, and have been shown to have anticancer and antioxidant properties. Flavonoids are compounds that have antioxidant and anti-inflammatory properties, and have been shown to reduce the risk of cardiovascular diseases and some types of cancer. Additionally, phenolic compounds in broccoli also play an important role in postharvest conservation. Broccoli is a highly perishable vegetable and sensitive to degradation, which can affect its quality and shelf life. It has been demonstrated that phenolic compounds in broccoli have antimicrobial and antioxidant properties, which can help reduce microbial activity and oxidation, thus prolonging the product's shelf life and improving its quality. After 21 days, there was a decrease in TPC in all treatments, but much greater in the Broc-Tomato treatment with a decrease of 68.06%. The broccoli from Broc-Control and Broc-Tom + $KMnO_4$ + UV-C + TiO_2 treatments with values of approximately 27 g mg^{-1} showed the lowest losses of TPC (25.36%), thus preserving higher nutritional quality (Table 3).

Chlorophyll is a green pigment found in plants and is essential for photosynthesis. In postharvest preservation of broccoli, chlorophyll plays an important role as an indicator of product quality and freshness because its degradation is associated with changes in appearance, flavor, and texture. As chlorophyll degrades, broccoli loses its bright green colour and turns yellowish, indicating a loss of freshness and quality. Therefore, measuring chlorophyll levels in broccoli can be a useful tool for evaluating product quality and shelf life. Specifically, three parameters were measured: chlorophyll a, chlorophyll b, and total chlorophyll. Chlorophyll at the end of the trial had the lowest values in the Broc-Tomato treatment (1.33 mL g^{-1}) and the highest values in the Broc-Control (1.81 mL g^{-1}) and Broc-Tom + $KMnO_4$ + UV-C + TiO_2 (1.80 mL g^{-1}) treatments (Table 3). The trends observed in chlorophyll b and total chlorophyll were the same, with lower values in Broc-Tomato treatment (5.49 and 9.87 mL g^{-1} respectively) and higher but significantly different values in Broc-Control (11.37 and 18.23 mL g^{-1} respectively) and Broc-Tom + $KMnO_4$ + UV-C + TiO_2 (9.08 and 15.41 mL g^{-1} respectively) treatments (Table 3).

Regarding color, the b* parameter is one of the three color parameters used in the CIELAB scale to measure the color of foods and other objects. The b* parameter describes positive values indicating a yellow component and negative values indicating a blue component. In postharvest conservation of broccoli, the b* parameter is important because it can be used to monitor changes in the colour of the product [42]. As indicated above when broccoli degrades and loses its quality, its bright green colour becomes more yellowish, which is reflected in higher values of the b* parameter. This response in b* was observed in this study with more positive value in Broc-Tomato (24.86) and less positive values in Broc-Control (14.45) and Broc-Tom + $KMnO_4$ + UV-C + TiO_2 (14.61) (Table 3). The evolution over time showed an equal behaviour in all treatments, but with a faster increase in positive values in the Broc-Tomato treatment (Supplementary Figure S2).

Moreover, a* parameter, which describes the red-green colour component of an object (positive values indicating a red component and negative values indicating a green component) has been more negative in Broc-Tomato (-15.26) and less negative values in Broc-Control (-8.17) and Broc-Tom + $KMnO_4$ + UV-C + TiO_2 (-8.48) (Table 3). The evolution over time showed a similar behaviour in all treatments, but with a faster increase in negative values in the Broc-Tomato treatment (Supplementary Figure S2). Finally, the colour parameter L* describes the brightness of an object, with higher values indicating greater brightness and lower values indicating lower brightness. During ethylene-mediated degradation of broccoli during postharvest storage, the decrease in chlorophyll can lead to an increase in brightness and, therefore, in L* values. This is because chlorophyll acts as a dark pigment, so its decrease makes the broccoli appear lighter and brighter. This response in L was observed in this study with more positive values in Broc-Tomato (49.63) and less positive values in Broc-Control (25.63) and Broc-Tom + $KMnO_4$ + UV-C + TiO_2 (26.11) (Table 3). The evolution over time showed equal behavior in all treatments, except in the Broc-Tomato treatment which had a faster increase in positive values (Supplementary Figure S2).

Other researchers have analyzed the same parameters and ethylene scavengers. For instance, Emadpour et al. [43] observed a weight loss reduction of only 3% during storage with potassium permanganate (without specifying the concentration). Mansourbahmani et al. [18] recorded a 2% weight loss reduction in 'Valouro' tomatoes with the application of 20% potassium permanganate mixed with zeolite in a 1:2 ratio, after 35 days of storage. According to Tilahun et al. [44], tissue degradation occurs during ripening, leading to the production of reactive oxygen species (ROS). These substances are eliminated by total phenolic compounds (TPC) and other components that contribute to the fruit's antioxidant capacity. Mansourbahmani et al. [18] observed that the TPC data after 35 days of treatment by applying 20% potassium permanganate mixed with zeolite in a 1:2 ratio were 35% higher than for untreated tomatoes. Ghosh et al. [45], in 2022, applied photoactivated titanium dioxide and chitosan to create a film for coating 'Tejaswani' peppers stored at room temperature (25 °C). The treated peppers exhibited maintained soluble solid content (SSC) along with enhanced color. However, none of these trials adhered to the experimental design planned in this study, which involves growing an ethylene-sensitive vegetable such as broccoli and an ethylene-producing vegetable such as tomato in the same storage chamber. Furthermore, we applied a triple combination of ethylene scavengers, making it challenging to compare our results with those of other researchers.

In summary, in terms of the evolution of the different physicochemical parameters analyzed, the ones that were most affected by the presence of ethylene during storage were MI, SSC, TPC, and total chlorophyll (Table 4).

Table 4. Summary table of the effect of ethylene on physico-chemical parameters. Mature index (MI); solid soluble content (SSC); Total phenol contents (TPC); Total acidity (TA); colour parameters as a*, b*, and L. F values express sensibility to ethylene. Higher values are correlated with higher sensitivity.

Parameters	F
MI	320.83 ***
SSC	306.50 ***
TPC	215.00 ***
Total chlorophyll	132.27 ***
TA	70.90 ***
Chlorophyll b	63.29 ***
L	53.74 ***
b*	51.16 ***
pH	34.46 ***
Weight	20.29 **
a*	19.43 **
Chlorophyll a	2.31 n.s.

, *, significant at $p < 0.01$, and 0.001, respectively. n.s., no significant.

3.3. Sensory Analysis

Table 5 displays the results of the descriptive sensory analysis conducted on broccoli samples. Significant differences were observed in 20 out of the 30 sensory descriptors studied.

Table 5. Descriptive sensory analysis of broccoli.

Sensory Descriptor	ANOVA ‡	Day 0 Broc-Control	Day 21 Broc-Control	Day 21 Broc-Tomato	Day 21 Broc-Tom + KMnO$_4$	Day 21 Broc-Tom + KMnO$_4$ + UV-C	Day 21 Broc-Tom + KMnO$_4$ + UV-C + TiO$_2$
COLOR							
Green color	***	9.5 b	5.5 a	2.5 c	8.5 b	8.5 b	8.5 b
Yellow color	***	0.5 d	1.5 c	6.0 a	2.5 b	2.5 b	1.5 c
Colour homogeneity	***	8.6 a	7.3 c	5.0 d	7.5 bc	7.8 abc	8.5 ab
External broccoli ID	***	9.0 a	2.7 c	3.2 c	6.7 b	8.0 ab	8.7 a
Inflorescences (closed)	***	9.3 ab	10.0 a	6.0 d	7.5 c	8.7 b	8.8 b
ODOR							
Broccoli ID	***	10.0 a	4.3 b	1.8 b	2.3 b	2.8 b	2.7 b
Green vegetable	***	9.5 a	2.6 b	1.0 b	2.1 b	2.0 b	2.0 b
Ripe vegetable	***	0.3 d	7.3 a	5.3 b	5.0 b	5.8 b	3.7 c
Earthy	NS	1.8	5.0	3.7	2.8	3.2	3.3
Fermented	NS	0.0	1.3	2.0	0.8	0.7	1.0
Sulfurous	**	8.0 a	4.3 ab	3.3 b	3.3 b	4.0 b	3.3 b
FLAVOR							
Broccoli ID	***	9.3 a	4.6 cd	3.0 d	6.5 bc	8.0 ab	5.8 c
Green vegetable	***	9.5 a	2.3 c	1.5 c	5.1 b	6.3 b	4.7 b
Ripe vegetable	***	0.1 b	7.6 a	6.0 a	4.8 ab	3.7 ab	4.3 ab
Earthy	*	0.7 b	3.6 a	3.5 a	2.0 b	1.3 b	1.5 b
Fermented	NS	0.0	0.8	1.5	0.0	0.3	1.0
Sulfurous	***	8.0 a	4.5 cd	2.7 d	5.8 bc	6.5 ab	5.5 bc
Woody	NS	0.0	0.8	1.0	0.0	0.5	0.0
Sweet	NS	3.0	4.0	3.5	5.3	4.3	4.3
Sour	NS	2.2	1.8	1.3	1.0	1.0	1.3
Bitter	NS	4.0	3.5	4.1	2.5	3.0	3.5
Astringency	NS	1.0	0.8	1.1	0.6	1.0	1.1
Aftertaste	**	8.3 a	4.8 c	4 c	6.5 b	5.8 b	6.3 b
TEXTURE							
Spicy	NS	2.7	1.8	1.3	2.1	2.5	2.7
Hardness	**	9.0 a	9.0 a	6.7 b	7.5 ab	8.5 a	9.5 a
Crunchiness	***	7.1 a	2.7 c	2.5 c	4.3 bc	6.1 ab	4.7 bc
Chewiness	***	8.0 b	9.3 a	9.7 a	8.1 b	8.6 ab	9.3 a
Juiciness	***	3.0 a	0.7 c	0.8 bc	2.0 abc	2.7 ab	1.7 abc
Residual particles	NS	5.0	6.0	6.5	6.3	5.5	6.5
Fibrousness	**	0.3 c	2.3 b	4.3 a	1.8 b	2.0 b	2.3 b

‡ NS = not significant at $p > 0.05$; *, **, ***. significant at $p < 0.05$, 0.01, and 0.001, respectively. Values (mean of three replications) followed by the same letter within the same sensory descriptor are not significantly different ($p > 0.05$) according to Tukey's least significant difference test.

Significant differences were found in the color of the samples under study. As expected, the sample stored for 21 days together with the tomato was the one with the least green color intensity and the most yellow color intensity. Initially, the broccoli had an intense green external colour that gradually turned yellow. Following this, the sample was stored for 21 days. In general, the samples in which the influence of the ethylene-regulating treatments was studied preserved the color of the original sample (fresh). Considering the general appearance of the sample, using a descriptor that encompassed color, presence, turgidity (visual), etc., the Broc-Tom + KMnO$_4$ + UV-C and the Broc-Tom + KMnO$_4$ + UV-C + TiO$_2$ treatments were the ones that best preserved the original appearance.

In the case of the smell of the samples, with reference to the characteristic smell of broccoli, none of the treatments studied managed to reproduce the smell of the fresh sample. All the studied treatments obtained much lower intensity values (~2–4, while the fresh sample had an intensity of 10). However, differences were observed in terms of ripe smell. In this case, the Broc-Tom + KMnO$_4$ + UV-C + TiO$_2$ treatment was the one that, together with the Broc-Control at day 0, presented the lowest intensity, compared with the 21-day treatment, which was the highest. The finding that the treatment effectively blocked the characteristic odor of the ripe product for an extended period highlights its efficacy. The fruit/vegetal aroma significantly influences the overall sensory quality and consumer preference for a fruit. Therefore, preserving the initial aroma of the fruit for a longer duration enhances its market potential [46].

No statistically significant differences were found in the basic flavors of the samples or in the astringency. However, the treatments studied did have an effect in the case of broccoli ID, green vegetable, brown vegetable, earthy, and sulfur flavors. In all cases, globally it could be observed that the ethylene-regulation treatments were able to stop the odors related to the maturity of the samples (mature, earthy, fermented vegetables) and maintain the characteristic odors (broccoli ID, green vegetable, sulfur). The compounds that are most related to the smell and taste of broccoli are isothiocyanates [47]. These give it its characteristic aroma and the longer they are preserved, the more the preservation of their quality can be related.

Upon analyzing the results of the texture analysis, no significant differences were observed in the content of residual particles nor the spiciness of the samples. Differences were apparent in hardness, crunchiness, chewiness, juiciness, and fibrousness. Similar to the case of the odor and taste of the broccoli samples, the ethylene-control treatments also worked to control the texture of the samples. With the use of these systems, all the descriptors related to the quality of the samples, such as hardness or chewiness, were maintained. That is, the sample better preserved its original turgor. In all the texture descriptors evaluated, the sample preserved with tomato was the one that obtained the worst results.

In view of these results, it can be pointed out that the panel of experts found more appreciable differences in the parameters related to color, firstly, and texture, secondly. In contrast, the sensory attributes related to flavor were not affected for the most part during the storage period under conditions of low ethylene concentration.

3.4. Principal Component Analysis

Furthermore, a principal component analysis (PCA) was performed to identify the variables that contributed the most to the overall variability in the experiment and to assess how the different treatments were distinguished from each other. The objective of this analysis was to derive a reduced number of linear combinations from the 12 variables examined (Weight, pH, SSC, TA, MI, TPC, chlorophyll a, chlorophyll b, total chlorophyll, a*, b*, and L*) that captured the most substantial variability present in the data. Two components were extracted since these two components had eigenvalues greater than or equal to 1.0. These components are referred to as principal component 1 (PC1), which explains 74.97% of the experiment's variability, and principal component 2 (PC2), which explains 8.00% of the experiment's variability. Together, they accounted for 82.97% of the variability in the original data (Supplementary Table S3 and Figure S3).

Subsequently, the focus shifted to identifying the variables that carried the most weight or exhibited greater importance within each extracted component. In PC1, the variables with the highest weights were determined to be as follows: MI > SSC > TPC > total chlorophyll > L > pH. Similarly, in PC2, the variable with the greatest weight was identified as chlorophyll a (Supplementary Table S4).

As mentioned earlier, another objective was to plot the treatments on a scatter diagram (Figure 3) or a biplot (Supplementary Figure S4). These figures were generated using the principal component table where the scores obtained for each component were represented for each treatment (5 per treatment, totaling 25 data points).

Additionally, the average score for each of the five treatments was included (Supplementary Table S5a). The scatter diagram demonstrated that the treatments were well-separated primarily along the first component (PC1) with a value of F = 116.12 ***, enabling the classification of treatments into five clusters (Supplementary Table S5b): the first cluster consisted of the Broc-Tomato treatment; the second cluster included the Broc-Tom + $KMnO_4$ treatment; the third cluster comprised the Broc-Tom + $KMnO_4$ + UV-C treatment; the fourth cluster contained the Broc-Tom + $KMnO_4$ + UV-C + TiO_2 treatment; the fifth cluster included the Broc-Control treatment (Supplementary Table S5c). In terms of PC2, the treatments did not form distinct clusters, with a value of F = 0.19 n.s. (Supplementary Table S5d,e).

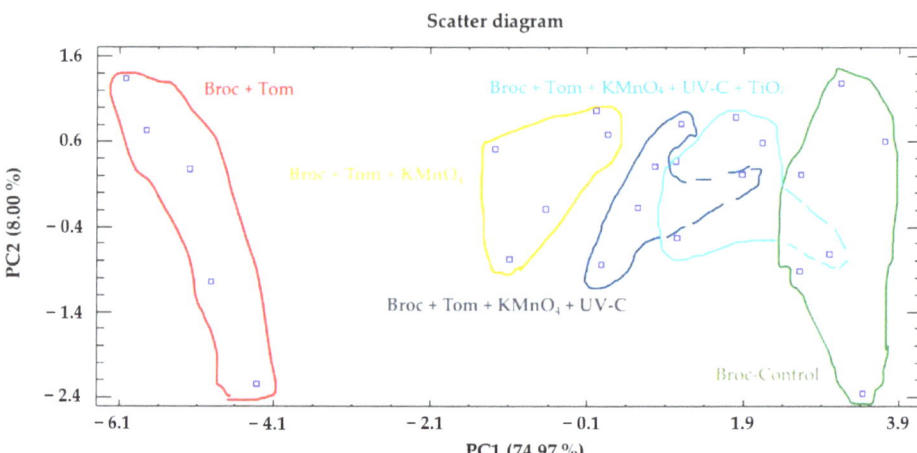

Figure 3. A principal component analysis applied to the different treatments (Broc-Control, Broc-Tomato, Broc-Tom + KMnO$_4$, Broc-Tom + KMnO$_4$ + UV-C, Broc-Tom + KMnO$_4$ + UV-C + TiO$_2$). Two principal components (PC1 and PC2) resulted in a model that explained 82.97% of the total variance. Number of replicates n = 5.

4. Conclusions

In this comprehensive study, we conducted a thorough assessment of ethylene-removal techniques, both individually and in combination, using KMnO$_4$, UV-C radiation, and TiO$_2$ to preserve the postharvest quality of broccoli. Furthermore, we examined the impact of ethylene produced by tomatoes on ethylene-sensitive broccoli through sensory analysis. The results obtained in this study have significant implications. The application of the aforementioned ethylene-elimination methods demonstrated remarkable efficacy in maintaining exceptionally low levels of this plant hormone, reaching values approaching zero. Notably, when evaluating the condition of the preserved broccoli, the triple combination system (Broc-Tom + KMnO$_4$ + UV-C + TiO$_2$) demonstrated comparable physicochemical quality to the Broc-Control treatment. This was evident in the increased weight, titratable acidity (TA), total phenolic compounds (TPC), and total chlorophyll content compared with the Broc-Tomato, Broc-Tom + KMnO$_4$, and Broc-Tom + KMnO$_4$ + UV-C treatments. Additionally, the Broc-Tom + KMnO$_4$ + UV-C + TiO$_2$ treatment exhibited lower levels of pH, soluble solid content (SSC), and internal browning (MI) compared with other treatments. These findings highlight the efficacy of the ethylene-elimination methods described in this study, particularly the novel triple combination with KMnO$_4$, UV-C, and TiO$_2$, in effectively delaying the postharvest ripening process of broccoli and extending its shelf life. By employing these innovative techniques, we have made significant strides in preserving the quality of broccoli during postharvest storage. The successful implementation of this approach can have far-reaching implications, including reducing food waste, enhancing marketability, and improving overall sustainability in the food industry.

Supplementary Materials: The following supporting information can be downloaded at: https://www.mdpi.com/article/10.3390/foods12122418/s1, Supplementary Figure S1: Evolution during storage time of weight, pH, SSC, TA, and MI expressed in broccoli subjected to different treatments (Broc-Control, Broc-Tomato, Broc-Tom + KMnO$_4$, Broc-Tom + KMnO$_4$ + UV-C and Broc-Tom + KMnO$_4$ + UV-C + TiO$_2$); Supplementary Figure S2: Evolution during storage time of the color parameters in broccoli subjected to different treatments (Broc-Control, Broc-Tomato, Broc-Tom + KMnO$_4$, Broc-Tom + KMnO$_4$ + UV-C and Broc-Tom + KMnO$_4$ + UV-C + TiO$_2$); Supplementary Figure S3: Sedimentation graph; Supplementary Figure S4: Graphical representation of the principal components marked with lines for each variable and with points for each score; Supplementary Table S1: Evolution during storage time of the physical variables in broccoli florets subjected to the different treatments: (Broc-Control, Broc-Tomato, Broc-Tom + $KMnO_4$, Broc-Tom + $KMnO_4$ + UV-C and Broc-Tom + $KMnO_4$ + UV-C + TiO_2); Supplementary Table S2: Evolution during storage time of the biochemical variables in broccoli florets subjected to different treatments: (Broc-Control, Broc-Tomato, Broc-Tom + $KMnO_4$, Broc-Tom + $KMnO_4$ + UV-C and Broc-Tom + $KMnO_4$ + UV-C + TiO_2); Supplementary Table S3: Principal component analysis; Supplementary Table S4: Table of component weights; Supplementary Table S5a: This table shows the scores of the principal components; Supplementary Table S5b: ANOVA table for the component 1 scores according to the treatments; Supplementary Table S5c: Multiple comparisons test for the component 1 scores by treatment using Tukey's HSD method; Supplementary Table S5d: ANOVA table for the component 2 scores according to the treatments; Supplementary Table S5e: Multiple comparisons test for the component 2 scores by treatment using Tukey's HSD method.

Author Contributions: Conceptualization. R.A.-S., J.R.A.-M., S.L.-M. and A.J.P.-L.; methodology. R.A.-S., J.R.A.-M., S.L.-M. and A.J.P.-L.; software. R.A.-S., J.R.A.-M. and L.N.-A.; validation. A.G.-B., E.N.-D. and Á.C.-B.; formal analysis. R.A.-S., J.R.A.-M., A.G.-B., S.L.-M. and A.J.P.-L.; investigation. R.A.-S., J.R.A.-M., A.G.-B., S.L.-M. and A.J.P.-L.; resources. J.R.A.-M., S.L.-M. and L.N.-A.; data curation. R.A.-S., J.R.A.-M., A.J.P.-L and L.N.-A.; writing—original draft preparation. R.A.-S., J.R.A.-M., S.L.-M. and A.J.P.-L.; writing—review and editing. R.A.-S., J.R.A.-M., S.L.-M. and A.J.P.-L.; visualization. A.J.P.-L., J.R.A.-M. and S.L.-M.; supervision. J.R.A.-M., S.L.-M. and Á.C.-B.; project administration. S.L.-M. and E.N.-D.; funding acquisition. E.N.-D. and J.R.A.-M. All authors have read and agreed to the published version of the manuscript.

Funding: Nuevas Tecnologías Agroalimentarias (KEEPCOOL): CFE/KE/76-19; "Cátedra Emprendimiento en el Ámbito Agroalimentario" from Universidad Católica San Antonio de Murcia (UCAM) and Banco Santander: CFE/KE/76-19.

Data Availability Statement: All related data and methods are presented in this paper. Additional inquiries should be addressed to the corresponding autor.

Acknowledgments: The authors gratefully acknowledge Antonio Cerdá (Cátedra UCAM-Banco Santander de Emprendimiento en el Ámbito Agroalimentario director), Hoyamar Sociedad Cooperativa from FECOAM ("Federación de Cooperativas Agrarias de Murcia"), especially Antonio Sanz and Lola Mondéjar for supplying the broccoli used in this study, and Miriam Monje for her help with figures.

Conflicts of Interest: The Doctoral Thesis (Ph.D.) of Ramiro Alonso Salinas, co-author of this work, is being co-financed by the company Nuevas Tecnologías Agroalimentarias (KEEPCOOL). within the UCAM Universidad Católica de Murcia Industrial Doctorate Program. The rest of the authors of the article declare that their contribution to this research was carried out in the absence of commercial or financial relationships that could be constructed as a possible conflict of interest.

References

1. Hegnsholt, E.; Unnikrishnan, S.; Pollmann-Larsen, M.; Askelsdottir, B.; Gerard, M. Tackling the 1.6-Billion-Ton Food Loss and Waste Crisis. *Boston Consult. Group* **2018**. Available online: https://www.bcg.com/publications/2018/tackling-1.6-billion-ton-food-loss-and-waste-crisis (accessed on 5 April 2023).
2. Shabir, I.; Dash, K.K.; Dar, A.H.; Pandey, V.K.; Fayaz, U.; Srivastava, S.; Nisha, R. Carbon footprints evaluation for sustainable food processing system development: A comprehensive review. *Future Foods* **2023**, *7*, 100215. [CrossRef]
3. Francisco, M.; Tortosa, M.; Martínez-Ballesta, M.C.; Velasco, P.; García-Viguera, C.; Moreno, D.A. Nutritional and phytochemical value of Brassica crops from the agri-food perspective. *Ann. Appl. Biol.* **2017**, *170*, 273–285. [CrossRef]
4. Conversa, G.; Lazzizera, C.; Bonasia, A.; Elia, A. Harvest season and genotype affect head quality and shelf-life of ready-to-use broccoli. *Agronomy* **2020**, *10*, 527. [CrossRef]
5. Alonso-Salinas, R.; López-Miranda, S.; Pérez-López, A.J.; Noguera-Artiaga, L.; Carbonell-Barrachina, A.; Núñez-Delicado, E.; Acosta-Motos, J.R. Novel combination of ethylene oxidisers to delay losses on postharvest quality. volatile compounds and sensorial analysis of tomato fruit. *LWT-Food Sci. Technol.* **2022**, *170*, 114054. [CrossRef]
6. Pereira-Lima, G.; Gómez-Gómez, H.; Seabra-Junior, S.; Maraschin, M.; Tecchio, M.A.; Vanz-Borges, C. Functional and nutraceutical compounds of tomatoes as affected by agronomic practices. Postharvest management and processing methods: A mini review. *Front. Nutr.* **2022**, *9*, 868492. [CrossRef]

7. Asoda, T.; Terai, H.; Kato, M.; Suzuki, Y. Effects of postharvest ethanol vapor treatment on ethylene responsiveness in broccoli *Postharvest Biol. Technol.* **2009**, *52*, 216–220. [CrossRef]
8. Cai, J.; Cheng, S.; Luo, F.; Zhao, Y.; Wei, B.; Zhou, Q.; Zhou, X.; Ji, S. Influence of ethylene on morphology and pigment changes in harvested broccoli. *Food Bioprocess Technol.* **2019**, *12*, 883–897. [CrossRef]
9. FAO (Food and Agriculture Organization). Faostat: Worldwide Tomato Production. 2020. Available online: https://www.fao.org/faostat/es/#data/QCL. (accessed on 5 April 2023).
10. Jeffery, E.H.; Brown, A.F.; Kurilich, A.C.; Keck, A.S.; Matusheski, N.; Klein, B.P.; Juvik, J.A. Variation in content of bioactive components in broccoli. *J. Food Compos. Anal.* **2003**, *16*, 323–330. [CrossRef]
11. Moreno, D.A.; Carvajal, M.; López-Berenguer, C.; García-Viguera, C. Chemical and biological characterisation of nutraceutical compounds of broccoli. *J. Pharm. Biomed. Anal.* **2006**, *41*, 1508–1522. [CrossRef]
12. Latté, K.P.; Appel, K.E.; Lampen, A. Health benefits and possible risks of broccoli—An overview. *Food Chem. Toxicol.* **2011**, *49*, 3287–3309. [CrossRef] [PubMed]
13. Yang, S.F.; Hoffman, N.E. Ethylene biosynthesis and its regulation in higher plants. *Annu. Rev. Plant Physiol.* **1984**, *35*, 155–189. [CrossRef]
14. Abeles, F.B.; Morgan, P.W.; Saltveit, M.E. Chapter 3—The biosynthesis of ethylene. In *Ethylene in Plant Biology*, 2nd ed.; Abeles, F.B., Morgan, P.W., Saltveit, M.E., Eds.; Academic Press: New York, NY, USA, 1992; pp. 26–55. [CrossRef]
15. Zhao, T.; Nakano, A.; Iwasaki, Y. Differences between ethylene emission characteristics of tomato cultivars in tomato production at plant factory. *J. Agric. Food Res.* **2021**, *5*, 100181. [CrossRef]
16. Ustun, H.; Dogan, A.; Peker, B.; Ural, C.; Cetin, M.; Ozyigit, Y.; Erkan, M. Determination of the relationship between respiration rate and ethylene production by fruit sizes of different tomato types. *J. Sci. Food Agric.* **2022**, *103*, 176–184. [CrossRef]
17. Janjarasskul, T.; Suppakul, P. Active and intelligent packaging: The indication of quality and safety. *Crit. Rev. Food Sci. Nutr.* **2018**, *58*, 808–831. [CrossRef]
18. Mansourbahmani, S.; Ghareyazie, B.; Zarinnia, V.; Kalatejari, S.; Mohammadi, R.S. Study on the efficiency of ethylene scavengers on the maintenance of postharvest quality of tomato fruit. *J. Food Meas. Charact.* **2018**, *12*, 691–701. [CrossRef]
19. Alonso-Salinas, R.; Acosta-Motos, J.R.; Núnez-Delicado, E.; Gabaldón, J.A.; López-Miranda, S. Combined effect of potassium permanganate and ultraviolet light as ethylene scavengers on post-Harvest quality of peach at optimal and stressful temperatures. *Agronomy* **2022**, *12*, 616. [CrossRef]
20. Bu, J.; Yu, Y.; Aisikaer, G.; Ying, T. Postharvest UV-C irradiation inhibits the production of ethylene and the activity of cell wall-degrading enzymes during softening of tomato (*Lycopersicon esculentum* L.) fruit. *Postharvest Biol. Technol.* **2013**, *86*, 337–345. [CrossRef]
21. Mabusela, B.P.; Belay, Z.A.; Godongwana, B.; Pathak, N.; Mahajan, P.V.; Caleb, O.J. Advances in vacuum ultraviolet photolysis in the postharvest management of fruit and vegetables along the value chains: A review. *Food Bioprocess Technol.* **2022**, *15*, 28–46. [CrossRef]
22. Li, W.; Liu, Z.; Li, X.; Li, X. Quality maintenance of 1-Methylcyclopropene combined with titanium dioxide photocatalytic reaction on postharvest cherry tomatoes. *J. Food Process. Preserv.* **2022**, *46*, e16500. [CrossRef]
23. Alves, M.J.; Nobias, M.C.; Soares, L.S.; Coelho, D.S.; Maraschin, M.; Basso, A.; Moreira, R.F.; José, H.J.; Montero, A.R. Physiological changes in green and red cherry tomatoes after photocatalytic ethylene degradation using continuous air flux. *Food Sci. Technol. Int.* **2023**, *29*, 3–12. [CrossRef]
24. Alonso-Salinas, R.; Acosta-Motos, J.R.; Pérez-López, A.J.; Noguera-Artiaga, L.; Núñez-Delicado, E.; Burló, F.; López-Miranda, S. Effect of combination of $KMnO_4$ oxidation and UV-C radiation on postharvest quality of refrigerated pears cv. 'Ercolini'. *Horticulturae* **2022**, *8*, 1078. [CrossRef]
25. Wei, H.; Seidi, F.; Zhang, T.; Jin, Y.; Xiao, H. Ethylene scavengers for the preservation of fruits and vegetables: A review. *Food Chem.* **2021**, *337*, 127750. [CrossRef] [PubMed]
26. Pathak, N.; Caleb, O.J.; Geyer, M.; Herppich, W.B.; Rauh, C.; Mahajan, P.V. Photocatalytic and photochemical oxidation of ethylene: Potential for storage of fresh produce—A review. *Food Bioprocess Technol.* **2017**, *10*, 982–1001. [CrossRef]
27. Kaewklin, P.; Siripatrawan, U.; Suwanagul, A.; Lee, Y.S. Active packaging from chitosan-titanium dioxide nanocomposite film for prolonging storage life of tomato fruit. *Int. J. Biol. Macromol.* **2018**, *112*, 523–529. [CrossRef] [PubMed]
28. Kim, S.; Jeong, G.H.; Kim, S.W. Ethylene gas decomposition using ZSM-5/WO_3-Pt-nanorod composites for fruit freshness. *ACS Sustain. Chem. Eng.* **2019**, *7*, 11250–11257. [CrossRef]
29. Álvarez-Hernández, M.H.; Artés-Hernández, F.; Ávalos-Belmontes, F.; Castillo-Campohermoso, M.A.; Contreras-Esquivel, J.C.; Ventura-Sobrevilla, J.M.; Martínez-Hernández, G.B. Current scenario of adsorbent materials used in ethylene scavenging systems to extend fruit and vegetable postharvest life. *Food Bioprocess Technol.* **2018**, *11*, 511–525. [CrossRef]
30. Guo, Y.; Wang, L.; Chen, Y.; Yun, L.; Liu, S.; Li, Y. Stalk length affects the mineral distribution and floret quality of broccoli (*Brassica oleracea* L. var. *italica*) heads during storage. *Postharvest Biol. Technol.* **2018**, *145*, 166–171. [CrossRef]
31. Phuong, N.; Uchino, T.; Tanaka, F. Effect of packing films on the quality of broccoli. *J. Fac. Agric. Kyushu Univ.* **2018**, *63*, 339–346. [CrossRef]
32. Zhang, B.; Peng, B.; Zhang, C.; Song, Z.; Ma, R. Determination of fruit maturity and its prediction model based on the pericarp index of absorbance difference (I_{AD}) for peaches. *PLoS ONE* **2017**, *12*, e0177511. [CrossRef]
33. Kidron, M.; Harel, E.; Mayer, A.M. Catechol oxidase activity in grapes and wine. *Am. J. Enol. Vitic.* **1978**, *29*, 30–35. [CrossRef]

34. Noguera-Artiaga, L.; Salvador, M.D.; Fregapane, G.; Collado-González, J.; Wojdyło, A.; López-Lluch, D.; Carbonell-Barrachina, A. Functional and sensory properties of pistachio nuts as affected by cultivar. *J. Sci. Food Agric.* **2019**, *99*, 6696–6705. [CrossRef] [PubMed]
35. Sammi, S.; Masud, T. Effect of different packaging systems on the quality of tomato (*Lycopersicon esculentum* Var. Rio Grande) fruits during storage. *Int. J. Food Sci. Technol.* **2009**, *44*, 918–926. [CrossRef]
36. Pathak, N. *Photocatalysis and Vacuum Ultraviolet Light Photolysis as Ethylene Removal Techniques for Potential Application in Fruit Storage*; Technische Universität Berlin: Berlin, Germany, 2019.
37. Gaikwad, K.K.; Singh, S.; Negi, Y.S. Ethylene scavengers for active packaging of fresh food produce. *Environ. Chem. Lett.* **2020**, *18*, 269–284. [CrossRef]
38. Álvarez-Hernández, M.H.; Martínez-Hernández, G.B.; Ávalos-Belmontes, F.; Miranda-Molina, F.D.; Artés-Hernández, F. Postharvest quality retention of apricots by using a novel sepiolite–loaded potassium permanganate ethylene scavenger. *Postharvest Biol. Technol.* **2020**, *160*, 111061. [CrossRef]
39. Fonseca, J.M.; Pabon, N.Y.L.; Nandi, L.G.; Valencia, G.A.; Moreira, R.F.P.M.; Monteiro, A.R. Gelatin-TiO$_2$-coated expanded polyethylene foam nets as ethylene scavengers for fruit postharvest application. *Postharvest Biol. Technol.* **2021**, *180*, 111602. [CrossRef]
40. de Chiara, M.L.; Pal, S.; Licciulli, A.; Amodio, M.L.; Colelli, G. Photocatalytic degradation of ethylene on mesoporous TiO$_2$/SiO$_2$ nanocomposites: Effects on the ripening of mature green tomatoes. *Biosyst. Eng.* **2015**, *132*, 61–70. [CrossRef]
41. Li, X.; Meng, Z.; Malik, A.U.; Zhang, S.; Wang, Q. Maintaining the quality of postharvest broccoli by inhibiting ethylene accumulation using diacetyl. *Front. Nutr.* **2022**, *9*, 1055651. [CrossRef]
42. Upadhyay, A.; Kumar, P.; Kardam, S.K.; Gaikwad, K.K. Ethylene scavenging film based on corn starch-gum acacia impregnated with sepiolite clay and its effect on quality of fresh broccoli florets. *Food Biosci.* **2022**, *46*, 101556. [CrossRef]
43. Emadpour, M.; Ghareyazie, B.; Kalaj, Y.R.; Entesari, M.; Bouzari, N. Effect of the potassium permanganate coated zeolite nanoparticles on the quality characteristic and shelf life of peach and nectarine. *Int. J. Agric. Technol.* **2015**, *11*, 1411–1421.
44. Tilahun, S.; Park, D.S.; Taye, A.M.; Jeong, C.S. Effect of ripening conditions on the physicochemical and antioxidant properties of tomato (*Lycopersicon esculentum* Mill.). *Food Sci. Biotechnol.* **2017**, *26*, 473–479. [CrossRef] [PubMed]
45. Ghosh, A.; Saha, I.; Fujita, M.; Debnath, S.C.; Hazra, A.K.; Adak, M.K.; Hasanuzzaman, M. Photoactivated TiO$_2$ nanocomposite delays the postharvest ripening phenomenon through ethylene metabolism and related physiological changes in *Capsicum* fruit. *Plants* **2022**, *11*, 513. [CrossRef] [PubMed]
46. Willner, B.; Granvogl, M.; Schieberle, P. Characterization of the key aroma compounds in bartlett pear brandies by means of the sensomics concept. *J. Agric. Food Chem.* **2013**, *61*, 9583–9593. [CrossRef] [PubMed]
47. Baky, M.H.; Shamma, S.N.; Xiao, J.; Farag, M.A. Comparative aroma and nutrients profiling in six edible versus nonedible cruciferous vegetables using MS based metabolomics. *Food Chem.* **2022**, *383*, 132374. [CrossRef] [PubMed]

Disclaimer/Publisher's Note: The statements, opinions and data contained in all publications are solely those of the individual author(s) and contributor(s) and not of MDPI and/or the editor(s). MDPI and/or the editor(s) disclaim responsibility for any injury to people or property resulting from any ideas, methods, instructions or products referred to in the content.

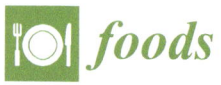

Article

Effect of CO₂ Laser Microperforation Pretreatment on the Dehydration of Apple Slices during Refractive Window Drying

Helena Núñez [1,2,*], Aldonza Jaques [1], Karyn Belmonte [1], Andrés Córdova [2,3], German Lafuente [1] and Cristian Ramírez [1]

[1] Departamento de Ingeniería Química y Ambiental, Universidad Técnica Federico Santa María, Valparaíso 2390123, Chile; aldonza.jaques@usm.cl (A.J.); karyn.belmonte.12@sansano.usm.cl (K.B.); german.lafuente.14@sansano.usm.cl (G.L.); cristian.ramirez@usm.cl (C.R.)
[2] Programa de Doctorado de Ciencias Agroalimentarias, Facultad de Ciencias Agronómicas y de los Alimentos Pontifica Universidad Católica de Valparaíso, Valparaíso 2360100, Chile; andres.cordova@pucv.cl
[3] Escuela de Alimentos, Pontificia Universidad Católica de Valparaíso, Valparaíso 2360100, Chile
* Correspondence: helena.nunez@usm.cl

Abstract: This research studied the use of CO_2 LASER microperforation as a pretreatment for the refractive window (RW) drying of apple slices with respect to total polyphenol content (TPC), antioxidant capacity, color ΔE, and product stability under accelerated storage. For this purpose, the processing variables assessed were pore size (200–600 μm), pore density (9–25 pores/cm²), and drying temperature (70–90 °C). As baseline criteria, a comparison with respect to the control without microperforations and samples subjected to conventional tunnel and lyophilization were also considered. The increase in the pore size from 200 to 600 μm resulted in shorter drying times (≤40 min), minimal change in color (ΔE) and loss of TPC, while DPPH was negatively affected by the combined effect of the pore density and the drying temperature. In general, the use of RW with CO_2 resulted in apples of higher quality than those obtained in conventional drying and comparable to those obtained through the use of freeze-drying. Finally, during accelerated storage, quality attributes decreased significantly for samples dried at 90 °C regardless of whether microperforations were used, suggesting that a compromise between drying temperature and pore size must be weighed to reduce processing time and to avoid further quality losses during storage.

Keywords: CO_2 laser microperforation; refractive window drying; bioactive compounds

Citation: Núñez, H.; Jaques, A.; Belmonte, K.; Córdova, A.; Lafuente, G.; Ramírez, C. Effect of CO₂ Laser Microperforation Pretreatment on the Dehydration of Apple Slices during Refractive Window Drying. *Foods* **2023**, *12*, 2187. https://doi.org/10.3390/foods12112187

Academic Editors: Antonio José Pérez-López and Luis Noguera-Artiaga

Received: 29 April 2023
Revised: 20 May 2023
Accepted: 24 May 2023
Published: 29 May 2023

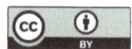

Copyright: © 2023 by the authors. Licensee MDPI, Basel, Switzerland. This article is an open access article distributed under the terms and conditions of the Creative Commons Attribution (CC BY) license (https://creativecommons.org/licenses/by/4.0/).

1. Introduction

Fruits provide basic nutrition along with significant health benefits for humans, but many of these fruits are produced seasonally and therefore may not be available to consumers year-round. For this reason, dried fruits represent an opportunity for consumers, since by eliminating the greatest amount of water content through various drying techniques, storage and transportation costs are reduced, and their shelf lives are increased because their stability to chemical reactions and microbial activity is improved [1]. Since the application of high temperatures during drying adversely affects the quality of dry products, it is important to select the appropriate technology [2]. Currently, the most common process of industrial food drying is convection drying or conventional drying [3]. These drying methods present long drying times and low thermal efficiency, which in turn results in lower quality products [1]. On the other hand, freeze-drying uses low-temperature operation [4], and it does not produce degradation of the food components due to thermal exposure, so nutritional reduction or sensory degradation is minimized [5]; however, it presents high capital and operational costs. The refractive window (RW) process is a fourth-generation drying technology in which hot water is used as the heating medium and circulates through the reservoir on a flexible polyester film (e.g., Mylar), where food material (pulp, juice, or sliced food) is placed. In this process, drying takes place by means of conduction and radiation, as the thermal energy is transferred from hot water to the food material through the film. Furthermore, moisture removed from the food material in the form of water vapor is carried away by a flow of air [6]. This technology has high thermal efficiency and higher heat and mass transfer rates [1,6,7] and decreased drying times, which has a positive impact on the retention of bioactive compounds and sensory properties and results in high retention of product quality [2,8,9].

Regardless of the drying method, the reduction in operating times is key to improving the productivity of any industry, which is why several technologies have been studied to improve mass and heat transfer, such as vacuum impregnation [10–13], pulsed electric fields [14–17], and ultimately, CO_2 laser microperforation [18–25].

The CO_2 laser is a device that generates a monochromatic, coherent, and directional beam of light that allows small holes to be made along a surface, thus causing minimal damage, without mechanical contact with the material [26]. This technology is an interesting proposal for the food industry since it allows a wavelength, whose energy is absorbed in large quantities by water, does not generate cross-contamination and allows an increase in the mass and heat transfer area during drying without damaging adjacent areas where it is applied [21]. Araya et al. [18] studied the effect of CO_2 laser microperforation pretreatment on the dehydration of apple slices at 70 °C in drying techniques with an osmotic dehydration pretreatment. Promising results were obtained by significantly reducing the drying time compared to the control treatment (conventional drying) by more than 50%; however, the effect of microperforation pretreatment and different drying temperatures on bioactive compounds and their antioxidant capacities was not studied. Chen et al. [27] studied the effect of CO_2 laser perforation as a pretreatment for blueberry skin before infrared freeze-drying. Laser perforation effectively increased drying speed, helped reduce shrinkage, increased rehydration capacity, and enhanced total phenolic compounds in dehydrated fruits.

The objective of this research is to determine the effect of microperforations with CO_2 laser technology as a pretreatment in the drying of apple slices (Granny smith) in refractive window technology in terms of total polyphenols, antioxidant capacity, color, drying times, and product stability under accelerated storage. As baseline criteria, comparison with conventional tunnel drying and lyophilization has also been considered. The study was performed using Granny smith apple slices as a model food, considering tissue and maturity homogeneity.

2. Materials and Methods
2.1. Materials

Granny Smith (GS) apples (*Malus domestica*) were purchased from a local supermarket in Valparaíso, Chile, and they were refrigerated at 2 ± 0.5 °C until use. Apples with 11 ± 1° Brix and slices were obtained exclusively from the parenchymatic tissue based on the work ok Ramírez et al. [28]. A solution with 2% and 1% citric and ascorbic acid, respectively, was prepared to avoid enzymatic browning of the apple samples after microperforations. All of the reagents were purchased from G.A. Sales. Apple slices were cut using a kitchen mandolin and cork borer to provide a sample thickness and diameter of 0.004 ± 0.0001 m thickness and 0.040 ± 0.001 m diameter, respectively, and each slice had an average weight of 0.003 ± 0.00048 kg.

2.2. Experimental Design

To determine the effect of microperforations on the total polyphenols, antioxidant capacity, and color as response variables, an experimental design was carried out. The variables were the operating temperature of the RW (from 70 to 90 °C), the pore diameter (from 200 to 600 µm), and the pore density (9 to 25 pores/cm^2) in the slice. The experimental variables were combined in a Box–Behnken design (BBD). RW drying at 70, 80, and 90 °C without microperforations was used as a control experiment. In addition, hot air drying in a tunnel at 70 °C and lyophilization were used for comparison to commercial existing drying processes. Figure 1 presents the proposed experimental design.

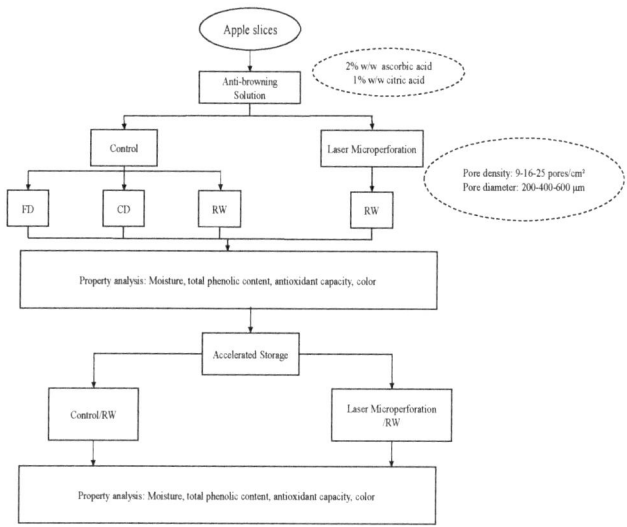

Figure 1. Experimental design.

2.2.1. CO_2 Laser Microperforations

The laser microperforations (LMP) were applied to the samples using a SYNRAD TI100 CO_2 laser (Firestar t100, Synrad Inc. Mukilteo, WA, USA) with a 125 nm lens, which was linked to the computer with WinMarkPro Laser Making Software, allowing for its configuration and adjustment. The parameters of residence time, number of pulses and power were established to pass through 100% of the sample, according to Araya et al. [18] (Table 1). The pore density (PD, the number of pores per unit area) configuration was conducted in honeycomb arrangements using 9, 16, and 25 pores/cm². The pore size generated was measured by optical microscopy (H 600 LL HP 100, Hund Wetzlar, Wetzlar, Germany) using the uEye Cockpit software from Imaging Development Systems 113 (IDS) and Image-Pro Plus, which allows for capturing a photo of a microscopic observation [20].

Table 1. Different configurations of power, residence time, and number of pulses were used to obtain the three pore sizes (PS) tested.

	Pore Size (PS)		
Parameter	PS1 203.25 ± 23.05 μm	PS2 417.89 ± 6.14 μm	PS3 623.41 ± 7.50 μm
Power (%) (based on 100 W)	10	25	75
Residence Time (μs)	2	1	1
Number of pulses	120	120	120

2.2.2. Conventional Drying (CD)

The conventional drying equipment (CD) used was a hot-air drying tunnel that was 2.7 m long and 0.4 m wide (15 KW, 80 V). On one side, there is a fan that drives the air at an average speed of 1.53 ± 0.25 m/s. The equipment capacity was 48 samples per drying process, which were placed on a support that was in the middle of the tunnel. The drying temperature was 70 °C for 135 min (the water activity attained for the dried samples was 0.316 ± 0.026).

2.2.3. Refractance Window™ (RW™)

The refractive window was made up of a thermoregulated water bath (Mermmet, model WND), in which a Mylar® sheet (thicknesses 0.1 mm) measuring 0.3 m wide by 0.5 m long was placed over the water, as according to Hernández et al. [29]. Sixty apple slices were placed on the Mylar sheet. The relative humidity in the laboratory was 47 ± 8%. The process ended when the samples reached a water activity (a_w) below 0.4. At $a_w < 0.4$, foods do not show microorganism spoilage [30]; furthermore, apple browning is reduced [31].

2.2.4. Freeze-Drying (FD)

All experiments were carried out in a Martin Christ freeze-dryer, model Alpha 2-4 LSCplus (Martin Christ Gefriertrocknungsanlagen, Osterode, Germany), which can operate at a total vacuum pressure of up to 0.3 mbar, provided with an MKS Baratron 622 capacitance manometer (MKS Instruments) and a condenser that can operate at temperatures as low as −85 °C. The apple slices were frozen in the freezer (Haier ULT Freezer, model DW-86W100J, China) at −85 °C for 24 h before being freeze-dried. The apple samples were placed onto the three shelves, considering a total load of 18 units. The drying temperature in the freeze dryer was 30 °C.

2.3. Determination of Moisture Content and Water Activity

The moisture content was determined by drying 5 g of the sample under vacuum conditions in an oven at 70 °C for 24 h and recording the final constant weight (AOAC method no. 934.06) [32]. The moisture content was calculated using Equation (1), where X^W corresponds to the mass fraction of water (g water/g sample), and m_0 and m_f are the masses of the initial and dry samples, respectively (g).

$$X^W = \frac{m_0 - m_f}{m_0} \qquad (1)$$

Water activity was determined using a dew-point hygrometer Aqualab series 4 TE (Decagon Devices, Inc., Pullman, Washington, DC, USA) with a resolution of 0.0001 a_w.

2.4. Determination of Color

The color of the samples was evaluated using a colorimeter (model CR-410, Konica Minolta, Tokyo, Japan) to measure the coordinates of the CIEL*a*b* uniform color space, where L^* is the luminosity, a^* is the red–green hue, and b^* is the yellow–blue hue. The type of illuminant is D65, and the degrees of the observer is 2°. The color difference was calculated using Equation (2), where ΔE indicates the magnitude of the color change between the initial (L_0^*, a_0^* y b_0^*) and final (L_f^*, a_f^* y b_f^*) parameters of the sample to be compared [33]. ΔE was obtained for all cases using a fresh apple and the dried controls for comparison with the dried samples.

$$\Delta E = \sqrt{\Delta L^{*2} + \Delta a^{*2} + \Delta b^{*2}} \qquad (2)$$

2.5. Determination of Total Polyphenol Content (TPC) and Antioxidant Activity

The extraction of polyphenols was performed by extracting two grams of the ground sample (fresh or dried) with 20 mL of an 80% methanol solution using a homogenizer at room temperature and protected from light for 1 h. The supernatant was filtered through Whatman paper No. 2 and stored at −20 °C.

The total polyphenol content in the extracts was determined using the Folin–Ciocalteu method [34] and expressed as gallic acid equivalents (GAEs) in mg/g dry matter.

The antioxidant capacity was determined using DPPH (2,2-diphenyl-2-picryl-hydrazyl) as performed by Galaz et al. [34]. The results were expressed as Trolox equivalents in μmol/g dry matter.

The total polyphenol content and antioxidant capacity were obtained using a Genesys 5 spectrophotometer (Spectronic Instrument, Inc., model 336001, New York, NY, USA) by measuring the absorbance at 765 and 517 nm, respectively.

2.6. Accelerated Storage Test

Accelerated storage tests were carried out in an oven with humidity control (Memmert, model HCP-108). The dehydrated apples were kept in aluminum Ziploc bags (11 × 16 × 3 m). The packaged samples were stored at 45 °C under constant accelerated relative humidity (75%) conditions for 4 weeks. The samples were analyzed for selected quality attributes, namely, antioxidant capacity (AC) (µmol/g dry matter), total phenolic content (TPC) (mg gallic acid equivalents (GAE)/g dry matter), moisture content (MC) (g water/g sample), and total color change (ΔE).

2.7. Experimental Design and Statistical Analysis

All of the data were reported as the means of three replicas and their respective standard deviations. The effect of microperforations on the RW was analyzed using a response surface methodology based on a Box–Behnken design (BBD) with three center points, Table 2 shows the values of each variable with their respective level in the proposed experimental design. The significance test of the results was performed with an analysis of variance (ANOVA) and Duncan's multiple range tests with a significance of 95% using the STATGRAPHIC Centurion XVIII software, Statpoint Inc.®, 2018.

Table 2. Box–Behnken design for surface analysis with 15 treatments in total, including 3 central points.

Experiments	Temperature	Pore Size	Pore Density
1	1	−1	0
2	1	1	0
3	−1	1	0
4	−1	−1	0
5	1	0	−1
6	1	0	1
7	−1	0	1
8	−1	0	−1
9	0	−1	−1
10	0	−1	1
11	0	1	1
12	0	1	−1
13	0	0	0
14	0	0	0
15	0	0	0
FACTORS	−1	0	+1
T_i (°C)	70	80	90
dpi (µm)	200	400	600
Dpi (pores/cm^2)	9	17	25

Where T_i, dpi and Dpi correspond to the variables of temperature, pore diameter and pore density, respectively, for the corresponding level i.

3. Results and Discussion

3.1. Color

Color is an important attribute that plays a significant role in food acceptance [35]. Table 3 shows the measured color parameters of fresh and dried apple slices. The fresh apple slice had a value of $L^* = 74.77 \pm 1.17$, $a^* = -5.47 \pm 0.70$ and $b^* = 19.69 \pm 2.09$, similar to reports from Araya et al. [18], Henríquez et al. [36] and Hernández et al. [29].

Table 3. Mean values of moisture and color parameters for fresh apple and all treatments dried.

	Experiment	Moisture (g Water/g Sample)	ΔE
	Fresh	0.866 ± 0.002 [a]	
	CD	0.023 ± 0.002 [b]	13.26 ± 0.15 [a]
	FD	0.011 ± 0.001 [c]	11.77 ± 0.05 [b]
70 °C	Control RW	0.038 ± 0.001 [d,e]	12.06 ± 0.17 [a,b]
	3 (17 pores/cm², 600 μm)	0.044 ± 0.001 [d,e,f]	5.89 ± 0.39 [c]
	4 (17 pores/cm², 200 μm)	0.103 ± 0.011 [g,h]	11.35 ± 1.11 [b,d]
	7 (25 pores/cm², 400 μm)	0.063 ± 0.007 [i]	6.92 ± 0.50 [c,j]
	8 (9 pores/cm², 400 μm)	0.096 ± 0.001 [g]	11.09 ± 0.66 [b,k]
80 °C	Control RW	0.035 ± 0.002 [d]	11.26 ± 1.26 [b]
	9 (9 pores/cm², 200 μm)	0.014 ± 0.001 [b,c]	8.90 ± 1.21 [e,f,i]
	10 (25 pores/cm², 200 μm)	0.094 ± 0.015 [g]	8.75 ± 0.44 [f,i]
	11 (25 pores/cm², 600 μm)	0.055 ± 0.002 [f,i]	8.22 ± 1.46 [e,f,g,i]
	12 (9 pores/cm², 600 μm)	0.057 ± 0.002 [i]	8.98 ± 0.90 [e,f,i]
	13 (17 pores/cm², 400 μm)	0.097 ± 0.007 [g]	8.48 ± 1.21 [e,f,h,i]
	14 (17 pores/cm², 400 μm)	0.067 ± 0.006 [i]	8.83 ± 1.04 [e,f,i]
	15 (17 pores/cm², 400 μm)	0.055 ± 0.003 [f,i]	9.65 ± 0.94 [e,f]
90 °C	Control RW	0.049 ± 0.001 [e,f]	12.56 ± 0.91 [a,b,d]
	1 (17 pores/cm², 200 μm)	0.065 ± 0.002 [i]	7.19 ± 0.89 [c,g,h,i]
	2 (17 pores/cm², 600 μm)	0.048 ± 0.002 [e,f]	5.89 ± 1.62 [c]
	5 (9 pores/cm², 400 μm)	0.092 ± 0.007 [g]	9.63 ± 0.07 [f,k]
	6 (25 pores/cm², 400 μm)	0.111 ± 0.005 [h]	7.76 ± 0.04 [i,j]

Means with different superscripts within a column differ significantly ($p < 0.05$).

With respect to delta color, comparing the results obtained between the control treatments, the value ΔE for the RW technique is slightly lower than that obtained for conventional drying; nevertheless, there are no significant differences between the different temperatures ($p < 0.05$). Similar results were obtained by other researchers, Franco et al. [37] and Hernández et al. [29]. In addition, when compared with the freeze-drying process, no significant differences were found ($p < 0.05$), similar to Caparino et al. [38] in mango and Puente et al. [39] in goldenberry. In the cases without microperforations, ΔE was between 11.26 and 12.56, and for the treatments with microperforations, ΔE presented values between 5.89 and 11.35.

The ΔE values were, in most cases, significantly lower when laser microperforations were applied in comparison to the control samples. The smallest color differences (ΔE = 5.89) were obtained in treatments 2 and 3 (17 pores/cm², 600 μm) at 70 and 90 °C, respectively. In general, microperforation pretreatments resulted in products that indicated lower degradation of the color, probably due to a reduction in process time with respect to the control. Table 4 shows the drying time; for the three temperatures, a decrease in drying times was observed, and the case of 70 °C, the application of different combinations of pore densities with different pore diameters presented a decrease of approximately 20% in the processing time. At 80 °C, the reduction in drying time was between 5 and 25% compared to the control treatment, while at 90 °C, the reduction values were between 2 and 13%, and the degradation of the product's original color appeared after long drying time exposure [37,40,41]. In general, there are no significant differences between the treatments with microperforations; however, it is possible to obtain a product with a similar delta color but with less processing time.

Table 4. Mean values (with standard deviation) of water activity (a_w).

	Experiment Refractance Window	a_w	Time (min)
70 °C	Control	0.361 ± 0.027 [a,b,c]	120 ± 6.4 [a]
	3 (17 pores/cm², 600 µm)	0.286 ± 0.019 [d,e]	93 ± 9.2 [b]
	4 (17 pores/cm², 200 µm)	0.357 ± 0.015 [a,b,c]	90 ± 0.71 [b]
	7 (25 pores/cm², 400 µm)	0.321 ± 0.031 [a,d,e]	90 ± 6.4 [b]
	8 (9 pores/cm², 400 µm)	0.388 ± 0.012 [b,c]	95 ± 1.4 [b]
80 °C	Control	0.376 ± 0.009 [a,b,c]	80 ± 4.2 [c]
	9 (9 pores/cm², 200 µm)	0.361 ± 0.027 [a,b,c]	76 ± 2.8 [c,d]
	10 (25 pores/cm², 200 µm)	0.222 ± 0.024 [f]	70 ± 4.2 [d,e]
	11 (25 pores/cm², 600 µm)	0.264 ± 0.022 [d,f]	60 ± 4.9 [f]
	12 (9 pores/cm², 600 µm)	0.361 ± 0.033 [a,b,c]	63 ± 3.5 [e,f]
	13-14-15 (17 pores/cm², 400 µm)	0.342 ± 0.060 [a,b,e]	60 ± 4.2 [f]
90 °C	Control	0.360 ± 0.033 [a,b,c]	45 ± 3.5 [g]
	1 (17 pores/cm², 200 µm)	0.358 ± 0.029 [a,b,c]	43 ± 2.1 [h]
	2 (17 pores/cm², 600 µm)	0.378 ± 0.016 [a,b,c]	37 ± 1.4 [h]
	5 (9 pores/cm², 400 µm)	0.353 ± 0.026 [a,b,c]	44 ± 2.8 [h]
	6 (25 pores/cm², 400 µm)	0.408 ± 0.014 [c]	39 ± 2.1 [h]

Means with different superscripts within a column differ significantly ($p < 0.05$).

3.2. Total Phenolic Content (TPC)

The fresh raw material had a total polyphenol content of 16.79 ± 0.56 mg GAE/g_{bs} (2.25 mg GAE/g_{bh}) with similar results to those reported in Mitić et al. [42] in Granny smith apples (1.97 mg GAE/g_{bh}). Figure 2A shows the results of the total polyphenol content obtained from the control experiments. There were no significant differences ($p < 0.05$) between the freeze-drying process and the RW at 90 °C. The greater retention of TPC in dehydrated samples at higher temperatures (90 °C) could be explained by the significant decrease in drying time (45 min), which decreases the thermal and oxidative degradation of phenolic compounds [43]. As already mentioned, during conventional drying at 70 °C, the drying time took place in 135 min, but despite the use of RW at 70 °C and 80 °C reducing the drying time to 120 and 80 min, respectively, such decreases were not enough to prevent spoilage of the bioactive compounds, as they presented similar concentrations ($p \leq 0.05$). The same trend has been reported through a comparison of RW at different temperatures with conventional drying of banana puree [44]. The difference in processing time can be explained by the drying mechanisms; the main process of freeze-drying is the sublimation and subsequent diffusion of water within the product in a vacuum environment; however, it requires a large consumption of energy and time. In the case of conventional drying (conduction and convection), they cause a decrease in the quality of the product in terms of nutritional, color, and functional properties due to the drying temperatures and processing times [45], while the RW drying can be performed at higher temperatures, because during the RW drying process, the three heat transfer mechanisms occur: conduction, convection and radiation. As the product loses moisture, the "window" closes and begins to "refract" the infrared radiation towards the water source, increasing the reflexivity [46]. At this stage, heat transfer through conduction is predominant, and evaporation is maintained until reaching the critical moisture content of the product. In the last stages of drying, a reduction in heat transfer occurs, which protects the product from overheating, thanks to the effects of evaporative cooling [47].

The results show that the minimum value corresponds to Experiment 1 (17 pores/cm², 200 µm, 90 °C), 6.59 ± 0.25 mg GAE/gbs, and the maximum TPC retention was in the case of Experiment 12 (9 pores/cm2, 600 µm, 80 °C), 12.49 ± 0.41 mg GAE/gbs. When comparing the control treatments and those with microperforations, significant differences in TPC were observed when a larger pore size (600 µm) was used for the cases of 70 and 80 °C, obtaining higher values in the case of the treatments with microperforations. In this regard, the Pareto chart (Figure 3a) shows that the pore diameter is the main variable that has a significant effect on the TPC. Figure 4 shows the interrelationship between the drying temperature, pore size, and TPC content of apple fruits. The figure results clearly show that increasing the pore size promotes the retention of polyphenols, and then the TPC content increases. Table 4 shows the a_w values of all treatments; in general, there are no significant differences ($p < 0.05$) in the different treatments, with the exception of treatments 3, 10 and 11, which present lower values. a_w is a key factor affecting the stability of polyphenols [48]. Tonon et al. [49] studied the anthocyanin stability of spray-dried açai juice and found that increased water activity resulted in greater degradation. This was attributed to the higher molecular mobility, which allows easier diffusion of oxygen, thus accelerating oxidation reactions. The water content (Table 3) is one of the most influential factors in nutrient degradation. As water is extracted and the food material shrinks, the chemical concentration increases, but certain water-soluble compounds may serve as decomposition catalysts [50]. Additionally, the degradation of TPC is well known to be related to the duration and intensity of heating; therefore, the time–temperature regime during the process should be considered apart from the pore diameter to retain them as high as possible. The response surface methodology analysis showed that the lack of fit was not significant for all response variables ($p > 0.05$), and the R-squared statistic for the response surface model was 90.75, while the R^2_{adj} value was 74.09, which indicates its ability to explain the effect of microperforations pretreatments on the retention of TPC.

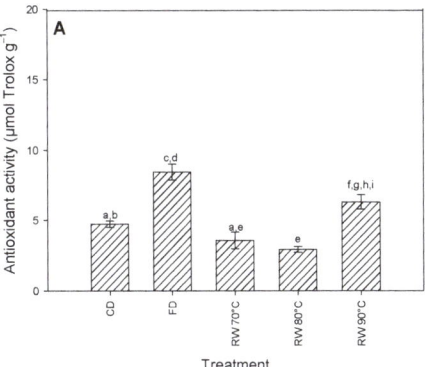
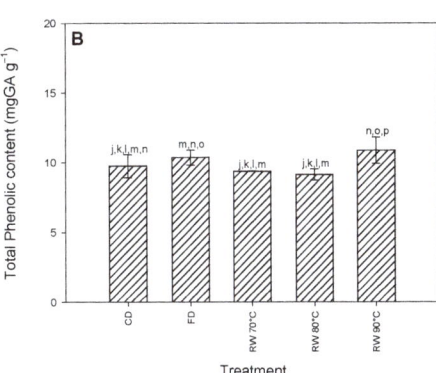

Figure 2. Effect of drying on (**A**) antioxidant activity and (**B**) total phenolic content (CD: conventional drying; FD: freeze drying; RW: refractance window). a–i: Different lowercase letters show that the results are statistically significantly different ($p < 0.05$) for antioxidant activity. j–p: Different lowercase letters show that the results are statistically significantly different ($p < 0.05$) for total phenolic content.

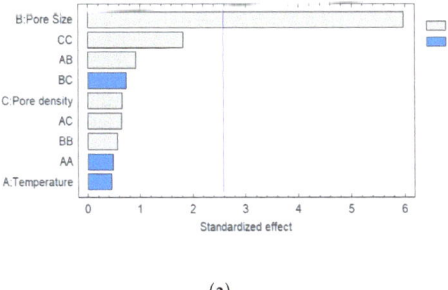
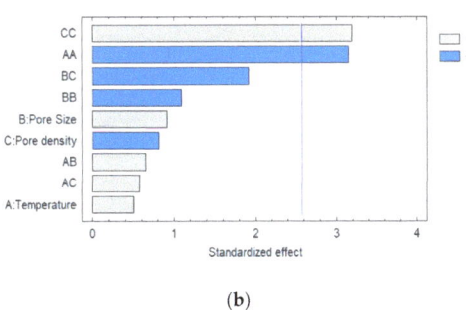

(**a**) (**b**)

Figure 3. Standardized Pareto charts ($\alpha = 0.05$) of effects of pore size, pore density, and temperature for (**a**) TPC and (**b**) antioxidant capacity.

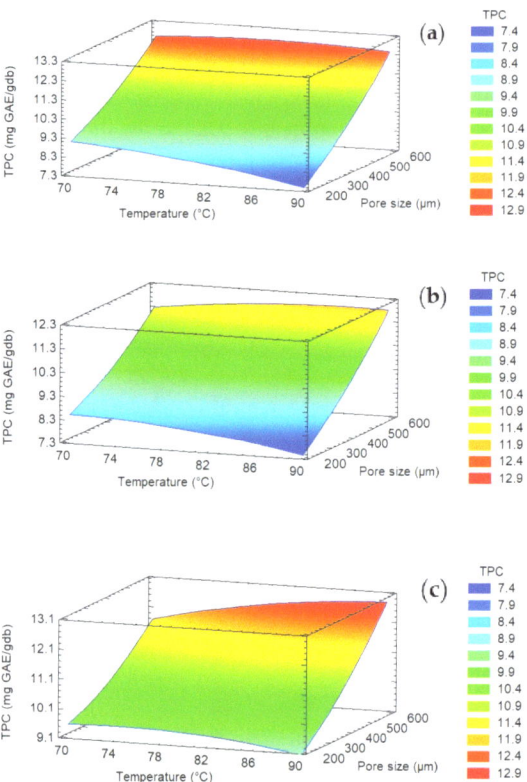

Figure 4. Surface response of the effects of pore size, pore density, and temperature on the TFC (**a**) pore density = 9 pores/cm^2, (**b**) pore density = 17 pores/cm^2, (**c**) pore density = 25 pores/cm^2.

3.3. Antioxidant Activity

The fresh raw material had an antioxidant capacity of 15.08 ± 0.73 µmol Trolox/gbs Figure 2B shows the results of the antioxidant capacity for the control experiments. In the control experiments, freeze-drying was the best method to retain the antioxidant activity with respect to the raw material, attaining a value of 8.42 ± 0.57 µmol Trolox/g$_{db}$. The drying tunnel and the refractive window at 70 and 80 °C present the lowest antioxidant capacity of the series of experiments carried out with values of 4.75 ± 0.22, 3.58 ± 0.58, and 2.94 ± 0.52 µmol Trolox/g$_{db}$, respectively. On the other hand, the refractive window at 90 °C (6.29 ± 0.22 µmol Trolox/g$_{db}$) presents a higher retention of antioxidant capacity compared to conventional drying; however, significant differences are evident with freeze-drying Baeghbali et al. [51] reported that there are no significant differences between drying in a refractive window at 91 °C of pomegranate juice and freeze-drying. On the other hand, Nayak et al. [52] presented the results of drying flakes of various colored potatoes through different drying methods, such as a refractive window at 95 °C, drum drying with steam at 145 °C, and freeze-drying. The results obtained concerning antioxidant capacity showed that there was no significant difference between the drying methods. Galaz et al. [34] used a combination of high temperatures and short processing time during the drying of pomegranate peel using a drum dryer. The combination of temperature–time allowed for the removal of dried products of pomegranate peel that maintain their antioxidant activity Therefore, the time–temperature relationship is a determining factor in the retention of the antioxidant capacity.

Laser microperforation allowed antioxidant capacity to be obtained in several treatments without significant differences in comparison with the freeze-drying process

($p > 0.05$). For example, at 70 °C, treatment 8 (9 pores/cm^2, 400 µm) was 7.21 ± 0.26 µmol Trolox/gdb; at 80 °C, treatments 11 (25 pores/cm^2, 600 µm) and 12 (9 pores/cm^2, 600 µm) were 7.68 ± 1.98 µmol Trolox/gdb and 8.87 ± 0.21 µmol Trolox/gdb, respectively, and at 90 °C, treatment 6 (25 pores/cm^2, 400 µm) was 7.15 ± 1.02 µmol Trolox/gdb. These results suggest that the combination of drying temperature, pore size, and pore density favors the retention of antioxidant capacity, with values higher than those of the control treatments and not presenting significant differences with freeze drying.

According to the results (Figure 3b), the factors with the largest effects on antioxidant activity were the quadratic effects terms temperature and pore density. Figure 5 presents the surface plot for the interaction effect between the pore size and temperature on the antioxidant capacity. The results showed that the maximum antioxidant capacity was attained at a temperature of 80 °C, a range of pore sizes larger than 400 µm, and a density of 9 pores/cm^2 (Figure 5).

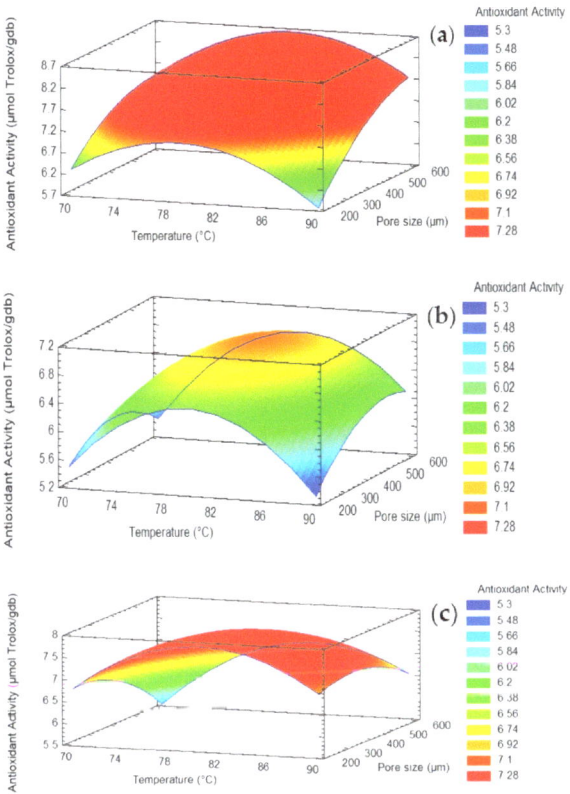

Figure 5. Surface response of the effects of pore size, pore density and temperature on the antioxidant activity. (**a**) pore density = 9 pores/cm^2, (**b**) pore density = 17 pores/cm^2, (**c**) pore density = 25 pores/cm^2.

3.4. Accelerated Storage Test

The accelerated storage tests apply the principles of chemical kinetics to quantify the effects that extrinsic factors such as temperature, humidity, and light have on the rate of deterioration reactions. By exposing food to controlled environments in which one or more of the extrinsic factors are held at a higher-than-normal level, spoilage rates are accelerated, resulting in a shorter-than-normal time for the product to fail [53]. Although the use of microperforations tended to retain the concentration of TPC in comparison to the control treatments, it is interesting to evaluate the effect on these compounds during storage. Hence, an accelerated storage study was carried out. The quality parameters and bioactive properties of the control cases (RW at 70, 80 and 90 °C) and of the two best experiments with perforation were analyzed according to the results obtained for color difference, antioxidant activity, TPC, and moisture (Table 5). The accelerated storage study was carried out for 4 weeks, comparing the results at the beginning and end of the period. Based on the results, Experiment 2 was chosen because it presents the lowest value of color difference. In addition, Experiment 6 was chosen because it presents one of the highest antioxidant capacity profiles and total polyphenol content among the series of experiments.

Table 5. Average values of moisture, ΔE, TPC and antioxidant activity for samples stored over time.

	Experiment	Moisture (g Water/g Sample)	ΔE	TPC	Antioxidant Capacity
Week 0	Control 70 °C	0.038 ± 0.001 [Aa]	-	9.365 ± 0.020 [Aa]	3.575 ± 0.582 [Aa]
	Control 80 °C	0.035 ± 0.002 [Aa]	-	9.128 ± 0.403 [Aa]	2.935 ± 0.265 [Aa]
	Control 90 °C	0.049 ± 0.001 [Ba]	-	10.883 ± 0.970 [Ba]	6.292 ± 0.519 [BCa]
	2 (17 pores/cm^2, 600 μm)	0.048 ± 0.002 [Ba]	-	11.672 ± 1.305 [Ba]	7.154 ± 1.012 [Ba]
	6 (25 pores/cm^2, 400 μm)	0.111 ± 0.006 [Ca]	-	11.254 ± 0.315 [Ba]	5.494 ± 1.059 [Ca]
Week 4	Control 70 °C	0.087 ± 0.001 [Ab]	32.93 ± 1.21 [A]	8.015 ± 0.190 [ABb]	3.408 ± 0.447 [Aa]
	Control 80 °C	0.118 ± 0.001 [Bb]	29.54 ± 1.56 [B]	7.587 ± 0.363 [Ab]	3.333 ± 0.365 [Aba]
	Control 90 °C	0.092 ± 0.001 [Cb]	37.11 ± 2.34 [C]	8.059 ± 0.191 [ABb]	3.052 ± 0.763 [Abb]
	2 (17 pores/cm^2, 600 μm)	0.118 ± 0.001 [Bb]	26.29 ± 0.95 [D]	8.568 ± 0.418 [Bb]	2.546 ± 0.087 [BCb]
	6 (25 pores/cm^2, 400 μm)	0.150 ± 0.001 [Db]	36.89 ± 1.18 [C]	7.906 ± 0.221 [Ab]	2.256 ± 0.251 [Cb]

A–D: Different uppercase letters within the same column and week show that the results are statistically significantly different ($p < 0.05$). a,b: Different lowercase letters within the same column and experiment show that the results are statistically significantly different ($p < 0.05$).

The results show a significant increase in the moisture content ($p < 0.05$) between weeks 0 and 4. Although the packaging may serve as a protective material against food spoilage, there will always be gas and water permeability, which are increased at high storage temperatures, such as in the current case, but other factors, such as pH, oxygen, material porosity and light, may also be affected [54]. In fact, it has been observed that dried apples can be stable and result in a good source of antioxidant compounds as long as packing materials with a high barrier against moisture sorption are used, resulting in the latter being the most detrimental factor [55,56]. The results from Table 5 also show that TPC degradation increased with increasing drying temperature ($p < 0.05$). For instance, at 70 °C and 80 °C, TPC retention was on average ~84%, while at 80 °C and 90 °C, TPC retention was ~72% regardless of whether microperforation pretreatments were performed. Regarding the antioxidant activity values of apple slices, no significant changes were observed after storage for controls at 70 °C and 80 °C; however, the increase in drying temperature at 90 °C resulted in ~42% retention regardless of whether microperforation pretreatment was used or not. This situation may be explained because the use of higher temperatures during processing may result in further autocatalytic reactions, especially in products subjected to concentrations where there is also the presence of sugars and reduced a_w [57]. The color difference (ΔE^*) between the dried apple slices at weeks 0 and 4 was determined. The results (Table 5) show that there were significant differences ($p < 0.05$) between the cases studied, except for the control at 90 °C in Experiment 6. At the end of the accelerated storage, the samples present high values of ΔE^*, ranging between 26.29 and 37.11, with Experiment 2 being the one that obtained the least color variation. The control samples present a lower color change ratio, which may be because the matrix without perforations protects from the reactions produced by the enzymes, the presence of water and the temperature during storage, avoiding, in the short term, more significant browning than in the perforated samples. Another observation is that the control samples, at a higher drying temperature, produce a lower color difference, but in storage, the samples dried at 90 °C show a greater color change than the samples at other temperatures. This may be because the samples dried at 90 °C present a greater retention of the bioactive components, which are more likely to react with ambient conditions and to reactivate enzymes (for example, polyphenol oxidase).

Regarding the perforated samples, an increase in the color difference greater than the control samples was observed. This behavior could be explained due to the presence of micropores that allow to increase the surface area in which bioactive compounds can react with oxygen. At 4 weeks, all samples exposed to the assay reached a similar order of magnitude in color difference, although a greater difference was observed in samples that were perforated.

4. Conclusions

For apple slices dried using RW, the application of laser microperforation allowed for the color retention, total polyphenol content, and antioxidant capacity to be comparable to those obtained through the freeze-drying process. Regarding the drying time required to get an a_w lower than 0.4, it was significantly lower in microperforated samples, attaining a time reduction in the range of 2–25% (which depends on drying temperature) compared with non-perforated samples. The pore size is a relevant variable in the retention of bioactive compounds, obtaining higher polyphenols content as pore size increased. In accelerated storage, the microperforated samples presented a higher loss of bioactive compounds, which could be explained due to an increase in the mass transfer area due to the presence of pores. However, an adequate design of pore size and distribution must be performed in order to create a pore that, during drying, remains open, allowing water migration, but, as drying occurs, closes. Therefore, this would avoid the loss of bioactive compounds due to increases in mass transfer area during drying.

Author Contributions: Experimental research, G.L.; formal Analysis, H.N., C.R., A.J., A.C., G.L. and K.B.; investigation, H.N. and C.R.; writing—Review and editing, C.R., A.C., K.B. and H.N.; project administration, H.N.; writing original draft, H.N., A.C. and K.B.; conceptualization, H.N., A.J. and C.R.; funding acquisition, C.R. All authors have read and agreed to the published version of the manuscript.

Funding: This research was funded by ANID through FONDECYT, project numbers 1230506 and 1211980 and scholarship number 21211634.

Data Availability Statement: The data presented in this study are available on request from the corresponding author.

Conflicts of Interest: The authors declare no conflict of interest.

References

1. Raghavi, L.M.; Moses, J.A.; Anandharamakrishnan, C. Refractance window drying of foods: A review. *J. Food Eng.* **2018**, *222*, 267–275. [CrossRef]
2. Ochoa-Martínez, C.I.; Quintero, P.T.; Ayala, A.A.; Ortiz, M.J. Drying characteristics of mango slices using the refractance window™ technique. *J. Food Eng.* **2012**, *109*, 69–75. [CrossRef]
3. Zarein, M.; Samadi, S.H.; Ghobadian, B. Investigation of microwave dryer effect on energy efficiency during drying of apple slices. *J. Saudi Soc. Agric. Sci.* **2015**, *14*, 41–47. [CrossRef]
4. Vega-Mercado, H.; Góngora-Nieto, M.M.; Barbosa-Cánovas, G.V. Advances in dehydration of foods. *J. Food Eng.* **2001**, *49*, 271–289. [CrossRef]
5. Ratti, C. Hot air and freeze-drying of high-value foods: A review. *J. Food Eng.* **2001**, *49*, 311–319. [CrossRef]
6. Nindo, C.I.; Tang, J. Refractance window dehydration technology: A novel contact drying method. *Dry. Technol. Int. J.* **2007**, *25*, 37–48. [CrossRef]
7. Tontul, I.; Eroğlu, E.; Topuz, A. Convective and refractance window drying of cornelian cherry pulp: Effect on physicochemical properties. *J. Food Process Eng.* **2018**, *41*, e12917. [CrossRef]
8. Mahanti, N.K.; Chakraborty, S.K.; Sudhakar, A.; Verma, D.K.; Shankar, S.; Thakur, M.; Singh, S.; Tripathy, S.; Gupta, A.K.; Srivastav, P.P. Refractance window™-drying vs. other drying methods and effect of different process parameters on quality of foods: A comprehensive review of trends and technological developments. *Future Foods* **2021**, *3*, 100024. [CrossRef]
9. Shende, D.; Datta, A.K. Refractance window drying of fruits and vegetables: A review. *J. Sci. Food Agric.* **2019**, *99*, 1449–1456. [CrossRef]

10. Bampi, M.; Domschke, N.N.; Schmidt, F.C.; Laurindo, J.B. Influence of vacuum application, acid addition and partial replacement of NaCl by KCl on the mass transfer during salting of beef cuts. *LWT Food Sci. Technol.* **2016**, *74*, 26–33. [CrossRef]
11. González-Pérez, J.E.; Jiménez-González, O.; Ramírez-Corona, N.; Guerrero-Beltrán, J.A.; López-Malo, A. Vacuum impregnation on apples with grape juice concentrate: Effects of pressure, processing time, and juice concentration. *Innov. Food Sci. Emerg. Technol.* **2022**, *77*, 102981. [CrossRef]
12. Pasławska, M.; Stepien, B.; Nawirska-Olszanska, A.; Sala, K. Studies on the effect of mass transfer in vacuum impregnation on the bioactive potential of apples. *Molecules* **2019**, *24*, 3533. [CrossRef] [PubMed]
13. Erihemu; Hironaka, K.; Oda, Y.; Koaze, H. Iron enrichment of whole potato tuber by vacuum impregnation. *LWT-Food Sci. Technol* **2014**, *59*, 504–509. [CrossRef]
14. Aamir, M.; Jittanit, W. Ohmic heating treatment for gac aril oil extraction: Effects on extraction efficiency, physical properties and some bioactive compounds. *Innov. Food Sci. Emerg. Technol.* **2017**, *41*, 224–234. [CrossRef]
15. Kusnadi, C.; Sastry, S.K. Effect of moderate electric fields on salt diffusion into vegetable tissue. *J. Food Eng.* **2012**, *110*, 329–336. [CrossRef]
16. Moreno, J.; Espinoza, C.; Simpson, R.; Petzold, G.; Nuñez, H.; Gianelli, M.P. Application of ohmic heating/vacuum impregnation treatments and air drying to develop an apple snack enriched in folic acid. *Innov. Food Sci. Emerg. Technol.* **2016**, *33*, 381–386 [CrossRef]
17. Simpson, R.; Ramírez, C.; Birchmeier, V.; Almonacid, A.; Moreno, J.; Nuñez, H.; Jaques, A. Diffusion mechanisms during the osmotic dehydration of Granny Smith apples subjected to a moderate electric field. *J. Food Eng.* **2015**, *166*, 204–211. [CrossRef]
18. Araya, E.; Nuñez, H.; Ramírez, N.; Jaques, A.; Simpson, R.; Escobar, M.; Escalona, P.; Vega-Castro, O.; Ramírez, C. Exploring the potential acceleration of Granny Smith apple drying by pre-treatment with CO_2 laser microperforation. *Food Bioprocess Technol.* **2022**, *15*, 391–406. [CrossRef]
19. Ferraz, A.C.O.; Mittal, G.S.; Bilanski, W.K.; Abdullah, H.A. Mathematical modeling of laser based potato cutting and peeling *BioSystems* **2007**, *90*, 602–613. [CrossRef]
20. Figueroa, C.; Ramírez, C.; Núñez, H.; Jaques, A.; Simpson, R. Application of vacuum impregnation and CO_2-laser microperforations in the potential acceleration of the pork marinating process. *Innov. Food Sci. Emerg. Technol.* **2020**, *66*, 102500 [CrossRef]
21. Fujimaru, T.; Ling, Q.; Morrissey, M.T. Effects of carbon dioxide (CO_2) laserperforation as skin pretreatment to improve sugar infusion process of frozen blueberries. *J. Food Sci.* **2012**, *77*, E45–E51. [CrossRef] [PubMed]
22. Olivares, J.; Nuñez, H.; Ramírez, C.; Jaques, A.; Pinto, M.; Fuentes, L.; Almonacid, S.; Vega-Castro, O.; Simpson, R. Application of moderate electric fields and CO_2-laser microperforations for the acceleration of the salting process of Atlantic salmon (*Salmo salar*). *Food Bioprod. Process.* **2021**, *125*, 105–112. [CrossRef]
23. Teng, X.; Zhang, M.; Mujumdar, A.S. Potential application of laser technology in food processing. *Trends Food Sci. Technol.* **2021**, *118*, 711–722. [CrossRef]
24. Veloso, G.; Simpson, R.; Núñez, H.; Ramírez, C.; Almonacid, S.; Jaques, A. Exploring the potential acceleration of the osmotic dehydration process via pretreatment with CO_2-laser microperforations. *J. Food Eng.* **2021**, *306*, 110610. [CrossRef]
25. Silva-Vera, W.; Avendaño-Muñoz, N.; Nuñez, H.; Ramírez, C.; Almonacid, S.; Simpson, R. CO_2 laser drilling coupled with moderate electric fields for enhancement of the mass transfer phenomenon in a tomato (*Lycopersicon esculentum*) peeling process *J. Food Eng.* **2020**, *276*, 109870. [CrossRef]
26. Tanzi, E.L.; Lupton, J.R.; Alster, T.S. Lasers in dermatology: Four decades of progress. *J. Am. Acad. Dermatol.* **2003**, *49*, 1–34 [CrossRef]
27. Chen, F.; Zhang, M.; Devahastin, S.; Yu, D. Comparative evaluation of the properties of deep-frozen blueberries dried by vacuum infrared freeze drying with the use of CO_2 laser perforation, ultrasound, and freezing–thawing as pretreatments. *Food Bioprocess Technol.* **2021**, *14*, 1805–1816. [CrossRef]
28. Ramírez, C.; Troncoso, E.; Muñoz, J.; Aguilera, J.M. Microstructure analysis on pre-treated apple slices and its effect on water release during air drying. *J. Food Eng.* **2011**, *106*, 253–261. [CrossRef]
29. Hernández, Y.; Ramírez, C.; Moreno, J.; Núñez, H.; Vega, O.; Almonacid, S.; Pinto, M.; Fuentes, L.; Simpson, R. Effect of refractance window on dehydration of osmotically pretreated apple slices: Color and texture evaluation. *J. Food Process Eng.* **2020**, *43*, e13304 [CrossRef]
30. Nieto, A.B.; Vicente, S.; Hodara, K.; Castro, M.A.; Alzamora, S.M. Osmotic dehydration of apple: Influence of sugar and water activity on tissue structure, rheological properties and water mobility. *J. Food Eng.* **2013**, *119*, 104–114. [CrossRef]
31. Moraga, G.; Talens, P.; Moraga, M.J.; Martínez-Navarrete, N. Implication of water activity and glass transition on the mechanical and optical properties of freeze-dried apple and banana slices. *J. Food Eng.* **2011**, *106*, 212–219. [CrossRef]
32. AOAC. *Official Methods of Analysis of AOAC International*, 19th ed.; AOAC International: Gaithersburg, MD, USA, 2016.
33. Sturm, B.; Nunez Vega, A.M.; Hofacker, W.C. Influence of process control strategies on drying kinetics, colour and shrinkage of air dried apples. *Appl. Therm. Eng.* **2014**, *62*, 455–460. [CrossRef]
34. Galaz, P.; Valdenegro, M.; Ramírez, C.; Nuñez, H.; Almonacid, S.; Simpson, R. Effect of drum drying temperature on drying kinetic and polyphenol contents in pomegranate peel. *J. Food Eng.* **2017**, *208*, 19–27. [CrossRef]
35. Rajoriya, D.; Shewale, S.R.; Hebbar, H.U. Refractance window drying of apple slices: Mass transfer phenomena and quality parameters. *Food Bioprocess Technol.* **2019**, *12*, 1646–1658. [CrossRef]

36. Henríquez, C.; Almonacid, S.; Chiffelle, I.; Valenzuela, T.; Araya, M.; Cabezas, L.; Simpson, R.; Speisky, H. Determination of antioxidant capacity, total phenolic content and mineral composition of different fruit tissue of five apple cultivars grown in Chile. *Chil. J. Agric. Res.* **2010**, *70*, 523–536. [CrossRef]
37. Franco, S.; Jaques, A.; Pinto, M.; Fardella, M.; Valencia, P.; Núñez, H.; Ramírez, C.; Simpson, R. Dehydration of salmon (*Atlantic salmon*), beef, and apple (Granny Smith) using refractance window™: Effect on diffusion behavior, texture, and color changes. *Innov. Food Sci. Emerg. Technol.* **2019**, *52*, 8–16. [CrossRef]
38. Caparino, O.A.; Tang, J.; Nindo, C.I.; Sablani, S.S.; Powers, J.R.; Fellman, J.K. Effect of drying methods on the physical properties and microstructures of mango (*Philippine "Carabao"* var.) powder. *J. Food Eng.* **2012**, *111*, 135–148. [CrossRef]
39. Puente, L.; Vega-Gálvez, A.; Ah-Hen, K.S.; Rodríguez, A.; Pasten, A.; Poblete, J.; Pardo-Orellana, C.; Muñoz, M. Refractance window drying of goldenberry (*Physalis peruviana* L.) pulp: A comparison of quality characteristics with respect to other drying techniques. *LWT-Food Sci. Technol.* **2020**, *131*, 109772. [CrossRef]
40. Calín-Sánchez, Á.; Lipan, L.; Cano-Lamadrid, M.; Kharaghani, A.; Masztalerz, K.; Carbonell-Barrachina, Á.A.; Figiel, A. Comparison of traditional and novel drying techniques and its effect on quality of fruits, vegetables and aromatic herbs. *Foods* **2020**, *9*, 1261. [CrossRef]
41. Wojdyło, A.; Figiel, A.; Legua, P.; Lech, K.; Carbonell-Barrachina, Á.A.; Hernández, F. Chemical composition, antioxidant capacity, and sensory quality of dried jujube fruits as affected by cultivar and drying method. *Food Chem.* **2016**, *207*, 170–179. [CrossRef]
42. Mitić, S.S.; Stojanović, B.T.; Stojković, M.B.; Mitić, M.N.; Pavlović, J.L. Total phenolics, flavonoids and antioxidant activity of different apple cultivars. *Bulg. Chem. Commun.* **2013**, *45*, 326–331.
43. Rajoriya, D.; Shewale, S.R.; Bhavya, M.L.; Hebbar, H.U. Far infrared assisted refractance window drying of apple slices: Comparative study on flavour, nutrient retention and drying characteristics. *Innov. Food Sci. Emerg. Technol.* **2020**, *66*, 102530. [CrossRef]
44. Rajoriya, D.; Bhavya, M.L.; Hebbar, H.U. Impact of process parameters on drying behaviour, mass transfer and quality profile of refractance window dried banana puree. *LWT-Food Sci. Technol.* **2021**, *145*, 111330. [CrossRef]
45. Moses, J.A.; Norton, T.; Alagusundaram, K.; Tiwari, B.K. Novel drying techniques for the food industry. *Food Eng. Rev.* **2014**, *6*, 43–55. [CrossRef]
46. Zotarelli, M.F.; Carciofi, B.A.M.; Laurindo, J.B. Effect of process variables on the drying rate of mango pulp by refractance window. *Food Res. Int.* **2015**, *69*, 410–417. [CrossRef]
47. Ortiz-Jerez, M.J.; Gulati, T.; Datta, A.K.; Ochoa-Martínez, C.I. Quantitative understanding of refractance window™ drying. *Food Bioprod. Process.* **2015**, *95*, 237–253. [CrossRef]
48. Rocha-Parra, D.F.; Lanari, M.C.; Zamora, M.C.; Chirife, J. Influence of storage conditions on phenolic compounds stability, antioxidant capacity and colour of freeze-dried encapsulated red wine. *LWT-Food Sci. Technol.* **2016**, *70*, 162–170. [CrossRef]
49. Tonon, R.V.; Brabet, C.; Hubinger, M.D. Anthocyanin stability and antioxidant activity of spray-dried açai (*Euterpe oleracea* Mart.) juice produced with different carrier agents. *Food Res. Int.* **2010**, *43*, 907–914. [CrossRef]
50. Henríquez, C.; Córdova, A.; Almonacid, S.; Saavedra, J. Kinetic modeling of phenolic compound degradation during drum-drying of apple peel by-products. *J. Food Eng.* **2014**, *143*, 146–153. [CrossRef]
51. Baeghbali, V.; Niakousari, M.; Farahnaky, A. Refractance window drying of pomegranate juice: Quality retention and energy efficiency. *LWT-Food Sci. Technol.* **2016**, *66*, 34–40. [CrossRef]
52. Nayak, B.; Berrios, J.D.J.; Powers, J.R.; Tang, J. Effect of extrusion on the antioxidant capacity and color attributes of expanded extrudates prepared from purple potato and yellow pea flour mixes. *J. Food Sci.* **2011**, *76*, C874–C883. [CrossRef] [PubMed]
53. Robertson, G.L. Food packaging and shelf life. In *Food Packaging and Shelf Life*; Robertson, G.L., Ed.; CRC Press: Boca Raton, FL, USA, 2010; pp. 1–16. ISBN 2013206534.
54. Sablani, S.S. Drying of fruits and vegetables: Retention of nutritional/functional quality. *Dry. Technol.* **2006**, *24*, 123–135. [CrossRef]
55. Lavelli, V.; Vantaggi, C. Rate of antioxidant degradation and color variations in dehydrated apples as related to water activity. *J. Agric. Food Chem.* **2009**, *57*, 4733–4738. [CrossRef] [PubMed]
56. Henríquez, M.; Almonacid, S.; Lutz, M.; Simpson, R.; Valdenegro, M. Comparison of three drying processes to obtain an apple peel food ingredient. *CYTA-J. Food* **2013**, *11*, 127–135. [CrossRef]
57. Bonazzi, C.; Dumoulin, E. Quality changes in food materials as influenced by drying processes. *Mod. Dry. Technol.* **2014**, *3*, 1–20.

Disclaimer/Publisher's Note: The statements, opinions and data contained in all publications are solely those of the individual author(s) and contributor(s) and not of MDPI and/or the editor(s). MDPI and/or the editor(s) disclaim responsibility for any injury to people or property resulting from any ideas, methods, instructions or products referred to in the content.

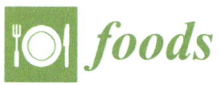

Article

Assessing the Impact of Roasting Temperatures on Biochemical and Sensory Quality of Macadamia Nuts (*Macadamia integrifolia*)

Noluthando Noxolo Aruwajoye [1], Nana Millicent Duduzile Buthelezi [2], Asanda Mditshwa [1], Samson Zeray Tesfay [1,*] and Lembe Samukelo Magwaza [1]

[1] Discipline of Crop and Horticultural Science, School of Agricultural, Earth and Environmental Sciences, University of KwaZulu-Natal, Private Bag X01, Scottsville, Pietermaritzburg 3209, South Africa
[2] Department of Biology and Environmental Sciences, Sefako Makgatho Health Sciences University, P.O. Box 235, Medunsa, Ga-Rankuwa 0204, South Africa
* Correspondence: tesfay@ukzn.ac.za

Abstract: Depending on the temperature regime used during roasting, the biochemical and sensory characteristics of macadamia nuts can change. 'A4' and 'Beaumont' were used as model cultivars to examine how roasting temperatures affected the chemical and sensory quality of macadamia nuts. Using a hot air oven dryer, macadamia kernels were roasted at 50, 75, 100, 125, and 150 °C for 15 min. The quantity of phenols, flavonoids, and antioxidants in kernels roasted at 50, 75, and 100 °C was significant ($p < 0.001$); however, these kernels also had high levels of moisture content, oxidation-sensitive unsaturated fatty acids (UFAs), and peroxide value (PV), and poor sensory quality. Low moisture content, flavonoids, phenols, antioxidants, fatty acid (FA) compositions, high PV, and poor sensory quality—i.e., excessive browning, an exceptionally crunchy texture, and a bitter flavor—were all characteristics of kernels roasted at 150 °C. With a perfect crispy texture, a rich brown color, and a strong nutty flavor, kernels roasted at 125 °C had lower PV; higher oxidation-resistant UFA compositions; considerable concentrations of flavonoids, phenols, and antioxidants; and good sensory quality. Therefore, 'A4' and 'Beaumont' kernels could be roasted at 125 °C for use in the industry to improve kernel quality and palatability.

Keywords: peroxide value; fatty acids; flavonoids; phenols; antioxidants activity; sensory evaluation

1. Introduction

According to [1,2], macadamia (*Macadamia integrifolia*) is the top-ranking nut in the world and is frequently consumed either roasted or as an ingredient in different confectionery items. The widespread intake of macadamia nuts may be attributed to its high nutritional value and alleged health benefits, which include reducing the risk of type 2 diabetes and cardiovascular disease [3–5]. These health advantages are linked to low cholesterol levels, a high oil content (69–78%) that is rich in monounsaturated fatty acids (80%), primarily oleic (60%) and palmitoleic (20%) acids, and antioxidants due to a number of phytochemicals and polyphenols also present in kernels [2,5–9]. The beneficial macronutrients protein, dietary fiber, vital minerals, vitamin E, and plant sterols are also abundant in macadamia [10]. Macadamia nuts are especially sensitive to hydrolytic and oxidative rancidity when they contain significant levels of free moisture because they have a high proportion of monounsaturated fatty acids [11,12].

According to [13,14], roasting is one of the best processing techniques for maintaining the quality of nuts and increasing their overall palatability. Kernels underwent sensory and chemical modifications as a result of this processing technique [15]. Through nonenzymatic reactions such as Maillard browning, it enhances the color, flavor, aroma, and texture of the nuts [16–18]. The pyrazines and pyridine compounds that give roasted nuts

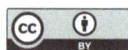

their characteristic brown color are byproducts of the Maillard reaction, which requires reducing sugars to react with amino acids to produce browning products [12,16,19].

The Maillard process occurs during roasting and produces a variety of volatile chemicals that give kernels their flavor and aroma [15,20]. According to [21], pyrazines, furans, and pyrroles are crucial elements of the scent of roasted kernels. Pyrazines are produced during heating by Strecker degradation and Maillard sugar–amine reactions [12]. Pyrazines feature nutty and roasted odors. Compared to raw kernels, roasted kernels have a crispier texture and a more delicate, distinctively nutty flavor that makes them more popular for consumption [13,22]. Additionally, roasting deactivates the oxidative enzyme system (lipoxygenic enzymes), lowers moisture content, and, as a result, gets rid of germs while minimizing degradative reactions such as lipid oxidation, which has antioxidant activity [18,22].

The sensory attributes, nutritional value, and lipid quality of nuts can all be impacted by roasting, despite the fact that roasting has numerous positive effects [23]. Furthermore, excessive roasting or high temperatures can promote lipid oxidation and non-enzymatic browning reactions, which can decrease the nutritional value of food by causing the loss of essential fatty acids, essential amino acids, and carbohydrates [23,24]. Additionally, this may hasten the occurrence of lipid oxidation, sometimes referred to as oxidative rancidity. According to [25], these chemical modification reactions may lead to the production of hazardous chemicals in nuts that may be harmful to consumers' health. Due to their high fat content and susceptibility to oxidation, macadamia nuts require low roasting temperatures [5,26]. The nut industry defines mild temperature as a range of 30 to 180 °C, during which roasting is performed for 15 to 60 min using a variety of techniques, including infrared heating, radio frequency and microwave dielectric processes, commercial electrical ovens, and so on [22,23,27]. However, little is known about the effect of mild roasting temperatures on the sensory and chemical quality of macadamia kernels. Therefore, the objective of this study was to evaluate the impact of different roasting temperatures on the sensory and biochemical quality of macadamia nuts.

2. Materials and Methods

2.1. Macadamia Samples

'Beaumont' and 'A4', two hybrids of Australian-bred *Macadamia integrifolia* cultivars, were taken from Elliot Farm's commercial orchards in Port Shepstone, KwaZulu-Natal, South Africa (latitude: 30°44′28″ S, longitude: 30°27′17″ E, and elevation: 36 m). According to standard industry procedure, nuts were harvested during the early season (May 2017) and the late season (June 2017). For further processing, approximately 20 kg of nuts from each cultivar were gathered on each sample day and brought to the Ukulinga Research Farm of the University of KwaZulu-Natal (UKZN).

2.2. Dehusking, Drying, and Cracking Process

At UKZN's Ukulinga Research Farm, dehusking was carried out on the same day as harvesting using a 01-one-lane dehusker from WMC Sheet Metal Works in Tzaneen, South Africa. Nuts-in-shell (NIS) were dried using a mechanical convection oven (RY-FB-550, Rongyao factory, Wuhan, China) at the UKZN Postharvest Research Laboratory for three days in a row, starting at 35 °C on the first day, 38 °C for the second day, and 50 °C for the third day, according to a method described by [28] with minor modifications. To prevent quality deterioration, these drying temperatures were chosen in accordance with nut industry practices [22,29]. The moisture level of the dried nuts was monitored, and they were only taken out of the oven when it reached 1.5%. Based on the initial and final (dry) weights, the moisture content of nuts was determined. According to [30], dry basis (db) calculations of moisture content in nuts were made using mass changes. According to [31], the moisture content was calculated as follows:

$$MC_{db} = \frac{W_i - W_d}{W_d} \times 100 \qquad (1)$$

where MC_{db} is moisture content on a dry mass basis, and W_i and W_d are the initial and the dry sample weights, respectively. Additionally, using a commercial mechanical macadamia nutcracker (TZ-150 macadamia nut cracker, Alibaba Group Houlding (PTY) LTD, Hangzhou, China), macadamia nuts were mechanically cracked into wholes, halves and bits. Only whole kernels were utilized in the experiment, and the shell and kernel were manually separated. The percentage of kernel recovery was computed and expressed as a percentage weight of the nut that is a kernel at 1.5% moisture content, with the rest being a shell (Equation (2)). Raw kernels are nuts that have been dried to a kernel moisture level of 1.5% for the purpose of dehusking and cracking [32].

$$KR = \frac{NIS - Shell}{NIS} \times 100 \qquad (2)$$

where KR is kernel recovery and NIS is nut-in-shell.

2.3. Roasting Process

The roasting process was carried out in accordance with [19] with minor modifications. Roasting temperatures were also selected based on industry norms for nuts in order to prevent quality degradation [18,22,23]. 'A4' and 'Beaumont' were used as two distinct cultivars during the early and late harvesting seasons. Only complete kernels with no visible faults were used for sampling. The kernels were roasted using a convection oven (RY-EB-550, Rongyao manufacture, Wuhan, China) for 15 min at 5 different temperatures, i.e., 50, 75, 100, 125, and 150 °C, at the Department of Horticultural Science Postharvest Laboratory of UKZN, South Africa. Raw kernels were used as the benchmark. For postharvest storage trials, commercial brown paper bags were filled with a randomly selected set of kernels, each weighing 2 kg and consisting of 15 replicates of each treatment, cultivar, and harvest season. After roasting, the sensory quality of the kernels was immediately assessed. The same day, the roasted kernels were ground into a fine powder and stored at -20 °C for future analysis using a Brabantia-table blender (BBEK 1051, Massdiscounter (Pty) Limited, Johannesburg, South Africa).

2.4. Quantification of Peroxide Value

Using a Brabantia-table blender (BBEK 1051, Massdiscounter (Pty) Limited, Johannesburg, South Africa), kernels were ground into a fine powder after roasting. The amount of kernel oil was quantified from ground sample material using a method similar to that of [33] with a few minor adjustments. Three grams of ground kernel sample were placed in a test tube with hexane (9.0 mL) before the test tube was immersed in an ultrasonic bath (Labotec, Model No. 132, Labotec (PTY) LTD, Johannesburg, South Africa) for 10 min. The test tube's residual received another 6 mL of hexane after the supernatant was vacuum-filtered. The test tube was then filled with the Buchner funnel after being left for 5 min. Following filtering, the supernatant was dried with 15 mL of hexane using a GenVac® concentrator (SPScientific, Genevac LTD, Suffolk, UK) while maintaining the sample's oil content. The remaining oil was measured and reported using its dry weight.

With a few minor adjustments, the peroxide value (PV) was calculated in accordance with [29]. In total, 20 mL of acetic acid/chloroform (3:2 v/v) was used to dissolve a 1 g sample of oil, and then a burette was used to add 1 mL of a saturated potassium iodide solution. Iodine was created after the reaction had occurred. Deionized water (50 mL) was added. Using a burette, iodine was titrated with $Na_2S_2O_3$. The following formula was used to compute the peroxide value (expressed as milliequivalents of peroxide per kilogram of sample):

$$PV \text{ (meq per kg)} = \frac{(S - B) \times N \times 1000}{Sample\ wt\ (g) \times 1000} \qquad (3)$$

where S = sample titration (µL); B = blank titration; N = normality of $Na_2S_2O_3$.

2.5. Quantification of Fatty Acid Profile

With minor changes, the method described by [5,34] was used to determine fatty acids (FAs). First, 2 mL of hexane was added after the sample was weighed at 100 mg. As an internal standard, heptadecanoic (C17) was added (50 µL of 1000 ppm). The sample combination received 1 mL of 20% sulfuric acid in methanol solution. The mixture was then incubated for one hour in an oven that was kept at a temperature of 80 °C. The mixture was allowed to cool at room temperature after incubation. In order to extract the fatty acid methyl esters (FAMEs), 3 mL of 20% (w/v) NaCl was added. To facilitate phase separation, the materials were agitated firmly and then centrifuged. The upper hexane phase (hexane containing FAMEs) was transferred to a gas chromatograph (GC) vial.

GC (Trace1300, Thermo Scientific, Austin, Texas, USA) connected to a flame ionization detector (FID) was used to separate the FAMEs. A GC-FID system and a CTC Analytics PAL autosampler were connected. On a non-polar Stabil wax (60 m, 0.32 mm ID, 0.25 m film thickness), FAs were separated. In this experiment, 1 mL/min of helium was employed as the carrier gas. At 240 °C, the injector temperature was maintained. A 5:1 split ratio was used to inject 1 L of the material. The oven's temperature was set to 50 °C for 2 min, then increased to 180 °C at a rate of 25 °C per minute and held for 2 min, 200 °C at a rate of 3 °C per minute and held for 5 min, and lastly 240 °C at a rate of 4 °C per minute and kept for 15 min. Using the Chrom-Card data system version 2.3 software for Windows (Thermo Electron, Rodano, Italy), each FA in the chromatogram was identified by comparing the retention times with certified standard mixes (Grain FAME Mix Supelco, Bellefonte, PA, USA; Catalog No: 47801) and quantified by the peak areas on the chromatogram. In terms of g of FA per g of total FAs, the results were expressed. The total fatty acids (TFA), the ratio of saturated to unsaturated fatty acids (SFA/MUFA), and the ratio of monounsaturated to polyunsaturated fatty acids (MUFA/PUFA) were all calculated using the fatty acid composition that was obtained [22].

2.6. Quantification of Free and Membrane-Bound Phenols

Phenols were identified using [35] as a guide, with a few minor modifications. One gram of each sample of roasted kernels was combined with ten milliliters of 99.8% (v/v) methanol and vortexed for thirty seconds. The mixture was then agitated for an additional night at room temperature in order to remove the free phenols. Following centrifugation of the mixture, the supernatant was filtered through Whatman® no. 1 filter paper, and the sample was once again washed with 10 mL of solvent until the solvent was clear. The remaining kernel residue was then effectively released from cell wall-bound phenols using acid hydrolysis. Each sample received 10 mL of 60% aqueous methanol that had been acidified (2 M hydrochloric acid) before being submerged in a hot water bath for 90 min. Supernatants were filtered through a 0.45 m filter after being allowed to cool in glass tubes. Gallic acid monohydrate was used as a standard in the spectrophotometric determination of the total phenolic concentration, and the result was expressed as mg OF gallic acid equivalents (GAE) kg^{-1} of sample dry weight (5 mL of distilled water + 1 mL of extract + 1 mL Folin–Ciocalteu reagent + 10 mL of 7% Na_2CO_3 + 8 mL of distilled water, left at room temperature overnight).

2.7. Quantification of Total Flavonoids Concentration

Using quercetin as a standard, the total flavonoid concentration was measured using aluminum chloride ($AlCl_3$) in accordance with an established procedure (kernel extract prepared for phenolic concentration determination). This procedure was based on that provided by [36], with a few minor adjustments. In a glass tube, 0.10 mL of the kernel extract was added. The reaction mixture was then added, and 5% $NaNO_2$ (0.03 mL) was added after that. It was let to stand at room temperature for 5 min. Then, 0.03 mL of 10% $AlCl_3$ was added and allowed to react for 6 min before being mixed with 0.2 mL of 1 mM NaOH and diluted to 1 mL with purified water. At 510 nm, the absorbance of the reaction mixture was measured in comparison to methanol, which served as a blank. In terms of sample dry weight, the results were represented as mg quercetin kg^{-1}.

2.8. Quantification of Total Antioxidants Activity

2.8.1. Free Radical Scavenging Capacity

The 2,2′-diphenyl-1-picrylhydrazyl (DPPH) free radical scavenging activity was assessed with some minor modifications from [37]. First, 1.94 mg of DPPH was dissolved in 50 mL of methanol to create the stock solution of the radical, which was then stored at −20 °C until usage. The DPPH stock solution was diluted with methanol to produce the working solution for the radical, which had an absorbance of around 0.98 (0.02) at 517 nm. In a polystyrene 4.5 mL cuvette, 20 L of gallic acid or sample extract was measured Following the addition of 1 mL of 0.1 mM DPPH solution, which was carried out in the dark and covered with aluminum foil, the mixture received 800 L of 100% methanol and was left to remain at room temperature for 60 min. The results were represented as mg DPPH GAE kg^{-1} of sample dry weight after the absorbance was measured at 517 nm against an absolute methanol blank in low light.

2.8.2. 2,2′-Azinobis-3-ethylbenzothiazoline-6-sulfonic Acid (ABTS) Assay

The 2,2′-azinobis-3-ethylbenzothiazoline-6-sulfonic acid (ABTS) concentration was calculated using [38] with a few minor adjustments. For evaluating the hydrophilic and lipophilic antioxidant fractions, respectively, a 7 mM solution of 2,2′-azinobis-3-ethylbenzothiazoline-6-sulfonic acid was made. The 7 mM ABTS solution was combined with 2.45 mM ammonium persulfate to create the ABTS radical cation (ABTS.+), which was then left to sit in the dark at room temperature for 3 to 6 h. After that, 10 mL of sample solution made from roasted material extracts in acetate buffer (pH 4.0) was added together with 1.0 mL of activated ABTS solution (A734 nm = 0.700 ± 0.5). The decrease in absorbance at 734 nm was recorded after 6 min and the results were expressed as mg ABTS GAE kg^{-1} of sample dry weight.

2.9. Sensory Evaluation

A randomized set of macadamia kernels were examined raw and immediately after roasting (50, 75, 100, 125 and 150 °C at the Department of Horticultural Science Postharvest Laboratory of UKZN. Samples were given to trained panelists ranging from the age of 25 to 44 to assess the quality of 'A4' and 'Beaumont'kernels in terms of their texture, colour and taste [13,26,39]. The trained panelists employed in this study were 5 males and 5 females as described by similar studies where the panelists ranged between 7 and 12 in number [40–42] Moreover, according to [13,39] with some minor modifications, the texture, colour, and taste of the kernels were evaluated using a 5-point scale as follows:Texture, where 1 denotes very hard, 2: hard, 3: slightly crispy, 4: crispy, and 5: very crispy; Colour, where 1 denotes very light, 2: light, 3: slightly brown, 4: brown, and 5: extremely brown and; Taste, where 1 denotes very nutty, 2: nutty, 3: slightly bitter, 4: bitter, and 5: extremely bitter.

2.10. Statistical Analysis

The collected data were subjected to analysis of variance (ANOVA) using GenStat statistical software (GenStat®, 18.1 edition, VSN International, Hemel Hempstead, UK) 18.1 Least significant difference values (LSD; $p < 0.001$) were calculated for mean separation.

3. Results and Discussion

3.1. Moisture Content

The 'A4' and 'Beaumont' cultivars' kernel moisture content considerably ($p < 0.001$) reduced as the roasting temperature rose (Figure 1). 'A4' and 'Beaumont' kernels roasted at 50, 75, 100, and 125 °C exhibited substantial drops in moisture content of 1.474% and 1.432%, 1.429% and 1.4%, 1.393% and 1.318%, and 1.319% and 1.211%, respectively, whereas kernels roasted at 150 °C had the lowest moisture content of 1.218% and 1.025%, respectively

This might be caused by convectional roasting processes, where moisture is first removed from the kernel's surface and then lost when water diffuses from the kernel's inside to the dried surface [43]. Additionally, excessive moisture evaporation and the loss of volatile compounds may be due to the significant decrease in kernel moisture content at 150 °C. This problem is made worse by the reaction of free amino acids and short-chain peptides with free mono- and disaccharides during nonenzymatic browning, as well as the potential for protein denaturation and degradation when roasting nuts at temperatures above 130 °C [27]. These chemical alterations may have an impact on the sensory and chemical quality of the kernel [18,22,44]. As a result of using higher temperatures (150 °C) during roasting, Refs. [13,14,26] reported similar significant decreases in kernel moisture content from 2.4% to 1%.

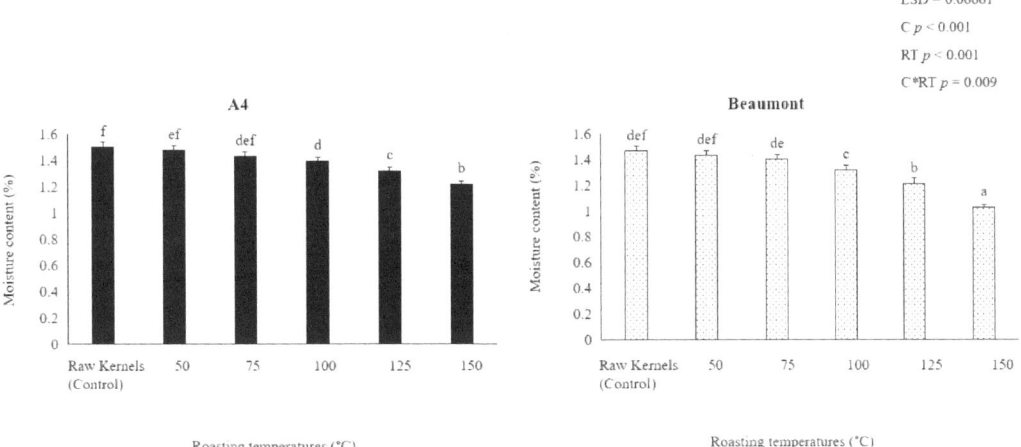

Figure 1. Moisture content of 'A4' and 'Beaumont' at different roasting temperatures. Different lowercase letters (a–f) indicate significant differences ($p < 0.01$) between the different roasting temperatures.

3.2. Peroxide Value (PV)

The most-used metric to assess the degree of primary oxidation products, mostly hydroperoxides in edible oils, is the peroxide value [12,23]. According to [25,29], a number of variables, such as roasting temperature, levels of unsaturated fatty acids, the presence of enzymes, and antioxidant levels, may have an impact on the peroxide value, which is a sign of autoxidation (free radical reaction). Nut rancidity results from a reaction between the hydroperoxides produced by autoxidation and other nut components such as proteins and amino acids [45].

From Figure 2, it can be observed that the PV of 'A4' and 'Beaumont' kernels roasted at 50 °C (2.203 and 1.303 meq O_2 kg^{-1}), 75 °C (1.72 and 1.232 meq O_2 kg^{-1}), 100 °C (1.569 and 1.011 meq O_2 kg^{-1}), and 125 °C (1.161 and 0.947 meq O_2 kg^{-1}) significantly ($p < 0.001$) declined with increasing roasting temperatures. It is thought that kernels roasted at 125 °C have reduced PV, which is a sign of high quality. A high-quality macadamia product is defined by a low peroxide value of less than 1 meq O_2 kg^{-1}, which is deemed acceptable for a freshly refined fat and is categorized by a low oxidation state, according to [24,46]. Our findings are in line with those of [45], who found that when roasting temperature increased (from 110 to 120 °C), the PV of Canariumindicum L. (Burseraceae) kernels drastically dropped from 1.30 to 1 meq O_2 kg^{-1}.

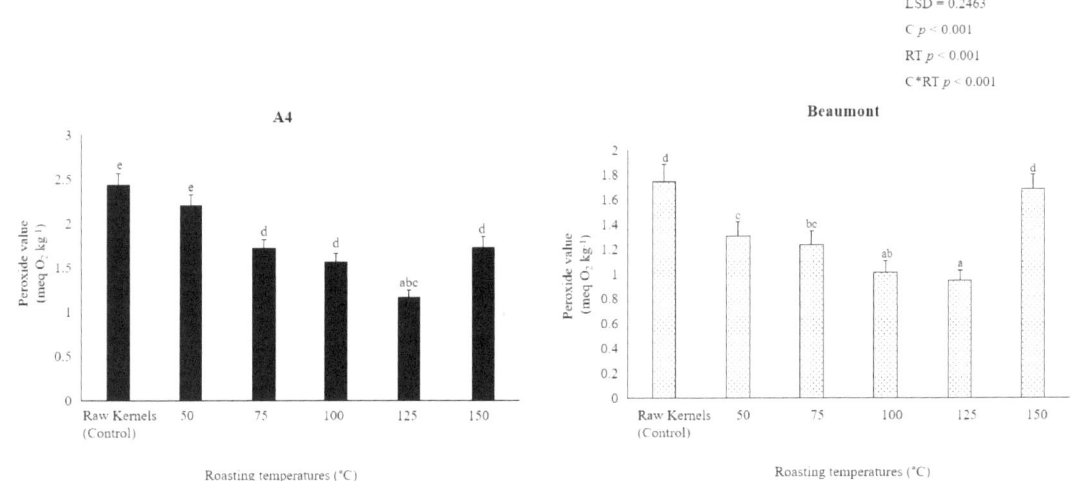

Figure 2. Peroxide value of 'A4' and 'Beaumont' at different roasting temperatures. Different lower case letters (a–e) indicate significant differences ($p < 0.01$) between the different roasting temperatures.

Both cultivars 'A4' (1.727 meq O_2 kg^{-1}) and 'Beaumont' (1.682 meq O_2 kg^{-1}) saw an increase in PV after being roasted at 150 °C. This could be attributable to greater temperatures, which encourage the peroxide's breakdown and polymerization into a variety of secondary compounds such as aldehydes and ketones [47]. According to [25] temperature has a significant impact on the rate at which edible oils oxidize and produce rancidity; the higher the temperature, the faster rancidity develops. Our findings concur with those of [23,44], who claimed that the increase in PV caused by thermal processing in sesame and walnuts, respectively, could be attributed to the rise in hydroperoxides caused by free radicals attacking the unsaturated fatty acids of oil. Our results indicate that roasting 'A4' and 'Beaumont' kernels at 150 °C should be avoided since [24,47] showed that the increase in PV may result in the development of detectable off-flavors.

3.3. Fatty Acids (FAs)

The FAME analysis of raw (control) and roasted kernels of 'A4' and 'Beaumont macadamia nuts identified a total of thirteen individual FAs, among which oleic acid (C18:1n9c) and palmitoleic acid (C16:1) were predominant, followed by palmitic acid (C16:0), omega-6 (n-6), linoleic acid (C18:2n6c), stearic acid (C18:0), and cis-11-Eicosenoic acid (C20:1) (Tables 1 and 2). Additionally, Tables 1 and 2 display the total amount of fatty acids (TFAs) found in 'A4' and 'Beaumont' kernels. 'A4' had the highest concentration of TFAs. The majority of the fatty acids in both cultivars were monounsaturated fatty acids (MUFA), followed by polyunsaturated fatty acids (PUFAs) and saturated fatty acids (STAs). Moreover, ($\sum$ n-6)/($\sum$ n-3) was high in both cultivars. The ratio of $\sum$ PUFA:$\sum$ SFA was low in both cultivars. These findings are in agreement with [5,22], who reported these major FAs in raw and roasted kernels of macadamia nuts and hazelnuts, respectively.

Table 1. Fatty acid compositions (μg/g) of 'A4' macadamia kernels with different roasting temperature treatments.

RT	Lauric Acid (C12:0)	Miristic Acid (C14:0)	Palmitic Acid (C16:0)	Stearic Acid (C18:0)	Arachidic Acid (C20:0)	Palmitoleic Acid (C16:1)	Oleic Acid (C18:1n9c)
Control	1.99 ± 0.03 a	8.43 ± 0.58 c	83.31 ± 44.22 b	42.67 ± 5.92 b	27.25 ± 4.08 c	469.71 ± 26.86 c	709.66 ± 56.78 c
50 °C	1.91 ± 0.67 a	7.06 ± 0.71 bc	93.01 ± 28.95 b	33.75 ± 2.97 ab	20.98 ± 0.40 bc	384.59 ± 24.75 b	571.27 ± 28.00 b
75 °C	1.89 ± 0.09 a	7.03 ± 0.85 bc	94.29 ± 8.58 b	33.77 ± 818 ab	16.48 ± 3.07 ab	286.80 ± 33.47 a	496.32 ± 25.79 b
100 °C	2.69 ± 1.08 ab	6.40 ± 0.57 ab	94.10 ± 2.74 b	22.03 ± 2.89 a	16.74 ± 1.07 ab	248.90 ± 33.61 a	395.45 ± 28.17 a
125 °C	1.49 ± 0.06 a	5.33 ± 0.44 ab	96.28 ± 13.37 bc	21.22 ± 3.09 a	13.81 ± 1.77 ab	472.96 ± 13.79 c	800.97 ± 13.64 d
150 °C	1.45 ± 0.08 a	4.67 ± 0.400 a	63.71 ± 9.67 a	20.54 ± 2.27 a	12.22 ± 2.65 a	214.16 ± 17.37 a	357.42 ± 17.37 a
RT	Cis-11-Eicosenoic acid (C20:1)	Linoleic acid (C18:2n6c)	Dihomo-γlinolenic acid (C20:3n6)	Eicosatrienoic acid (C20:3n3)	Omega-6 (n-6)	Omega -3 (n-3)	(∑ n-6)/(∑ n-3)
Control	43.48 ± 5.92 c	64.34 ± 5.54 c	5.26 ± 0.96 c	2.14 ± 0.89 b	69.61 ± 6.45 d	2.14 ± 0.89 b	97.82 ± 46.57 c
50 °C	32.91 ± 1.72 bc	53.54 ± 6.52 bc	2.58 ± 0.40 b	1.05 ± 0.34 a	56.12 ± 6.21 cd	1.05 ± 0.34 ab	86.34 ± 34.47 c
75 °C	27.22 ± 1.87 ab	42.59 ± 1.21 ab	2.02 ± 0.57 b	0.83 ± 0.31 a	44.62 ± 1.04 bc	0.83 ± 0.31 ab	94.63 ± 39.57 c
100 °C	ND	34.67 ± 1.81 a	1.30 ± 0.13 ab	ND	34.25 ± 0.86 a	ND	ND
125 °C	22.68 ± 1.43 a	32.74 ± 1.89 a	1.38 ± 0.54 ab	1.55 ± 0.08 b	34.80 ± 1.88 ab	0.88 ± 0.08 ab	23.31 ± 1.14 a
150 °C	22.51 ± 1.17 a	33.83 ± 3.05 a	0.01 ± 0.60 a	1.56 ± 0.27 b	35.74 ± 3.08 ab	0.91 ± 0.27 ab	44.58 ± 12.77 b
RT	∑ PUFA:∑ SFA	∑ SFA	∑ MUFA	∑ PUFA	∑ TFA		
Control	0.65 ± 0.17 ab	136.40 ± 39.87 c	1250.10 ± 50.67 d	71.75 ± 7.21 c	1458.25 ± 37.18 e		
50 °C	0.48 ± 0.11 a	135.69 ± 27.83 c	1009.74 ± 28.97 c	57.17 ± 6.20 b	1202.61 ± 15.31 d		
75 °C	0.36 ± 0.03 a	127.74 ± 18.06 c	813.21 ± 25.38 b	45.45 ± 1.25 ab	986.40 ± 16.01 c		
100 °C	0.39 ± 0.02 a	92.72 ± 3.56 b	650.84 ± 16.37 a	35.64 ± 1.56 a	779.20 ± 17.30 b		
125 °C	0.55 ± 0.07 a	73.04 ± 11.84 a	651.27 ± 6.62 a	34.75 ± 1.93 a	631.51 ± 10.81 a		
150 °C	0.43 ± 0.08 a	90.41 ± 9.10 b	700.68 ± 19.24 ab	36.42 ± 3.28 ab	727.52 ± 14.62 b		

RT (roasting temperature), ∑ (sum), SFA (saturated fatty acids), MUFA (monounsaturated fatty acids), PUFA (polyunsaturated fatty acids), PUFA:SFA (ratio of polyunsaturated fatty acids to saturated fatty acids), TFA (total fatty acids), ND (not detected). Values are the mean ± SE. Means within a column of the same parameter with different letters are significantly different ($p < 0.001$).

Table 2. Fatty acid compositions (μg/g) of 'Beaumont' macadamia kernels with different roasting temperature treatments.

RT	Lauric Acid (C12:0)	Miristic Acid (C14:0)	Palmitic Acid (C16:0)	Stearic Acid (C18:0)	Arachidic Acid (C20:0)	Palmitoleic Acid (C16:1)	Oleic Acid (C18:1n9c)
Control	1.88 ± 0.16 a	7.61 ± 1.56 bc	94.27 ± 19.48 b	33.72 ± 4.76 bc	13.90 ± 2.75 b	336.75 ± 27.80 d	602.10 ± 45.62 de
50 °C	1.94 ± 0.06 a	8.92 ± 1.31 c	115.89 ± 44.35 b	35.97 ± 2.10 c	19.99 ± 2.16 c	271.77 ± 12.04 c	543.08 ± 26.45 cd
75 °C	1.57 ± 0.07 a	5.40 ± 0.51 ab	139.94 ± 89.08 bc	28.01 ± 2.66 b	20.61 ± 1.86 c	225.39 ± 24.22 bc	416.35 ± 22.58 b
100 °C	1.63 ± 0.04 a	4.65 ± 0.29 a	49.75 ± 0.83 a	16.53 ± 0.87 a	3.96 ± 0.36 a	200.94 ± 14.23 b	501.29 ± 5.23 c
125 °C	2.44 ± 0.98 ab	3.80 ± 0.26 a	37.24 ± 2.22 a	14.78 ± 0.69 a	4.00 ± 0.16 a	340.36 ± 4.55 de	624.92 ± 3.54 e
150 °C	1.36 ± 0.02 a	3.59 ± 0.13 a	36.82 ± 19.48 a	9.67 ± 1.71 a	2.74 ± 1.38 a	139.49 ± 10.59 a	291.03 ± 22.27 a
RT	cis-11-Eicosenoic acid (C20:1)	Linoleic acid (C18:2n6c)	Dihomo-γ linolenic acid (C20:3n6)	eicosatrienoic acid (C20:3n3)	Omega -6 (n-6)	Omega-3 (n-3)	(∑n-6)/(∑ n-3)
Control	27.73 ± 1.78 ab	52.70 ± 5.40 c	15.22 ± 14.09 c	0.62 ± 0.17 a	67.92 ± 15.59 cd	0.60 ± 0.18 a	113.77 ± 53.10 b
50 °C	35.99 ± 2.38 bc	52.46 ± 2.82 c	3.17 ± 0.92 a	1.81 ± 0.83 b	55.63 ± 2.90 c	1.81 ± 0.83 b	64.55 ± 27.93 ab
75 °C	30.68 ± 1.45 bc	43.06 ± 2.21 b	5.42 ± 1.02 b	3.63 ± 0.42 c	48.48 ± 2.80 bc	3.61 ± 0.42 c	13.74 ± 1.36 a
100 °C	30.50 ± 1.40 bc	30.41 ± 0.78 ab	0.55 ± 0.09 a	ND	30.96 ± 0.82 ab	ND	ND
125 °C	37.19 ± 1.7 c	22.02 ± 1.11 a	0.76 ± 0.09 a	ND	22.56 ± 1.29 a	ND	ND
150 °C	17.97 ± 1.90 a	29.63 ± 2.52 ab	0.09 ± 0.52 a	1.31 ± 0.45 ab	32.72 ± 2.33 ab	1.31 ± 0.45 ab	59.95 ± 37.5 ab
RT	∑ PUFA:∑ SFA	∑ SFA	∑ MUFA	∑ PUFA	∑ TFA		
Control	0.49 ± 0.04 ab	137.48 ± 22.48 c	959.68 ± 30.76 e	68.39 ± 15.58 dc	1165.55 ± 49.44 de		
50 °C	0.42 ± 0.08 ab	162.72 ± 47.72 d	861.84 ± 31.01 d	57.44 ± 3.16 c	1082.00 ± 68.90 d		
75 °C	0.49 ± 0.14 ab	174.91 ± 91.31 d	693.04 ± 8.73 c	52.11 ± 2.93 bc	920.06 ± 91.18 c		
100 °C	0.43 ± 0.01 ab	72.15 ± 1.16 b	518.69 ± 9.63 a	30.96 ± 0.82 a	621.80 ± 8.62 b		
125 °C	0.53 ± 0.03 b	58.26 ± 4.01 a	531.12 ± 6.06 ab	22.60 ± 1.05 a	419.06 ± 9.97 a		
150 °C	0.38 ± 0.12 a	82.89 ± 20.74 b	460.56 ± 16.97 b	34.03 ± 2.22 ab	577.48 ± 34.83 b		

RT (roasting temperature), ∑ (sum), SFA (saturated fatty acids), MUFA (monounsaturated fatty acids), PUFA (polyunsaturated fatty acids), PUFA:SFA (ratio of polyunsaturated fatty acids to saturated fatty acids), TFA (total fatty acids), ND (not detected). Values are the mean ± SE. Means within a column of the same parameter with different letters are significantly different ($p < 0.001$).

Tables 1 and 2 show that control kernels of 'A4' and 'Beaumont' significantly ($p < 0.001$) had the highest amounts of ∑ TFAs (1458.25 and 1165.55 μg/g), ∑ MUFAs (1250.10 and 959.68 μg/g), ∑ PUFAs (71.75 and 68.39), (∑ n-6)/(∑ n-3) (97.82 and 113.77 μg/g), linoleic acid (C18:2n6c) (64.34 and 52.70 μg/g), dihomo-γ-linolenic acid (C20:3n6) (5.26 and 15.22 μg/g), and omega-6 (n-6) (69.61 and 67.92 μg/g), respectively. The kernels are nutritious due to the large number of unsaturated fatty acids (UFAs), but they are also more prone to lipid peroxidation and rancidity, particularly when they have a high moisture content [5,48]. High kernel moisture content stimulates the breakdown of lipids into free fatty acids (FFAs), which leads to the creation of rancidity, as well as the growth of microfungi that produce deteriorating enzymes [49]. This is supported by Figures 1 and 2, which demonstrate that the control kernels of 'A4' and 'Beaumont' had significantly ($p < 0.001$) greater PV (2.432 and 1.741 meq O_2 kg^{-1}) and moisture content (1.5 and 1.46%), respectively. These values are within the acceptable range but indicate kernel susceptibility to the development of rancidity [11,48]. Moreover, control kernels of 'A4' and 'Beaumont had significantly ($p < 0.001$) high $\sum$ SFAs (136.40 and 137.48 µg/g) and lower $\sum$ PUFA: $\sum$ SFA (0.43 and 0.38 µg/g), respectively. Our findings are similar to [50], who reported a low ratio of $\sum$ USFA: $\sum$ SFA (0.11%) and high $\sum$ SFA (8.42%), attributed to the low content of linoleic acid content, probably as the result of its peroxidation [51].

With higher roasting temperatures, the fatty acid contents of 'A4' and 'Beaumont' kernels significantly ($p < 0.001$) reduced (Tables 1 and 2). This could be explained by the enzymes becoming inactive during roasting, which also results in a decrease in the activity of the lipase enzyme and moisture content [52]. Additionally, 'A4' and 'Beaumont' kernels roasted at 150 °C demonstrated a further drop and a smaller number of FA components. According to [52], excessive roasting at temperatures above 150 °C could hasten the oxidation of lipids. 'A4' and 'Beaumont' kernels roasted at 150 °C had considerably ($p < 0.001$) lower levels of linoleic acid (C18:2n6c) of 0.01 and 0.09 g/g, respectively. According to [43], the breakdown of linoleic acid during heating processes might result in the production of aliphatic aldehydes such as 2-heptenal and nonanal, which are to blame for the emergence of bad flavors and odors in nuts [49]. According to the Southern African Macadamia Growers Association (SAMAC), 1.73 and 1.69 meq O_2 kg^{-1} of the 'A4' and 'Beaumont' kernels, respectively, roasted at 150 °C had significantly ($p < 0.001$) higher PV, which is within the acceptable limit, but illustrates the vulnerability of kernels to the development of rancidity [48].

Additionally, 'A4' and 'Beaumont' kernels roasted at 125 °C exhibited considerably ($p < 0.001$) the largest concentrations of oleic acid (C18:1n9c) (751.97 and 624.92 g/g) and palmitoleic acid (C16:1) (472.96 and 340.36 g/g), respectively. This may be because some FAs are released when kernels are roasted at 125 °C, resulting in the synthesis of Maillard and caramelization browning products [18]. Oleic acid-rich oils are less likely to experience lipid oxidation [53]. 'A4' and 'Beaumont' kernels roasted at 125 °C contained significantly ($p < 0.001$) more oleic acid (C18:1n9c) (800.97 and 624.92 ug/g) and lower linoleic acid (C18:2n6c) (32.74 and 22.02 ug/g), respectively. Higher temperature during roasting can result to degradation of unsaturated fatty acids [54]. Ref. [55] observed from their study on the stability and change in fatty acids composition of several oils that oils rich in linoleic and linolenic acids are less heat-tolerant compared to those rich in oleic acid (C18:1). In their study, the oils rich in oleic acid remained relatively stable during heat treatment temperatures between 150 and 180°C [55]. Thus, this could be the case for the Oleic Acids and lower linolenic acids observed when nuts were roasted at 125 °C.

Moreover, 'A4' and 'Beaumont' kernel roasted at 125 °C are less prone to lipid oxidation and the formation of rancidity. 'A4' and 'Beaumont' kernels roasted at 125 °C had significantly ($p < 0.001$) reduced PV (1.16 and 0.95 meq O_2 kg^{-1}, respectively), proving this. These PV show that the kernels are fresh and do not taste rancid because they are within the minimal permissible level (1–3 meq O_2 kg^{-1}) [11,48].

3.4. Phenolic Concentration

Phenolic concentration was discovered to be inversely correlated with flavonoid concentration, with phenolic concentrations of 'A4' and 'Beaumont' roasted at 50 °C (0.096 and 0.143 mg GAE kg^{-1}), 75 °C (0.095 and 0.137 mg GAE kg^{-1}), 100 °C (0.089 and 0.130 mg GAE kg^{-1}), 125 °C (0.082 and 0.127 mg GAE kg^{-1}), and 150 °C (0.038 and 0.087 mg GAE kg^{-1}). The majority of phenolic chemicals, according to [56], are extremely unstable and may be lost during processing. In accordance with [44], who reported that roasting temperatures above 130 °C lead to a gradual decrease in total phenolic concentration as a result of thermal and oxidative degradation of polyphenols and intermediate products of the brown reaction, it can be seen from Figure 3 that roasting 'A4' and 'Beaumont' kernels at 150 °C further reduced phenolic concentration. In pine nuts roasted at 150 °C, Ref. [52] similarly found a comparable decline in total phenolics, which they hypothesized would be caused by heat stress-induced thermal breakdown of phenolic compounds. Additionally, Ref. [57] observed that rancidity, oxidation, and hydrolysis could all contribute to the breakdown of phenols at high roasting temperatures. This confirms our findings even more, as Figure 2 demonstrates that kernels roasted at 150 °C had high PV within the permissible range, but also suggests that these kernels are more prone to developing rancidity [24].

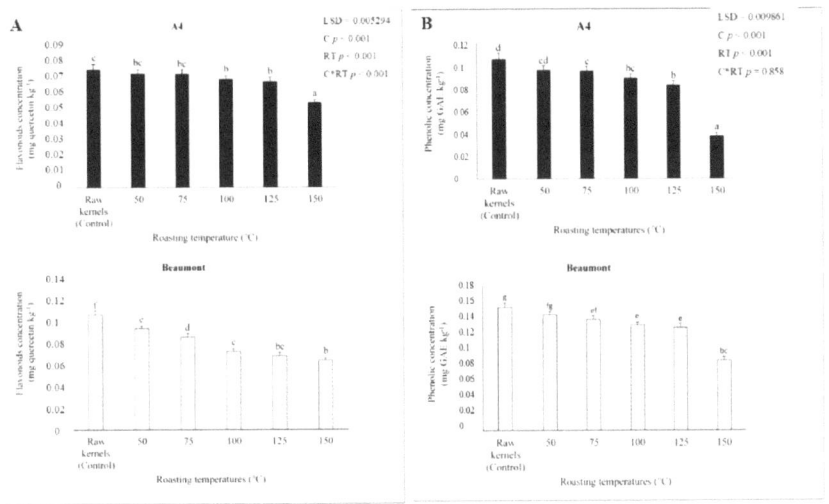

Figure 3. Flavonoid (**A**) and phenolic (**B**) concentrations of 'A4' and 'Beaumont' kernels at different roasting temperatures. Different lowercase letters (a–g) indicate significant differences ($p < 0.01$) between the different roasting temperatures.

3.5. Flavonoid Concentration

With increasing roasting temperature, the flavonoid concentrations of 'A4' and 'Beaumont' kernels decreased significantly ($p < 0.001$) (0.071 and 0.097 mg quercetin kg^{-1}, 0.071 and 0.089 mg quercetin kg^{-1}, 0.067 and 0.075 mg quercetin kg^{-1}, 0.066 and 0.071 mg quercetin kg^{-1}, and 0.053 and 0.067 mg quercetin kg^{-1}). According to [58], depending on the temperatures used to roast items, the concentration of flavonoids in food and their functional qualities may change during thermal processing [59,60]. According to [16], some antioxidants are lost during roasting as a result of chemical processes such as the Maillard browning reaction. In our study, roasting the 'A4' and 'Beaumont' kernels at 150 °C further decreased the flavonoid content (Figure 3). This may also be due to the kernels' vulnerability to rancidity after being roasted at 150 °C, as shown by their high PV levels (Figure 2), which may encourage nutritional loss and the emergence of bad flavors [61]. Given that the synthesis and polymerization of 5-hydroxymethylfurfural (HMF) are accelerated at low moisture content, the drop in flavonoid concentration at 150 °C may also be attributable to hydrolytic mechanisms. This is consistent with our findings, as Figure 1 demonstrates that the lowest moisture level was found in kernels roasted at 150 °C, which may have facilitated the loss of flavonoids during roasting. According to [62], high roasting temperatures may cause intracellular water to evaporate, resulting in significant changes in the chemical composition, including the formation of protein, amino acids, reducing sugars, sucrose, trigonelline, chlorogenic acid, and melanoidins, which are primarily caused by Maillard reactions. The loss of flavonoids could come from several chemical processes. Our results are consistent with those of [60], who found that apricot kernels roasted at 720 W (24.56 mg

CE/g DW) had lower flavonoid concentrations than those roasted at 540 W (32.41 mg CE/g DW), presumably due to heat stress.

3.6. Antioxidant Activity (DPPH (2,2'Diphenyl1-picrylhydrazyl) and ABTS (2,2'-Azinobis-3-ethylbenzothiazoline-6-sulfonic Acid) Assay)

The decrease in flavonoids and phenols was accompanied by changes in antioxidant activity (Figure 3). 'A4' and 'Beaumont' cultivars' antioxidant activity (DPPH and ABTS) significantly ($p < 0.001$) decreased with rising roasting temperature. Compared to kernels roasted at a higher temperature of 150 °C (0.003 and 0.005 ABTS mg GAE kg^{-1} and 0.001 and 0.006 DPPH mg GAE kg^{-1}, respectively), 'A4' and 'Beaumont' kernels roasted at 50 °C had a high concentration of antioxidants (0.017 and 0.017 ABTS mg GAE kg^{-1} and 0.005 and 0.007 DPPH mg GAE kg^{-1}). Ref. [63] reported a similar decrease in antioxidants in hazelnuts roasted at 180 °C, which may be due to the oxidation of phenols [64]. It is clear from Figure 4 that roasting 'A4' and 'Beaumont' kernels at 150 °C further reduced the antioxidant activity. Juhaimi et al. [60] showed that apricot kernels roasted at 720 W had decreased antioxidant activity, which may have been caused by phenolics being damaged by heat. Higher roasting temperatures, such as 160 °C, promote excessive browning in products commonly referred to as dark roast in beans and further reduce the total antioxidant activity due to oxidation, hydrolysis, decarboxylation, and other degradative chemical reactions, resulting in the degradation of the product's sensory and chemical quality, according to [65,66]. This further corroborates our observations because kernels roasted at 150 °C displayed a notable rise in PV (Figure 2).

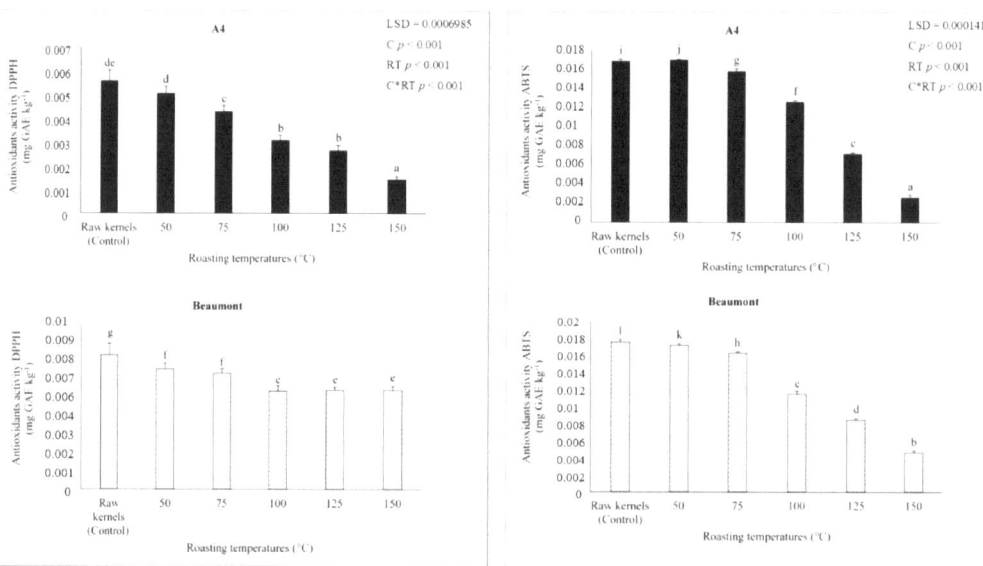

Figure 4. Antioxidant activity of 'A4' and 'Beaumont' at different roasting temperatures. Different lowercase letters (a–l) indicate significant differences ($p < 0.01$) between the different roasting temperatures.

3.7. Sensory Evaluation

3.7.1. Kernel Texture

As the roasting temperature increased, 'A4' and 'Beaumont' kernels became considerably ($p < 0.001$) more crispy, which is thought to be a fundamental property of roasted kernels [67]. This might be a result of heat permeating the kernels, which would reduce moisture content and make the kernels crispy [68]. According to [69,70], the internal microstructure of samples is altered during roasting, producing a texture that is typically more brittle, crispy, and/or crunchy. The appealing crispy texture of the roasted kernels at 125 °C won the panelists' favor. Our results are consistent with those of [71], who said that eight trained panelists preferred pistachio kernels that had been roasted at 120 °C because such kernels had the most appetizing crispy texture. According to [71–73], pistachio and soybean kernels roasted at lower temperatures (100 °C) had a hard texture that is less crispy. Figure 5A also demonstrates that kernels roasted at lower temperatures (50, 75, and 100 °C) had a hard texture. Heat stress caused unattractive excessive crispiness in 'A4' and 'Beaumont' kernels when they were roasted at 150 °C [13].

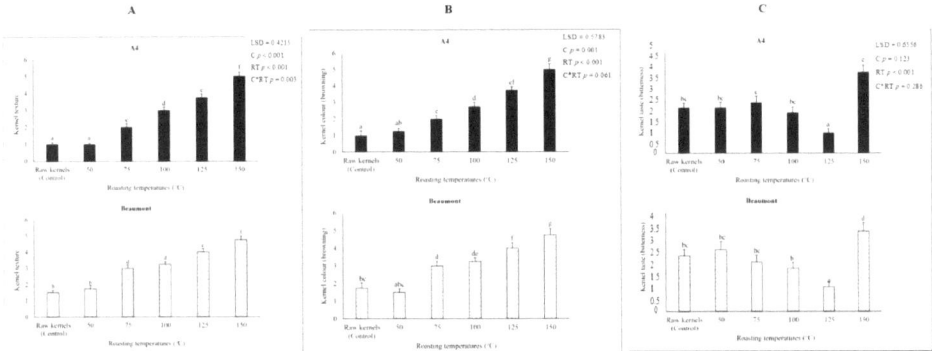

Figure 5. Kernel texture (**A**), color (**B**), and taste (**C**) of 'A4' and 'Beaumont' at different roasting temperatures. Different lowercase letters (a–g) indicate significant differences ($p < 0.01$) between the different roasting temperatures.

3.7.2. Kernel Color

Because brown pigments increase as the Maillard and caramelization reactions advance, color is one of the criteria that is employed for process control during roasting [71]. In addition, it serves as one of the most crucial characteristics of roasted nuts and a gauge of kernel flavor [67,68,74]. In our study, the panelists rated the color of the roasted kernels as poor because they had a light color, whereas roasting temperatures over 75 °C considerably ($p < 0.001$) improved the color of the kernels (Figure 5). The development of color due to pyrazines and pyridines compounds, which are recognizable products resulting from non-enzymatic browning reactions such as Maillard browning and caramelization, could be attributed to the browning of 'A4' and 'Beaumont' kernels with increasing temperatures [12,28,75]. Le Lagadec et al. [76] added that enzymatic and non-enzymatic processes that take place during roasting transform sucrose into the reducing sugars glucose and fructose. The Maillard reaction, which appears to be responsible for the browning of the kernels, is primarily made up of reducing sugars and amino acids [19]. According to our study, roasted kernels at 125 °C had the most desired brown color, whereas those at 150 °C were overly brown and therefore over-roasted [77]. Our results are consistent with those of [78], who found that roasting almond nuts over 150 °C caused the kernels to become darker in color. This darker color may be the consequence of a non-enzymatic reaction that happens when a reducing sugar and protein are cooked together [79].

3.7.3. Kernel Taste

The panelists felt that lower roasting temperatures of 50 and 75 °C lead to mildly nutty-tasting kernels, while roasting temperatures above 75 °C considerably ($p < 0.001$) improved kernel flavor (Figure 5). 'A4' and 'Beaumont' kernels roasted at 100 °C had a nutty taste, and kernels roasted at 125 °C had an extremely nutty taste, which might be related to the development of desired flavors through Maillard reactions during roasting [18,67]. According to [71], the chemical reactions that take place during roasting, such as the interaction of carbohydrates with proteins, lipids, and physiologically active compounds, result in the production of flavor and aroma. According to [17,76,80], benzaldehyde methylphenol, and alkylbenzenes are flavor and aromatic chemicals that are produced during roasting and provide nuts a more palatable, improved, and robust nutty-roasted flavor. Additionally, kernels roasted at 125 °C had the lowest PV, indicating that there were no discernible off-flavors in the kernels [11]. Although [71] showed that higher roasting temperatures (150 °C) induced an increase in bitterness in pistachio kernels, the 'A4' and 'Beaumont' kernels were assessed as being extremely bitter. High roasting temperatures cause proteins and carbohydrates to alter, lipids to oxidize, and the flavor of kernels to become bitter [71]. High roasting temperatures (>150 °C), according to [81], impairs the stability of the hazelnuts' proteins, carbohydrates, and oil. This reduces the overall palatability of the products and makes the kernels bitter. These findings are similar to those of Ref. [68], who observed that roasting peanuts at high temperatures (149 to 204 °C) caused a bitter taste because these temperatures cause the oxidation of secondary products such as aldehydes, ethanol, and ketones, which are linked to off-flavors. Additionally, kernels roasted at 150 °C had higher PV levels (Figure 2), an excessively crispy texture (Figure 5), and a dark brown color, all of which are signs of over-roasting and may lead to the development of unsavory compounds such as 5-hydroxymethylfurfural, which is linked to off-flavors or a bitter taste [18,71].

4. Conclusions

According to the results of the current study, although 'A4' and 'Beaumont' kernels roasted at low temperatures (50, 75, and 100 °C) had slightly elevated levels of flavonoids, phenols, and antioxidants, they also had higher moisture levels and FA composition, which promoted the development of rancidity, as indicated by higher levels of PV and poor kernel texture, color, and taste, as noted by trained panelists. The chemical and sensory qualities of macadamia nuts were greatly impacted by increasing roasting temperatures. 'A4' and 'Beaumont' kernels roasted at 125 °C had lower levels of rancidity (PV), high levels of oxidation-resistant FA compositions such as oleic acid, which delayed the rancidification process, and low levels of FA compositions, such as linoleic acid, which accelerated the oxidation process. Flavonoids, phenols, and antioxidants were significantly concentrated in the roasted kernels at 125 °C as well. Additionally, the judges said that roasted kernels at 125 °C had a perfectly crisp texture, a brown color, and were very nutty. However, a significant amount of rancidity; decreased content of flavonoids, phenols, and antioxidants; and an excessively crispy texture, a dark brown color, and a bitter flavor were present in kernels that were roasted at 150 °C. The results of this study, therefore, recommend roasting 'A4' and 'Beaumont' kernels at 125 °C to prevent rancidity and quality loss due to over-roasting. Additionally, because macadamia kernels quickly acquire rancidity, it is not advised to keep them fresh.

Author Contributions: Conceptualization, S.Z.T., L.S.M. and N.M.D.B.; Methodology, S.Z.T., L.S.M. and N.M.D.B.; Formal Analysis, N.M.D.B. Investigation, S.Z.T., L.S.M. and N.M.D.B.; Resources, S.Z.T. and L.S.M.; Writing—Original Draft Preparation, N.M.D.B.; Writing—Review and Editing, S.Z.T., L.S.M. and N.N.A.; Visualization, N.M.D.B. and N.N.A.; Supervision, S.Z.T., L.S.M. and A.M. All authors have read and agreed to the published version of the manuscript.

Funding: This work was funded by the National Research Foundation (NRF), South Africa, Grant number: 142060.

Institutional Review Board Statement: Not applicable.

Informed Consent Statement: Not applicable.

Data Availability Statement: Data is contained within the article.

Acknowledgments: The authors thank the National Research Foundation of South Africa for the financial support for this research project.

Conflicts of Interest: The authors declare no conflict of interest.

References

1. Eagappan, K.; Sasikumar, S. Research Article Therapeutic effects of nuts in various diseases. *Int. J. Recent Sci. Res.* **2014**, *5*, 191–192.
2. Navarro, S.L.B.; Rodrigues, C.E.C. Macadamia oil extraction methods and uses for the defatted meal byproduct. *Trends Food Sci. Technol.* **2016**, *54*, 148–154. [CrossRef]
3. Jiang, R.; Jacobs, D.R., Jr.; Mayer-Davis, E.; Szklo, M.; Herrington, D.; Jenny, N.S.; Kronmal, R.; Barr, R.G. Nut and seed consumption and inflammatory markers in the multi-ethnic study of atherosclerosis. *Am. J. Epidemiol.* **2005**, *163*, 222–231. [CrossRef] [PubMed]
4. Lovejoy, J.C. The impact of nuts on diabetes and diabetes risk. *Curr. Diab. Rep.* **2005**, *5*, 379–384. [CrossRef]
5. Rengel, A.; Pérez, E.; Piombo, G.; Ricci, J.; Servent, A.; Tapia, M.S.; Gibert, O.; Montet, D. Lipid profile and antioxidant activity of macadamia nuts (*Macadamia integrifolia*) cultivated in Venezuela. *Nat. Sci.* **2015**, *7*, 535–547.
6. Kaijser, A.; Dutta, P.; Savage, G. Oxidative stability and lipid composition of macadamia nuts grown in New Zealand. *Food Chem.* **2000**, *71*, 67–70. [CrossRef]
7. Moreno-Pérez, A.J.; Sánchez-García, A.; Salas, J.J.; Garcés, R.; Martínez-Force, E. Acyl-ACP thioesterases from macadamia (*Macadamia tetraphylla*) nuts: Cloning, characterization and their impact on oil composition. *Plant Physiol. Biochem.* **2011**, *49*, 82–87. [CrossRef]
8. Sinanoglou, V.J.; Kokkotou, K.; Fotakis, C.; Strati, I.; Proestos, C.; Zoumpoulakis, P. Monitoring the quality of γ-irradiated macadamia nuts based on lipid profile analysis and Chemometrics. Traceability models of irradiated samples. *Food Res. Int.* **2014**, *60*, 38–47. [CrossRef]
9. Oboh, G. Effect of blanching on the antioxidant properties of some tropical green leafy vegetables. *LWT-Food Sci. Technol.* **2005**, *38*, 513–517. [CrossRef]
10. Ros, E. Health benefits of nut consumption. *Nutrients* **2010**, *2*, 652–682. [CrossRef]
11. Borompichaichartkul, C.; Luengsode, K.; Chinprahast, N.; Devahastin, S. Improving quality of macadamia nut (*Macadamia integrifolia*) through the use of hybrid drying process. *J. Food Eng.* **2009**, *93*, 348–353. [CrossRef]
12. Phatanayindee, S.; Borompichaichartkul, C.; Srzednicki, G.; Craske, J.; Wootton, M. Changes of chemical and physical quality attributes of macadamia nuts during hybrid drying and processing. *Dry. Technol.* **2012**, *30*, 1870–1880. [CrossRef]
13. Nikzadeh, V.; Sedaghat, N. Physical and sensory changes in pistachio nuts as affected by roasting temperature and storage. *Am.-Eur. J. Agric. Environ. Sci.* **2008**, *4*, 478–483.
14. Shakerardekani, A.; Karim, R.; Ghazali, H.M.; Chin, N.L. Effect of roasting conditions on hardness, moisture content and colour of pistachio kernels. *Int. Food Res.* **2011**, *18*, 723–729. [CrossRef]
15. Saklar, S.; Katnas, S.; Ungan, S. Determination of optimum hazelnut roasting conditions. *Int. J. Food Sci. Technol.* **2001**, *36*, 271–281. [CrossRef]
16. McDaniel, K.A.; White, B.L.; Dean, L.L.; Sanders, T.H.; Davis, J.P. Compositional and mechanical properties of peanuts roasted to equivalent colors using different time/temperature combinations. *J. Food Sci.* **2012**, *77*, 1292–1298. [CrossRef]
17. Schlörmann, W.; Birringer, M.; Böhm, V.; Löber, K.; Jahreis, G.; Lorkowski, S.; Müller, A.K.; Schöne, F.; Glei, M. Influence of roasting conditions on health-related compounds in different nuts. *Food Chem.* **2015**, *180*, 77–85. [CrossRef]
18. Taş, N.G.; Gökmen, V. Maillard reaction and caramelization during hazelnut roasting: A multiresponse kinetic study. *Food Chem.* **2017**, *221*, 1911–1922.
19. Srichamnong, W.; Srzednicki, G. Internal discoloration of various varieties of Macadamia nuts as influenced by enzymatic browning and Maillard reaction. *Sci. Hortic.* **2015**, *192*, 180–186. [CrossRef]
20. Vázquez-Araújo, L.; Verdu, A.; Navarro, P.; Martínez-Sánchez, F.; Carbonell-Barrachina, Á.A. Changes in volatile compounds and sensory quality during toasting of Spanish almonds. *Int. J. Food Sci. Technol.* **2009**, *4*, 2225–2233. [CrossRef]
21. Vázquez-Araújo, L.; Enguix, L.; Verdú, A.; García-García, E.; Carbonell-Barrachina, A.A. Investigation of aromatic compounds in toasted almonds used for the manufacture of turrón. *Eur. Food Res. Technol.* **2008**, *227*, 243–254. [CrossRef]
22. Belviso, S.; Dal Bello, B.; Giacosa, S.; Bertolino, M.; Ghirardello, D.; Giordano, M.; Rolle, L.; Gerbi, V.; Zeppa, G. Chemical, mechanical and sensory monitoring of hot air-and infrared-roasted hazelnuts (*Corylus avellana* L.) during nine months of storage. *Food Chem.* **2017**, *217*, 398–408. [CrossRef] [PubMed]
23. Tonfack, D.F.; Selle, E.; Morfor, A.T.; Tiencheu, B.; Hako Touko, B.A.; Teboukeu Boungo, G.; Ndomou Houketchang, S.; Karuna, M.S.L.; Linder, M.; Ngoufack, F.Z. Effect of boiling and roasting on lipid quality, proximate composition, and mineral content of walnut seeds (*Tetracarpidium conophorum*) produced and commercialized in Kumba, South-West Region Cameroon. *Food Sci. Nutr.* **2018**, *6*, 417–423. [CrossRef] [PubMed]
24. Borompichaichartkul, C.; Chinprahast, N.; Devahastin, S.; Wiset, L.; Poomsa-Ad, N.; Ratchapo, T. Multistage heat pump drying of macadamia nut under modified atmosphere. *Int. Food Res. J.* **2013**, *20*, 2199–2203.
25. Süvari, M.; Sivri, G.T.; Öksüz, Ö. Effect of different roasting temperatures on acrylamide formation of some different nuts. *J. Environ. Sci. Toxicol. Food Technol.* **2017**, *4*, 38–43. [CrossRef]
26. Kita, A.; Figiel, A. Effect of roasting on properties of walnuts. *Pol. J. Food Nutr. Sci.* **2007**, *57*, 89–94.
27. Marzocchi, S.; Pasini, F.; Verardo, V.; Ciemniewska-Żytkiewicz, H.; Caboni, M.F.; Romani, S. Effects of different roasting conditions on physical-chemical properties of Polish hazelnuts (*Corylus avellana* L. var. Kataloński). *LWT-Food Sci. Technol.* **2017**, *77*, 440–448. [CrossRef]

28. Walton, D.A.; Randall, B.W.; Le Lagadec, M.D.; Wallace, H.M. Maintaining high moisture content of macadamia nuts-in-shell during storage induces brown centres in raw kernels. *J. Sci. Food Agric.* **2013**, *93*, 2953–2958. [CrossRef]
29. Walton, D.A.; Randall, B.W.; Poienou, M.; Nevenimo, T.; Moxon, J.; Wallace, H.M. Shelf life of tropical *Canarium* nut stored under ambient conditions. *Horticulturae* **2017**, *3*, 24. [CrossRef]
30. Wang, Y.; Zhang, L.; Johnson, J.; Gao, M.; Tang, J.; Powers, J.R.; Wang, S. Developing hot air-assisted radio frequency drying for in-shell macadamia nuts. *Food Bioprocess Technol.* **2014**, *7*, 278–288. [CrossRef]
31. Khir, R.; Pan, Z.; Salim, A.; Hartsough, B.R.; Mohamed, S. Moisture diffusivity of rough rice under infrared radiation drying *LWT-Food Sci. Technol.* **2011**, *44*, 1126–1132. [CrossRef]
32. Du Preez, A.B. Studies on Macadamia Nut Quality. Master's Thesis, University of Stellenbosch, Cape Town, South Africa, 2015
33. Meyer, M.D.; Terry, L.A. Development of a rapid method for the sequential extraction and subsequent quantification of fatty acids and sugars from avocado mesocarp tissue. *J. Agric. Food Chem.* **2008**, *56*, 7439–7445. [CrossRef]
34. Ling, B.; Hou, L.; Li, R.; Wang, S. Thermal treatment and storage condition effects on walnut paste quality associated with enzyme inactivation. *LWT-Food Sci. Technol.* **2014**, *59*, 786–793. [CrossRef]
35. Hertog, M.G.L.; Hollman, P.C.H.; Katan, M.B. Content of potentially anticarcinogenic flavonoids of 28 vegetables and 9 fruits commonly consumed in the Netherlands. *J. Agric. Food Chem.* **1992**, *40*, 2379–2383. [CrossRef]
36. Eghdami, A.; Sadeghi, F. Determination of total phenolic and flavonoids contents in methanolic and aqueous extract of *Achillea millefolium*. *Org. Chem. J.* **2010**, *2*, 81–84.
37. Ahmed, D.; Khan, M.M.; Saeed, R. Comparative analysis of phenolics, flavonoids, and antioxidant and antibacterial potential of methanolic, hexanic and aqueous extracts from *Adiantum caudatum* leaves. *Antioxidants* **2015**, *4*, 394–409. [CrossRef]
38. Tesfay, S.Z.; Bertling, I.; Bower, J.P. Effects of postharvest potassium silicate application on phenolics and other anti-oxidant systems aligned to avocado fruit quality. *Postharvest Biol. Technol.* **2011**, *60*, 92–99. [CrossRef]
39. Sanful, R.E. Production and sensory evaluation of tigernut beverages. *Pak. J. Nutr.* **2009**, *8*, 688–690. [CrossRef]
40. Srisawas, W.; Jindal, V.K. Sensory evaluation of cooked rice in relation to water-to-rice ratio and physicochemical properties. *J. Texture Stud.* **2007**, *38*, 21–41. [CrossRef]
41. De Angelis, D.; Kaleda, A.; Pasqualone, A.; Vaikma, H.; Tamm, M.; Tammik, M.L.; Summo, C. Physicochemical and sensory evaluation of meat analogues produced from dry-fractionated pea and oat proteins. *Foods* **2020**, *9*, 1754. [CrossRef]
42. Chen, Y.; Fu, Y.; Li, P.; Xi, H.; Zhao, W.; Wang, D.; Xie, J. Characterization of Traditional Chinese Sesame Oil by Using Headspace Solid-Phase Microextraction/Gas Chromatography–Mass Spectrometry, Electronic Nose, Sensory Evaluation, and RapidOxy. *Foods* **2020**, *11*, 3555. [CrossRef] [PubMed]
43. Hojjati, M.; Lipan, L.; Carbonell-Barrachina, A. Effect of roasting on physicochemical properties of wild Almonds (*Amygdalusscoparia*). *J. Am. Oil Chem. Soc.* **2016**, *93*, 1211–1220. [CrossRef]
44. Tenyang, N.; Ponka, R.; Tiencheu, B.; Djikeng, F.T.; Azmeera, T.; Karuna, M.S.L.; Prasad, R.B.N.; Womeni, H.M. Effects of boiling and roasting on proximate composition, lipid oxidation, fatty acid profile and mineral content of two sesame varieties commercialized and consumed in Far-North Region of Cameroon. *Food Chem.* **2017**, *221*, 1308–1316. [CrossRef]
45. Bai, S.H.; Darby, I.; Nevenimo, T.; Hannet, G.; Hannet, D.; Poienou, M.; Grant, E.; Brooks, P.; Walton, D.; Randall, B. Effects of roasting on kernel peroxide value, free fatty acid, fatty acid composition and crude protein content. *PLoS ONE* **2017**, *12*, e0184279.
46. Walton, D. Anatomy and Handling: Implications for Macadamia Nut Quality. Ph.D. Thesis, University of the Sunshine Coast, Sunshine Coast, Australia, 2005.
47. Makeri, M.U.; Bala, S.M.; Kassum, A.S. The effects of roasting temperatures on the rate of extraction and quality of locally-processed oil from two Nigerian peanut (*Arachis hypogea* L.) cultivars. *Afr. J. Food Sci.* **2011**, *5*, 194–199.
48. Canneddu, G.; Júnior, L.C.C.; Teixeira, G.H. Quality evaluation of shelled and unshelled macadamia nuts by means of near-infrared spectroscopy (NIR). *J. Food Sci.* **2016**, *81*, 1613–1621. [CrossRef]
49. Pannico, A.; Schouten, R.E.; Basile, B.; Romano, R.; Woltering, E.J.; Cirillo, C. Non-destructive detection of flawed hazelnut kernels and lipid oxidation assessment using NIR spectroscopy. *J. Food Eng.* **2015**, *160*, 42–48. [CrossRef]
50. Ghirardello, D.; Contessa, C.; Valentini, N.; Zeppa, G.; Rolle, L.; Gerbi, V.; Botta, R. Effect of storage conditions on chemical and physical characteristics of hazelnut (*Corylus avellana* L.). *Postharvest Biol. Technol.* **2013**, *81*, 37–43. [CrossRef]
51. Redondo-Cuevas, L.; Castellano, G.; Torrens, F.; Raikos, V. Revealing the relationship between vegetable oil composition and oxidative stability: A multifactorial approach. *J. Food Compos. Anal.* **2018**, *66*, 221–229. [CrossRef]
52. Cai, L.; Cao, A.; Aisikaer, G.; Ying, T. Influence of kernel roasting on bioactive components and oxidative stability of pine nut oil. *Eur. J. Lipid Sci. Technol.* **2013**, *115*, 556–563. [CrossRef]
53. Asibuo, J.Y.; Akromah, R.; Adu-Dapaah, H.K.; Safo-Kantanka, O. Evaluation of nutritional quality of groundnut (*Arachis hypogaea* L.) from ghana. *Afr. J. Food Agric. Nutr. Dev.* **2008**, *2*, 133–150. [CrossRef]
54. Cherif, A.; Slama, A. Stability and Change in Fatty Acids Composition of Soybean, Corn, and Sunflower Oils during the Heating Process. *J. Food Qual.* **2022**, *2022*, 6761029. [CrossRef]
55. Suri, K.; Singh, B.; Kaur, A.; Singh, N. Impact of roasting and extraction methods on chemical properties, oxidative stability and Maillard reaction products of peanut oils. *J. Food Sci. Technol.* **2019**, *56*, 2436–2445. [CrossRef]
56. Jinap, S.; Jamilah, B.; Nazamid, S. Sensory properties of cocoa liquor as affected by polyphenol concentration and duration of roasting. *Food Qual. Prefer.* **2004**, *15*, 403–409.

57. Kotsiou, K.; Tasioula-Margari, M. Monitoring the phenolic compounds of Greek extra-virgin olive oils during storage. *Food Chem.* **2016**, *200*, 255–262. [CrossRef]
58. Kunyanga, C.N.; Imungi, J.K.; Okoth, M.W.; Biesalski, H.K.; Vadivel, V. Flavonoid content in ethanolic extracts of selected raw and traditionally processed indigenous foods consumed by vulnerable groups of Kenya: Antioxidant and type II diabetes-related functional properties. *Int. J. Food Sci. Nutr.* **2011**, *62*, 465–473. [CrossRef]
59. Randhir, R.; Kwon, Y.I.; Shetty, K. Effect of thermal processing on phenolics, antioxidant activity and health-relevant functionality of select grain sprouts and seedlings. *Innov. Food Sci. Emerg. Technol.* **2008**, *9*, 355–364. [CrossRef]
60. Juhaimi, F.A.; Özcan, M.M.; Ghafoor, K.; Babiker, E.E. The effect of microwave roasting on bioactive compounds, antioxidant activity and fatty acid composition of apricot kernel and oils. *Food Chem.* **2018**, *243*, 414–419. [CrossRef]
61. Chutichudet, B.; Chutichudet, P. Shading application on controlling the activity of polyphenol 6 oxidase and leaf browning of grand rapids' lettuce. *Int. J. Agric. Res.* **2011**, *6*, 400–409. [CrossRef]
62. Duarte, S.M.d.S.; Abreu, C.M.P.d.; Menezes, H.C.d.; Santos, M.H.d.; Gouvêa, C.M.C.P. Effect of processing and roasting on the antioxidant activity of coffee brews. *Food Sci. Technol.* **2005**, *25*, 387–393. [CrossRef]
63. Açar, Ö.Ç.; Gökmen, V.; Pellegrini, N.; Fogliano, V. Direct evaluation of the total antioxidant capacity of raw and roasted pulses, nuts and seeds. *Eur. Food Res. Technol.* **2009**, *229*, 961–969. [CrossRef]
64. Ali, A.; Chong, C.H.; Mah, S.H.; Abdullah, L.C.; Choong, T.S.Y.; Chua, B.L. Impact of storage conditions on the stability of predominant phenolic constituents and antioxidant activity of dried Piper betle extracts. *Molecules* **2018**, *23*, 484. [CrossRef] [PubMed]
65. Votavová, L.; Voldrich, M.; Sevcik, R.; Cizkova, H.; Mlejnecka, J.; Stolar, M.; Fleisman, T. Changes of antioxidant capacity of robusta coffee during roasting. *Czech J. Food Sci.* **2009**, *27*, 49–52. [CrossRef]
66. Dybkowska, E.; Sadowska, A.; Rakowska, R.; Debowska, M.; Swiderski, F.; Swiader, K. Assessing polyphenols content and antioxidant activity in coffee beans according to origin and the degree of roasting. *Rocz. Państ. Zakł. Hig.* **2017**, *68*, 347–353.
67. Soleimanieh, S.M.; Eshaghi, M.; Vanak, Z.P. The effect of roasting method and conditions on physic chemicals and sensory properties of sunflower seed kernels. *Int. J. Biosci.* **2015**, *6*, 7–17.
68. Shi, X. Effects of Different Roasting Conditions on Peanut Quality. Ph.D. Thesis, North Carolina State University, Raleigh, NC, USA, 2015.
69. Lee, C.M.; Resurreccion, A.V.A. Predicting sensory attribute intensities and consumer acceptance of stored roasted peanuts using instrumental measurements. *J. Food Qual.* **2006**, *29*, 319–338. [CrossRef]
70. Boge, E.L.; Boylston, T.D.; Wilson, L.A. Effect of cultivar and roasting method on composition of roasted soybeans. *J. Sci. Food Agric.* **2009**, *89*, 821–826. [CrossRef]
71. Moghaddam, T.M.; Razavi, S.M.A.; Taghizadeh, M.; Sazgarnia, A. Sensory and instrumental texture assessment of roasted pistachio nut/kernel by partial least square (PLS) regression analysis: Effect of roasting conditions. *J. Food Sci. Technol.* **2016**, *53*, 370–380. [CrossRef]
72. Mridula, D.; Goyal, R.K.; Bhargav, V.K.; Manikantan, M.R. Effect of roasting on texture, colour and acceptability of soybean for making sattu. *Am. J. Food Technol.* **2007**, *2*, 265–272.
73. Jokanović, M.R.; Džinić, N.R.; Cvetković, B.R.; Grujić, S.; Odžaković, B. Changes of physical properties of coffee beans during roasting. *Acta Period. Technol.* **2012**, *43*, 21–31. [CrossRef]
74. Wang, S. Sensory and GC Profiles of Roasted Peanuts: Their Relationships to Consumer Acceptability and Changes during Short Storage. Ph.D. Thesis, University of Georgia, Athens, GA, USA, 2015.
75. Corzo-Martínez, M.; Corzo, N.; Villamiel, M.; Del Castillo, M.D. Browning reactions. *Food Biochem. Food Process.* **2012**, *4*, 56–83.
76. Le Lagadec, M.D. Kernel brown centres in macadamia: A review. *Crop Pasture Sci.* **2009**, *60*, 1117–1123. [CrossRef]
77. Borjian, B.M.; Goli, A.; Gharachourloo, M. Effect of roasted sesame oil on qualitative properties of frying oil during deep-fat frying. *J. Agric. Sci. Technol.* **2016**, *18*, 1531–1542.
78. Ng, S.; Lasekan, O.; Muhammad, K.; Sulaiman, R.; Hussain, N. Effect of roasting conditions on color development and Fourier transform infrared spectroscopy (FTIR-ATR) analysis of Malaysian-grown tropical almond nuts (*Terminalia catappa* L.). *Chem. Centr. J.* **2014**, *8*, 55. [CrossRef]
79. Kahyaoglu, T.; Kaya, S. Modeling of moisture, color and texture changes in sesame seeds during the conventional roasting. *J. Food Eng.* **2006**, *75*, 167–177. [CrossRef]
80. Xiao, L.; Lee, J.; Zhang, G.; Ebeler, S.E.; Wickramasinghe, N.; Seiber, J.; Mitchell, A.E. HS-SPME GC/MS characterization of volatiles in raw and dry-roasted almonds (*Prunus dulcis*). *Food Chem.* **2014**, *151*, 31–39. [CrossRef]
81. Özdemir, M. Mathematical Analysis of Color Changes and Chemical Parameters of Roasted Hazelnuts. Ph.D. Thesis, Istanbul Technical University, Institute of Science and Technology, Department of Food Engineering, Istanbul, Turkey, 2001.

Disclaimer/Publisher's Note: The statements, opinions and data contained in all publications are solely those of the individual author(s) and contributor(s) and not of MDPI and/or the editor(s). MDPI and/or the editor(s) disclaim responsibility for any injury to people or property resulting from any ideas, methods, instructions or products referred to in the content.

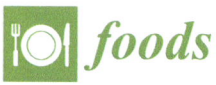

Article

Quality Improvement of Garlic Paste by Whey Protein Isolate Combined with High Hydrostatic Pressure Treatment

Baoyuan Zang, Zhichang Qiu, Zhenjia Zheng, Bin Zhang *,† and Xuguang Qiao †

Key Laboratory of Food Processing Technology and Quality Control of Shandong Higher Education Institutes, College of Food Science and Engineering, Shandong Agricultural University, 61 Daizong Street, Tai'an 271018, China; xgqiao@sdau.edu.cn (X.Q.)
* Correspondence: zbin@sdau.edu.cn
† These authors contributed equally to this work.

Abstract: Garlic, one of the most popular spices and medical herbs, has a unique pungent flavor and taste. Conventional homogenization and thermal treatment commonly lead to flavor and color deterioration in garlic paste, because allicin is highly susceptible to degradation and reaction. The present study was to investigate the effects of whey protein isolate (WPI) and different levels of high hydrostatic pressure (HHP, 200, 300, 400, 500, and 600 MPa) on the quality of garlic paste Results showed that the addition of WPI in the homogenization of garlic significantly prevented green discoloration. Furthermore, WPI plus HHP under 500 MPa could better protect the color of garlic paste. Higher pressure (600 MPa) led to WPI aggregation, resulting in higher green color chroma of garlic paste. GC-MS results revealed that the application of WPI and HHP in garlic paste increased the relative level of pungent flavor compounds and decreased those of unpleasant odor compounds. The correlation analysis results revealed that WPI efficiently prevented garlic green discoloration, which is attributed to the thiol group in WPI exchanging the sulfonyl groups in allicin In consideration of the microbial load, flavor and color quality of garlic paste, the optimal processing conditions were found at 500 MPa for 5 min with 2% WPI addition, extending shelf life to 25 days.

Keywords: whey protein isolate; high hydrostatic pressure; garlic paste; green discoloration; volatile compounds

Citation: Zang, B.; Qiu, Z.; Zheng, Z.; Zhang, B.; Qiao, X. Quality Improvement of Garlic Paste by Whey Protein Isolate Combined with High Hydrostatic Pressure Treatment. *Foods* **2023**, *12*, 1500. https://doi.org/10.3390/foods12071500

Academic Editors: Antonio José Pérez-López and Luis Noguera-Artiaga

Received: 7 February 2023
Revised: 27 March 2023
Accepted: 27 March 2023
Published: 3 April 2023

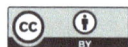

Copyright: © 2023 by the authors. Licensee MDPI, Basel, Switzerland. This article is an open access article distributed under the terms and conditions of the Creative Commons Attribution (CC BY) license (https://creativecommons.org/licenses/by/4.0/).

1. Introduction

Garlic (*Allium sativum* L.) contains abundant nutritional components (e.g., polysaccharides, proteins, lipids and organosulfur compounds) and has been widely used as a seasoning or herbal medicine around the world [1,2]. Previous studies have shown that the typical flavor of fresh garlic and numerous bioactive activities of garlic are mainly attributed to the organosulfur compounds [3]. Among them, allicin is the predominant constituent of organosulfur compounds (accounting for 70–80%) and, therefore, can be used as an indicator of the quality of garlic products [4]. However, allicin is unstable and easily decomposes into other, secondary sulfur-containing components, leading to flavor deterioration. In minced, crushed, sliced, pureed, or other mechanical disruption of garlic, intensely green pigments are often formed during processing, which represents the discoloration from a cream white to green color [5]. Allicin also plays a key role in garlic green discoloration. These problems of flavor deterioration and green discoloration greatly limit the development and consumption of processed garlic products [6].

In order to improve the stability of flavor and inhibit the discoloration of garlic products, some measures have been applied to garlic processing, such as blanching and the addition of chemical additives, which are applied to the intact garlic to kill alliinase [7]. Although the garlic products treated with thermal processing and pH adjustment can maintain good appearance, their pungent flavor and biological activities are completely lost [8,9]. Compared with thermal processing, high hydrostatic pressure (HHP) treatment minimized this effect on the physicochemical properties and biological activities of garlic products, but green discoloration still occurred [10,11]. The conjugation of allicin and cysteine was reported to enhance the stability of allicin, which was beneficial to its antioxidant and anticancer activities [12–14]. This is mainly due to the exchange of the thiol group in cysteine with the sulfonyl groups in allicin to produce stable disulfide bonds. However, the amount of cysteine is strictly limited as a food additive. For example, the maximum addition in flour-based foods must be less than 0.06 g/kg [15]. The excessive addition of cysteine may pose considerable risks in food. Considering that the reaction of thiol groups and sulfonyl groups can occur between allicin and proteins with free sulfonyl groups, proteins have high potential to stabilize allicin. Jiang et al. [15] reported that ultrasound-assisted binding of allicin and whey protein isolates exhibited better stability and emulsification. Huang et al. [16] found that allicin–soy protein isolate conjugates not only caused structural changes in the protein, but also increased the thermal stability and antioxidant activity of allicin. Therefore, it is of interest to investigate the effect of natural protein isolates on the quality of garlic products. Previous studies generally focused on the physiochemical properties and bioactivity of allicin–protein conjugates. To our knowledge, there are no studies that have reported the application of proteins in garlic products.

Whey protein isolate (WPI) is recognized as a high-quality animal protein because of its high digestion/absorption properties and great nutritional value [17]. In this study, the effect of WPI addition and HHP treatment on microbial load, color characteristics and allicin content in garlic paste were investigated. The results were used to prevent flavor deterioration and green discoloration of garlic paste. The flavor profiles of HPP-WPI treated garlic paste were evaluated by solid-phase microextraction-gas chromatography-mass spectrometry (SPME-GC-MS). The results revealed the interaction effects of WPI and HHP treatment on garlic quality and provided a valuable strategy for the improvement and quality control of garlic products.

2. Materials and Methods

2.1. Materials and Reagents

Garlic was purchased from Laiwu (Shandong, China). Diallyl disulfide (>98% purity, HPLC grade) was obtained from Sigma-Aldrich Co., Ltd. (Shanghai, China). Ascorbic acid (>99% purity) was purchased from Hualan Chemical Technology Co., Ltd. (Shanghai, China). Whey protein isolate (90% purity) was obtained from Maclin Co., Ltd. (Shanghai, China). Acetonitrile and methanol (HPLC grade) were purchased from Yuwang Chemical Co., Ltd. (Dezhou, China). All other chemicals were of analytical grade.

2.2. Preparation of Garlic Paste

The garlic paste was prepared according to the procedure of Jiang et al. [15], with some modifications. Briefly, a 2% WPI solution was sonicated (40 kHz, 25 W/L) at 60 °C for 15 min to increase the exposure of sulfhydryl groups. Then, peeled garlic was homogenized with 2% WPI (1:2, m/v) to obtain garlic paste. The pH of garlic paste was adjusted to 4.0 with 0.04 g/mL ascorbic acid solution. The final concentration of ascorbic acid in garlic paste was about 2.50 mg/g. The resulting garlic paste was packed (50 g for each pouch) and sealed, followed by HPP treatment at 200–600 MPa for 5–25 min (operated at 25 °C) to investigate its effect on the quality of the garlic paste. The HHP equipment (Bao Tou KeFa High Pressure Technology Co., Ltd., Baotou Inner Mongolia, China) was equipped with a reservoir volume of 3 L, and the pressure generated within the chamber was automatically adjusted by a digital computer. The garlic paste was freshly prepared using purified water to homogenize (pH 5.77), then treated with pH adjustment and HHP according to the above procedure to obtain the original garlic paste (GP) and HHP-GP.

2.3. Microbiological Analysis

As described in a previous report [6], 15 g garlic paste was homogenized with 135 mL sterile saline (8.5 g/L NaCl). The obtained sample was serially diluted 10-fold with sterile saline. Subsequently, 0.5 mL of diluent was fully mixed with 20 mL plate count agar medium in a sterile Petri dish and incubated upside-down at 36 °C for 48 h. The colony count was calculated and expressed as Log CFU/g.

2.4. Color Index Analysis

The color index of garlic paste was evaluated using a CR-10 Plus colorimeter (Kefeng Instrument Co., Ltd., Baoding, Hebei, China). The different garlic paste products were placed in Petri dishes for 6 h and directly measured at 25 °C. The L* value represents lightness, a* the degree of red (a* > 0) or green (a* < 0), and b* the degree of yellow (b* > 0) or blue (b* < 0). Saturation (chroma, C*) is used to represent the purity of the color, and color difference (ΔE) is used to represent the overall color change. C* and ΔE were calculated according to the following formulas:

$$C^* = \sqrt{a^{*2} + b^{*2}} \quad (1)$$

$$\Delta E^* = \sqrt{(\Delta L^*)^2 + (\Delta a^*)^2 + (\Delta b^*)^2} \quad (2)$$

where ΔL*, Δa* and Δb* indicates the color difference between the color indices of the processed garlic paste and the original garlic paste.

2.5. Allicin Content Analysis

The extraction and analysis of allicin was carried out according to Zhang et al. [18], as based on Tocmo's method [19]. Briefly, an equal volume (*v/w*) of n-hexane was added to 10.0 g garlic paste to extract allicin (3 times). The organic phases were combined and concentrated using an air stream at 25 °C. The final residue was dissolved in 60% methanol, filtered, and analyzed using high performance liquid chromatography (HPLC). Allicin content analysis was performed on a Shimadzu LC-20AT system (Kyoto, Japan) equipped with an InertSustain C18 (4.6 × 9 × 250 mm, 5 μm) column. The mobile phase was acetonitrile: water: methanol (50:41:9), and the flow rate was at 1.0 mL/min. To accurately determine allicin content, allicin external standards were synthesized and isolated according to our previous report [18].

2.6. Analysis of Free Sulfhydryl (SH) Content

The SH content was determined according to Ayim et al. [20] with some modification. Briefly, garlic paste was diluted with distilled water (1:5, *m/v*) to obtain garlic extract. Next, 0.5 mL garlic extract was mixed with 5 mL Tris-Gly buffer, then 20 μL Ellman's reagent was added. The final mixture was reacted at 25 °C for 30 min. After that, the absorbance was measured at 412 nm using a spectrophotometer (BioTek Instruments, Charlotte, VT, USA). A blank group was prepared using buffer instead of garlic extract. The SH group contents were calculated using Equation (3) [15]:

$$C_{SH} \text{ (μmol/g)} = (73.53 \times \Delta A_{412} \times D)/C \quad (3)$$

where D represents dilution coefficient, C represents the protein concentration in garlic extract (mg/mL), and ΔA_{412} is the differential between the treatment group and original garlic paste.

2.7. Analysis of Volatile Components

2.7.1. Extraction of Volatile Components

Briefly, 2.0 g garlic paste was exactly weighed and transferred into a 10 mL headspace vial, followed by air-tight sealing with a Teflon-coated rubber septum and an aluminum cap. A 75 μm DVB/CAR/PDMS SPME fiber was first conditioned at 250 °C for 3 min. Then, headspace extraction of the volatile compounds was carried out with the SPME fiber at 50 °C for 30 min. After that, the SPME fiber was immediately transferred to the inlet of GC, and volatile components were desorbed at 250 °C for 10 min.

2.7.2. GC-MS Analysis

GC-MS analysis was conducted following the method of Chen et al. [21] with some modifications on a Shimadzu TQ8030 GC–MS (Shimadzu Co., Ltd., Kyoto, Japan) coupled with an Agilent DB-5MS column (30.0 m × 0.25 mm i.d., 0.25 µm, Agilent Technologies, Santa Clara, CA). The oven temperature was initially held at 50 °C for 4 min, then increased to 65 °C (increase rate, 1 °C/min), 75 °C (increase rate, 10 °C/min), 90 °C (increase rate, 1 °C/min), 210 °C (increase rate, 3°C/min), and finally heated to 280 °C at a rate of 10 °C/min and held for 10 min. High-purity helium (99.99%) was used as the carrier gas at a fixed flow of 1.0 mL/min (split ratio, 1:30). The MS conditions were as follows: injector temperature of 280°C, ion source temperature of 230 °C, ionization voltage of 70 eV, scanning range of 30–450 m/z. The volatile compounds were identified using the NIST 11 mass spectrometry library. The characteristic flavor compounds in garlic (including diallyl sulfides and vinyl-dithiins) were identified by external standards prepared by our laboratory [18] and commercially available standards. The peak normalization method was used for calculating the relative abundance of each compound in the garlic paste.

2.8. Microbiological Stability

Garlic paste after processing (HHP-WP) was stored at 25 °C and 4 °C to determine its microbiological stability during storage. The colony count analysis was as described in Section 2.3. The SGompertz growth equation was used to describe microbial behavior and predict the shelf life of HHP-WP. The SGompertz model equation is derived from the Gompertz model, calculated using Equation (4):

$$\left[Log\left(\frac{Nt}{N0}\right)\right] = a \times \exp\{-\exp[-k(t-M)]\} \tag{4}$$

where N_t and N_0 represent the colony count on day t and day 0, respectively; a represents the logarithmic value of the total number of bacterial colonies as time increases. K represents the relative maximum growth rate; and M represents the time required to obtain the maximum growth rate [22].

2.9. Statistical Analysis

The results were expressed as mean values ± standard deviation, analyzed using SPSS 26.0 (IBM Corporation, Armonk, NY, USA). One-way analysis of variance (ANOVA) and Duncan's test ($p < 0.05$) were used to evaluate the statistical differences. All treatments were determined independently in triplicate.

3. Results

3.1. Effects of WPI and HHP Treatments on Microbial Load of Garlic Paste

Figure 1 shows the effect of HHP pressure and time on the total number of microbial colonies. The total number of colonies in the original garlic paste was 3.88 ± 0.22 Log (CFU/g), which was similar to that of the garlic paste supplemented with WPI (WP) ($p > 0.05$). This indicated that there was no significant effect on the microbial load of the garlic paste due to the addition of WPI. As shown in Figure 1A, the number of colonies showed a significant ($p < 0.05$) decrease as the HHP pressure was increased from 0 MPa to 500 MPa and held for 5 min. Further increases in HHP pressure only resulted in a slight decrease in the number of colonies ($p > 0.05$). The response of microbial load to HHP time followed a similar trend with HHP pressure (Figure 1B). The most effective treatment for microbial inactivation was achieved at 500 MPa for 25 min, with a total number of colonies of 2.47 ± 0.02 Log CFU/g. At a longer HHP times (>5 min), the decrease in the number of colonies was slower, which might have been due to the fact that pressure was not uniformly transmitted throughout the garlic paste [23]. In order to obtain the limited microbial index (3.70 Log CFU/g), the garlic paste was treated by HHP at 500 MPa for at least 5 min.

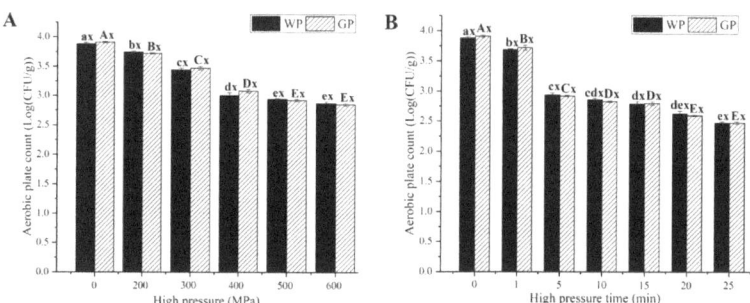

Figure 1. Effect of (**A**) HHP treatment and (**B**) pressure holding time at 500 MPa on microbial inactivation. "a–e" and "A–E" mean within WP and GP group, respectively, while different letters indicate a significant difference ($p < 0.05$). "x" means there was no significant difference ($p \geq 0.05$) between WP and GP under the same HHP condition.

3.2. Effects of WPI and HHP Treatments on Color Appearance

The color parameters and appearance of original and processed garlic paste were measured after incubating at 25 °C for 6 h (Figure 2). Freshly homogenized garlic paste was cream white. In Figure 2, the original garlic paste shows an a^* value of -7.4 ± 0.14 and C^* value of 38.20 ± 0.24, with a vivid green color by visual observation (Figure 2F). In comparison, the a^* value of WP was significantly increased to -1.37 ± 0.25 ($p < 0.05$) and appeared as a bright white appearance, which suggested that the treatment with WPI could effectively inhibit the greening of garlic paste. As the HHP pressure increased, the L^*, a^* and ΔE values of GP showed an increasing trend, while the b^* and C^* values gradually decreased, with significant differences between most of the different treatment groups ($p < 0.05$). As described in previous studies, the green discoloration began with a vivid green color, then the green color faded and turned to green-yellow [5,11]. Therefore, the above result indicated that HHP treatment effectively accelerated the green discoloration. Although the color parameters of WP had variation characteristics similar to those of GP at different HHP pressures, it usually had significantly lower b^*, C^* and ΔE values. Significantly higher L^* and a^* values were also observed at the same pressure between WP and GP (except for ΔE values at 500 MPa) ($p < 0.05$). Notably, the a^* value of WP was only -2.3 ± 0.13, considering that the a^* value had a higher chromaticity property that affected the color appearance [24]. The large visual difference in appearance can be seen in Figure 2F. These results indicate that WPI combined with HHP treatment can maintain the color of original garlic paste without storage. At 500 MPa, WP obtained the lowest a^* and C^* values and highest L^* values, presenting the whitest appearance (Figure 2F). The decrease in green color and increase in brightness could be attributed to the inactivation of polyphenol oxidase at 200–500 MPa [25]. Notably, further increases in HHP pressure led to an increase in chromaticity (C^*), which might have been caused by the occurrence of WPI aggregation at 600 MPa [26].

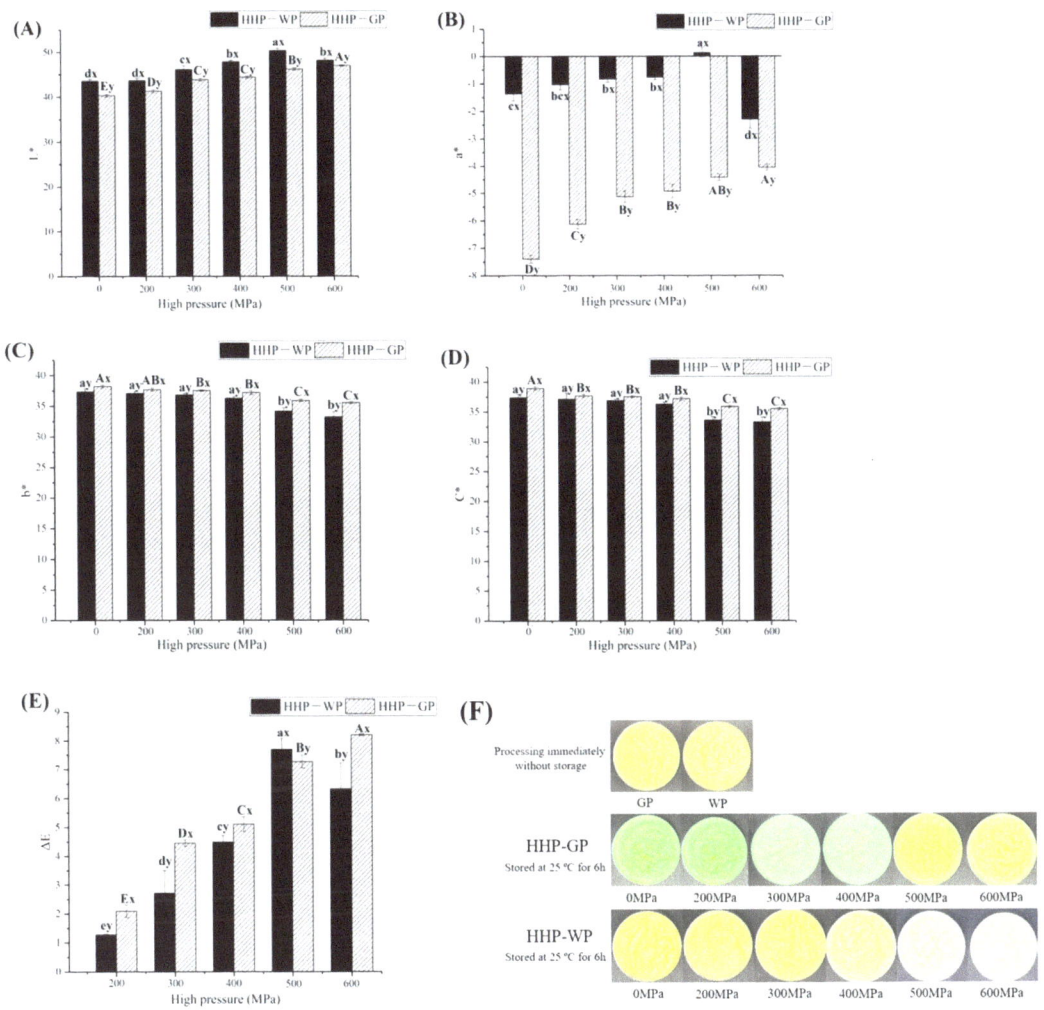

Figure 2. Effect of HHP treatment on garlic paste color indexes and appearances. (**A**) L*, (**B**) a*, (**C**) b*, (**D**) color chroma, C*, (**E**) total color difference, ΔE, (**F**) color appearance "a–e" and "A–E" mean within HHP-WP and HHP-GP group, respectively, while different letters indicate a significant difference ($p < 0.05$). "x-y" with different letters indicates a significant difference ($p \geq 0.05$) between HHP-WP and HHP-GP under the same HHP conditions.

As shown in Figure 3, for WP and GP treated with 500 MPa held for different treatment durations, the color parameters and visual appearance of garlic paste were monitored after incubating at 25 °C for 6 h. As the treatment time increased, the L*, a* and ΔE of WP and GP showed an increasing trend. Contrarily, both b* and C* decreased in WP and GP. For WP, the highest L* and a* values appeared at 20 min, and extending the processing time to 25 min resulted in a decrease in a* and C*, corresponding to light green color appearance in HHP-WP at 25 min (Figure 3F). This result suggests that HPP processing time above 25 min at 500 MPa might lead to the aggregation of WPI and be detrimental to the maintenance of the color of WP.

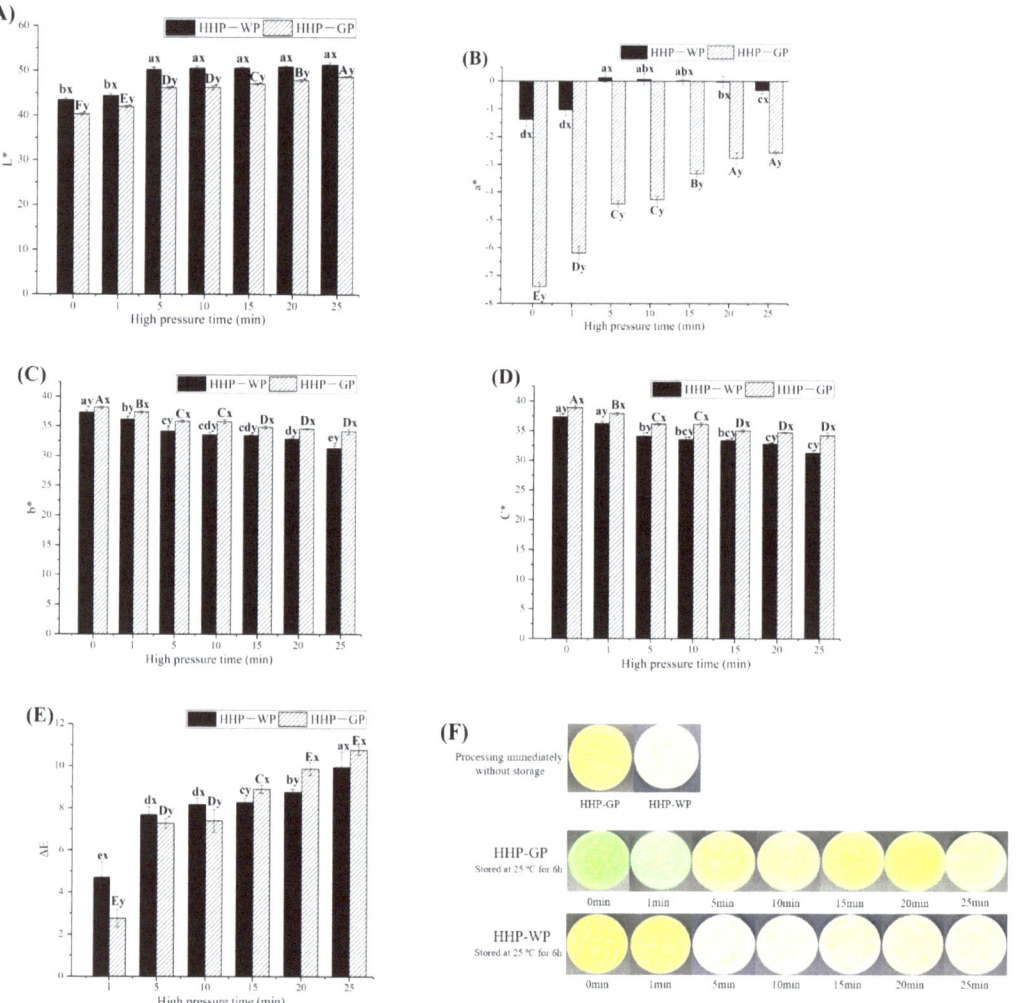

Figure 3. Effect of HHP time on garlic paste color indexes and appearances. (**A**) L*, (**B**) a*, (**C**) b*, (**D**) color chroma, C*, (**E**) total color difference, ΔE, (**F**) color appearance. "a–e" and "A–E" mean within HHP-WP and HHP-GP group, respectively, while different letters indicate a significant difference ($p < 0.05$). "x-y" with different letters indicates a significant difference ($p \geq 0.05$) between HHP-WP and HHP-GP under the same HHP conditions.

3.3. Effects of WPI and HHP Treatments on Allicin Content and Thiol Groups

The effects of WPI combined with different HHP levels on the content of allicin and free thiol (SH) groups are shown in Figure 4A. As shown in Figure 4A, in raw garlic, the allicin content was 3.41 ± 0.13 mg g^{-1}. After treating with WPI, the allicin content was sharply reduced, to 0.94 ± 0.12 mg g^{-1}. This result indicated that allicin reacted with the thiol groups in WPI [15]. With the increase in pressure, the allicin content in HHP-GP decreased continuously from 3.41–2.19 mg g^{-1}, whereas the SH groups increased continuously from 0.33–0.43 μmol g^{-1} (Figure 4A). It could be explained that HHP promotes green discoloration, in which allicin participated [11,27], and the increase in thiol groups was attributed to the ability of allicin to cleave disulfide under high pressure [28]. In HHP-WP, the minimal allicin content of 0.35 mg g^{-1} was achieved at 500 MPa, with a maximal SH content of 1.3 µmol g^{-1}. Carullo et al. [26] reported that 200–400 MPa HHP treatment contributed to trigger partial unfolding of WPI, resulting in unmasking of buried thiol groups. More severe HHP treatment (600 MPa) is commonly accompanied by the occurrence of protein aggregation, which leads to a decrease in free thiol groups [25,29]. Therefore, more allicin was used to bind WPI at 200–500 MPa, decreasing allicin content. In addition, the increase in allicin at 600 MPa might due to the reversibility of allicin binding to the residues, which was in agreement with allyl isothiocyanate binding β-lactoglobulin [30].

The changes in allicin content and thiol groups in HHP-WP under 500 MPa over processing time are shown in Figure 4B. With increasing HHP processing time, the allicin content decreased first, then increased, and the SH content showed a contrary trend of change. This indicated that longer processing time at 500 MPa also leads to WPI aggregation. The higher allicin content was achieved at 5, 10, and 15 min, corresponding 1.30, 1.32, and 1.32 mg g^{-1}, respectively, showing no significant difference ($p > 0.05$).

Based on the above results for microbial inactivation, color appearance and allicin content, additional investigations on the influence of WPI combined with HHP treatment on the flavor compounds in garlic paste, in comparison with untreated and only WPI treated samples, were performed, setting HHP parameters at 500 MPa for 5 min.

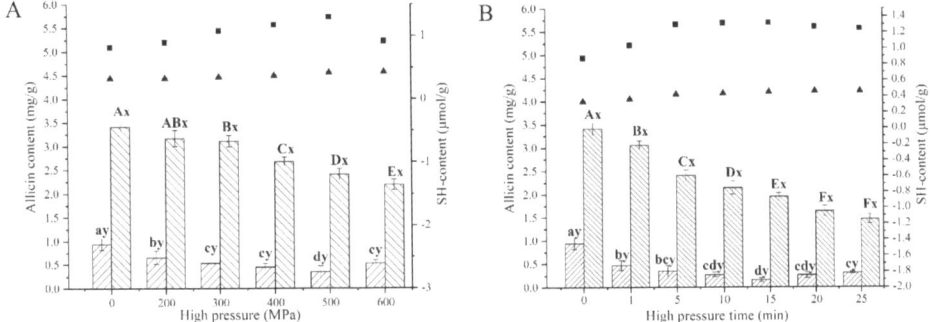

Figure 4. Effect of (**A**) HHP and (**B**) pressure holding time at 500 MPa on the contents of allicin and thiol groups. ▨ represents allicin content in HHP-WP; ▧ represents allicin content in HHP-GP; ■ represents the content of SH groups in HHP-WP; ▲ presents the content of SH groups in HHP-GP. "a–d" and "A–F" mean within HHP-WP and HHP-GP group, respectively, while different letters indicate a significant difference ($p < 0.05$). "x-y" with different letters indicates a significant difference ($p \geq 0.05$) between HHP-WP and HHP-GP under the same HHP conditions.

3.4. Effects of WPI and HHP Treatments on Flavor Compounds

SPME–GC–MS was conducted to study the influence of WPI and HHP treatments on the sensory aroma of garlic paste. A total of 38 compounds were identified in original garlic paste, as described in our previous report [6], and 41 components were observed in the WP. After HHP treatment, another new component was generated in HHP-WP. Moreover, the signal intensities of individual compounds among three samples showed significant differences, indicating that the aroma compounds were increased, decreased, or generated due to addition of WPI and HHP treatment.

As shown in Table 1, in original garlic paste, the highest relatively abundant volatile flavor component was diallyl disulfide (DADS, 19.36%), followed by diallyl trisulfide (DATS, 16.57%), 3-Vinyl-3,4-dihydro-1,2-dithiin (3-VDT, 11.45%), and 2-Vinyl-2,4-dihydro-1,3-Dithiin (2-VDT, 8.60%). Our results were in agreement with those of Ferioli et al. [31]. These organosulfur compounds were related to the typical garlic scent, garlic pungency and odor, as reported by previous studies [6,19,32]. Those predominant volatile compounds, linear polysulfides (DADS and DATS), have strong volatilities with a pungent smell [33]. It was reported that 2-VDT and 3-VDT were the major transformation products of allicin in GC analysis [19]. The dominant volatile compounds in WP and HHP-WP were similar to those in original garlic paste; however, the relative proportions showed significant differences. In WP and HHP-WP, DADS was increased to 23.50% and 28.91%, respectively. This result indicated that WPI combined with HHP treatment could maintain, even increase, the pungent smell of garlic. The 2-VDT and 3-VDT continuously decreased to 4.17% and 5.96%, respectively, after WPI combined with HHP treatment, which corresponded to a decrease in allicin.

The application of WPI combined with HHP treatment resulted in a significant decrease ($p < 0.05$) in methallyl disulfide, and a relative decrease in methallyl sulfide. These compounds were commonly recognized as breath metabolites of allicin with unpleasant smell [34]. Moreover, cyclotrisiloxane hexamethyl was observed in WP and HHP-WP and identified as the main bioactive compound in Dillenia scabrella leaves [35]. Additionally, 2,4-dimethyl-thiophene (0.244%) was generated during HHP treatment. Several thiophenes were identified in pyrolysis bio-oils, which were cyclic structures generated through free radical reactions by smaller sulfur compounds [36], recognized as the most stable sulfur-containing compounds. Thus, it is not surprising that the dimethyl thiophene were determined under high HHP.

In summary, WPI combined with HHP treatment increased the levels of the predominant volatile aroma components and decreased unpleasant odor. Additionally, the presence of four new compounds gave HHP-WP a richer and balanced odor.

Table 1. Changes in flavor compounds after WPI and HHP treatment.

Volatile	Relative Abundance (%)			Feature
	GP	WP	HHP-WP	
Diallyl disulfide	19.36	23.50	28.91	Pungency
Diallyl sulfide	1.19	1.13	0.69	Pungency
2-Vinyl-2,4-dihydro-1,3-Dithiin	8.60	5.57	4.17	Garlic scent
3-Vinyl-3,4-dihydro-1,2-dithiin	11.45	7.48	5.96	Garlic scent
Diallyl trisulfide	16.57	15.86	15.25	Pungency
Methallyl disulfide	1.27	0.21	0.19	Unpleasant smell
Diallyl tetrasulfide	0.82	0.67	0.71	Pungency
Methallyl sulfide	2.18	1.22	1.13	Unpleasant smell
2-Vinyl-2,4-dihydro-1,3-dithiin	0.16	0.13	0.14	-
1,3-Ditjiane	0.30	0.53	0.59	-
1,1'-Thiobis-1-propene	5.17	4.32	3.76	-
2-Mercapto-3,4-dimethyl-2,3-dihydrothiophene	0.36	1.00	1.02	-
(Z)-1-(Methylthio)-1-propene	0.25	0.19	0.18	-
2,4-Dimethyl-5,6-dithia-2,7-nonadienal	2.23	1.34	1.05	-
1,3-Benzenedithiol	0.25	0.15	0.13	-
1,2-Dithiolane	0.20	ND	ND	-
1-Propyl-2-(4-thiohept-2-en-5-yl)disulfide	ND	0.13	0.14	-
Cyclotrisiloxane, hexamethyl-	ND	0.89	0.73	-
Methyl allylthioacetate	ND	0.12	0.13	-
Thiophene,2,4-dimethyl-	ND	ND	0.24	-

ND: not detected.

3.5. Changes in the Microbial Count of Garlic Paste during Storage

The total number of colonies in freshly homogenized garlic paste was 3.91 ± 0.23 Log CFU/g, and 2.94 ± 0.17 Log CFU/g in garlic paste after WPI-HHP (500 MPa, 5 min) treatment. As shown in Figure 5, the total number of colonies presented a rising trend during storage at 4 °C and 25 °C. The total number of colonies increased to 3.62 ± 0.22 Log CFU/g at 25 °C on day 8, and increased to Log 3.80 ± 0.19 CFU/g after further storage (day 10), resulting in exceeding the limit level (3.70 Log CFU/g). However, under storage at 4 °C, the total number of colonies reached 3.49 ± 0.14 Log CFU/g at day 18. The SGompertz equation was used for fitting the growth of colonies. The SGompertz growth model parameters were $Y = 1.0928 \times \exp\{-\exp[-0.3014 \times (t - 5.4513)]\}$, $R^2 = 0.9947$ (25 °C), and $Y = 0.8601 \times \exp\{-\exp[-0.1592 \times (t - 12.9969)]\}$ $R^2 = 0.9980$ (4 °C). According to the equation, the garlic paste could be stored at 4 °C for 25 days. Therefore, our results indicated that HHP contributed to product preservation.

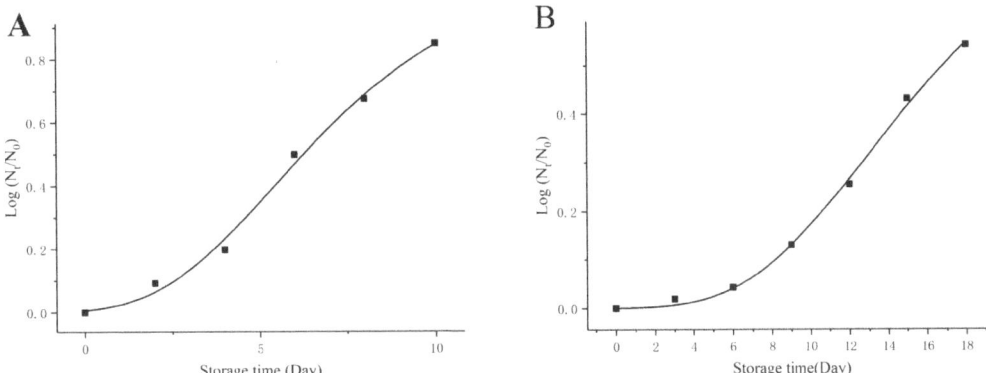

Figure 5. Changes in the number of colonies in HHP-WP during storage at 25 °C (**A**) and 4 °C (**B**). The scatter plots represent the number of colonies at different times, and the curve represents the fitting of the SGompertz model.

3.6. The Relationship between Color Indexes and Quality-Related Attributes

As shown in Figure 6, the color indexes and quality-related attributes of garlic paste after WPI and HHP treatment were analyzed using Pearson significant correlation analysis. For L* and a*, strong positive correlations were only obtained with DADS and thiol. In addition, it could be seen that allicin showed a strong negative correlation with thiol groups and DADS, while showing a positive correlation with 2-VDT, 3-VDT and methyl disulfide. DADS represented the decomposition level of allicin, and thiol groups were increased with WPI addition and unfolding. From these results, it can be assumed that the control of garlic green discoloration in the presence of WPI is attributed to the exchange of thiol groups with sulfonyl groups in allicin. Moreover, the chroma (C*) index showed a strong positive correlation with allicin content. Allicin played a vital role in green color generation in garlic paste, which was in agreement with previous studies [5,37]. Microorganism counts were positively correlated with methallyl disulfide, which indicated that HPP inactivated microorganisms and decreased the unpleasant odor with WPI unfolding in HPP treatment. Therefore, the WPI-HHP treatment was considered as a potential preservation method, facilitating the inactivation of microorganisms and obtaining a balanced aroma.

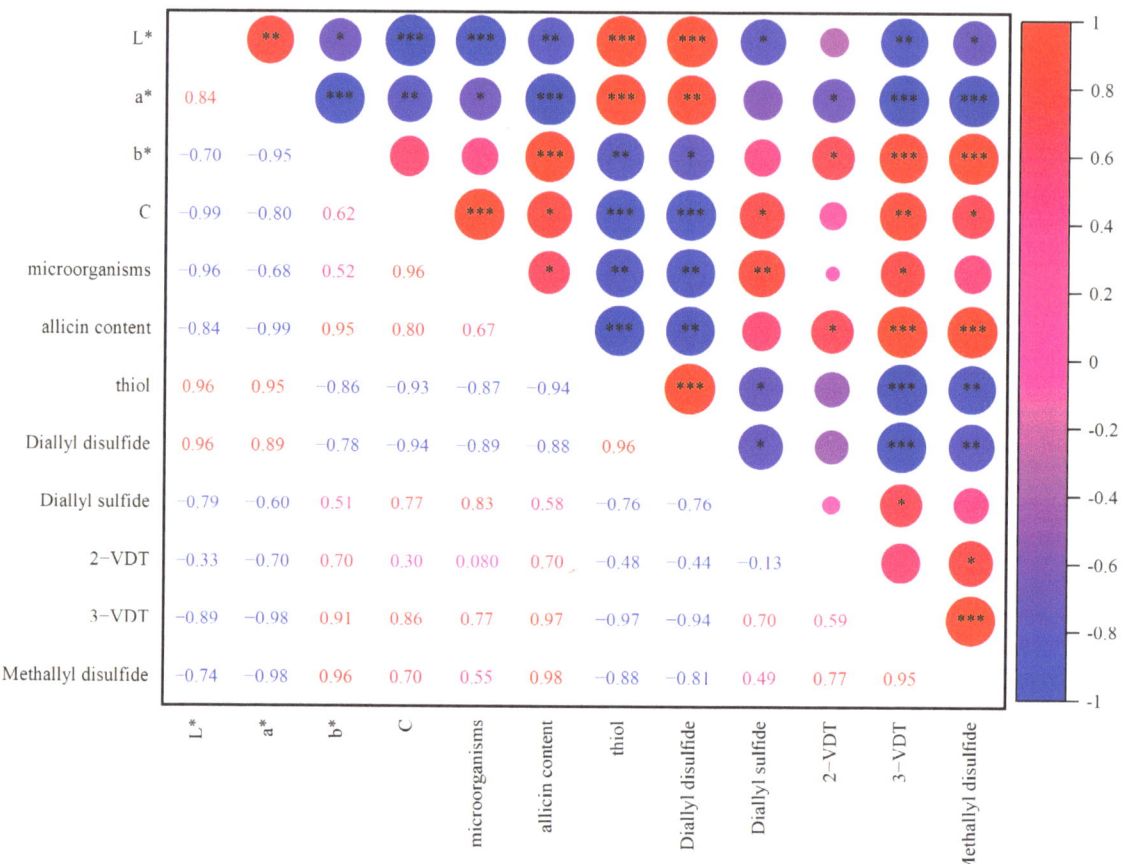

Figure 6. Correlation analysis of color indexes and quality-related attributes. * indicates $0.01 < p \leq 0.05$, ** indicates $0.001 < p \leq 0.01$, *** indicates $p \leq 0.001$, respectively.

4. Conclusions

The effects of WPI addition and HHP processing on the microbial inactivation, color parameters, bioactive compounds and volatile aroma profiles of garlic paste, as well as the storage stability, were investigated. Noticeable green discoloration was observed in original garlic paste when HHP processing was employed, corresponding with the changes in L*, a*, b*, and Chroma (C*). In contrast, the addition of WPI to garlic paste (WP) significantly inhibited the garlic's green discoloration. Further, the application HHP at 500 MPa to WP better preserved the color quality. In consideration of microbial inactivation, color appearance and allicin content of garlic paste, the optimal treatment was as follows: addition of 2% WPI, with HPP parameters of 500 MPa for 5 min. The shelf life of garlic paste with WPI-HHP treatment extended to 25 days. Moreover, GC-MS results revealed that WPI combined with HHP treatment could increase the relative level of the predominant volatile aroma component (diallyl disulfide), while reducing that of unpleasant odor components (methallyl sulfides). It is speculated that WPI reacts with allicin to prevent green discoloration through thiol groups in WPI. The results revealed that WPI combined with HHP treatment show advantages in maintaining garlic paste color quality and the sensory volatile aroma, which provide an important scientific basis for the development of the garlic industry.

Author Contributions: Conceptualization, Z.Z.; Data curation, B.Z. (Baoyuan Zang), Z.Q. and Z.Z.; Funding acquisition, X.Q.; Investigation, B.Z. (Baoyuan Zang) and Z.Q.; Project administration, B.Z. (Bin Zhang); Software, Z.Q.; Supervision, B.Z. (Bin Zhang) and X.Q.; Writing—original draft, B.Z. (Baoyuan Zang); Writing—review and editing, Z.Q., Z.Z., B.Z. (Bin Zhang) and X.Q. All authors have read and agreed to the published version of the manuscript.

Funding: This work was supported by the Special Fund for Leading Talent in Mount Tai of Shandong Province (No. tscy 20200121).

Data Availability Statement: All related data and methods are presented in this paper. Additional inquiries should be addressed to the corresponding author.

Conflicts of Interest: The authors declare no conflict of interest.

References

1. Qiu, Z.; Zheng, Z.; Zhang, B.; Sun-Waterhouse, D.; Qiao, X. Formation, nutritional value, and enhancement of characteristic components in black garlic: A review for maximizing the goodness to humans. *Compr. Rev. Food Sci. Food Saf.* **2020**, *19*, 801–834. [CrossRef]
2. Feng, Y.; Xu, B.; Yagoub, A.E.A.; Ma, H.; Sun, Y.; Xu, X.; Yu, X.; Zhou, C. Role of drying techniques on physical, rehydration, flavor, bioactive compounds and antioxidant characteristics of garlic. *Food Chem.* **2021**, *343*, 128404. [CrossRef] [PubMed]
3. Putnik, P.; Gabrić, D.; Roohinejad, S.; Barba, F.J.; Granato, D.; Mallikarjunan, K.; Lorenzo, J.M.; Kovačević, D.B. An overview of organosulfur compounds from *Allium* spp.: From processing and preservation to evaluation of their bioavailability, antimicrobial, and anti-inflammatory properties. *Food Chem.* **2019**, *276*, 680–691. [CrossRef] [PubMed]
4. Ramirez, D.A.; Locatelli, D.A.; González, R.E.; Cavagnaro, P.F.; Camargo, A.B. Analytical methods for bioactive sulfur compounds in *Allium*: An integrated review and future directions. *J. Food Compos. Anal.* **2017**, *61*, 4–19. [CrossRef]
5. Kubec, R.; Curko, P.; Urajova, P.; Rubert, J.; Hajšlová, J. *Allium* discoloration: Color compounds formed during greening of processed garlic. *J. Agric. Food Chem.* **2017**, *65*, 10615–10620. [CrossRef]
6. Qiu, Z.; Zhang, M.; Li, L.; Zhang, B.; Qiao, Y.; Zheng, Z. Effect of blend oil on the volatile aroma profile and storage quality of garlic paste. *Food Chem.* **2022**, *371*, 131160. [CrossRef]
7. Zhang, B.; Qiu, Z.; Zhao, R.; Zheng, Z.; Lu, X.; Qiao, X. Effect of blanching and freezing on the physical properties, bioactive compounds, and microstructure of garlic (*Allium sativum* L.). *J. Food Sci.* **2021**, *86*, 31–39. [CrossRef] [PubMed]
8. Ahmed, J.; Shivhare, U. Thermal kinetics of color change, rheology, and storage characteristics of garlic puree/paste. *J. Food Sci.* **2001**, *66*, 754–757. [CrossRef]
9. Zang, J.; Wang, D.; Zhao, G. Mechanism of discoloration in processed garlic and onion. *Trends Food Sci. Technol.* **2013**, *30*, 162–173. [CrossRef]
10. Kim, K.W.; Kim, Y.-T.; Kim, M.; Noh, B.-S.; Choi, W.-S. Effect of high hydrostatic pressure (HHP) treatment on flavor, physicochemical properties and biological functionalities of garlic. *LWT-Food Sci. Technol.* **2014**, *55*, 347–354. [CrossRef]
11. Hong, S.I.; Kim, D.M. Storage quality of chopped garlic as influenced by organic acids and high-pressure treatment. *J. Sci. Food Agric.* **2001**, *81*, 397–403. [CrossRef]
12. Lee, Y. Induction of apoptosis by S-allylmercapto-L-cysteine, a biotransformed garlic derivative, on a human gastric cancer cell line. *Int. J. Mol. Med.* **2008**, *21*, 765–770. [CrossRef] [PubMed]
13. Liang, D.; Qin, Y.; Zhao, W.; Zhai, X.; Guo, Z.; Wang, R.; Tong, L.; Lin, L.; Chen, H.; Wong, Y.-C. S-allylmercaptocysteine effectively inhibits the proliferation of colorectal cancer cells under in vitro and in vivo conditions. *Cancer Lett.* **2011**, *310*, 69–76. [CrossRef]
14. Zhang, G.; Parkin, K.L. A tissue homogenate method to prepare gram-scale *Allium* thiosulfinates and their disulfide conjugates with cysteine and glutathione. *J. Agric. Food Chem.* **2013**, *61*, 3030–3038. [CrossRef] [PubMed]
15. Jiang, H.; Xing, Z.; Wang, Y.; Zhang, Z.; Mintah, B.K.; Dabbour, M.; Li, Y.; He, R.; Huang, L.; Ma, H. Preparation of allicin-whey protein isolate conjugates: Allicin extraction by water, conjugates' ultrasound-assisted binding and its stability, solubility and emulsibility analysis. *Ultrason. Sonochem.* **2020**, *63*, 104981. [CrossRef] [PubMed]
16. Huang, L.; Jia, S.; Wu, R.; Chen, Y.; Ding, S.; Dai, C.; He, R. The structure, antioxidant and antibacterial properties of thiol-modified soy protein isolate induced by allicin. *Food Chem.* **2022**, *396*, 133713. [CrossRef]
17. Abd El-Salam, M.H.; El-Shibiny, S. Glycation of whey proteins: Technological and nutritional implications. *Int. J. Biol. Macromol.* **2018**, *112*, 83–92. [CrossRef]
18. Zhang, B.; Zheng, Z.; Liu, N.; Liu, P.; Qiu, Z.; Qiao, X. Effect of different combined mechanical and thermal treatments on the quality characteristics of garlic paste. *J. Food Sci. Technol.* **2021**, *58*, 1061–1071. [CrossRef]
19. Tocmo, R.; Wu, Y.; Liang, D.; Fogliano, V.; Huang, D. Boiling enriches the linear polysulfides and the hydrogen sulfide-releasing activity of garlic. *Food Chem.* **2017**, *221*, 1867–1873. [CrossRef]
20. Ayim, I.; Ma, H.; Alenyorege, E.A.; Ali, Z.; Donkor, P.O.; Zhou, C. Integration of ultrasonic treatment in biorefinery of tea residue: Protein structural characteristics and functionality, and the generation of by-products. *J. Food Meas. Charact.* **2018**, *12*, 2695–2707. [CrossRef]

21. Chen, X.; Chen, H.; Xiao, J.; Liu, J.; Tang, N.; Zhou, A. Variations of volatile flavour compounds in finger citron (*Citrus medica* L. var. *sarcodactylis*) pickling process revealed by E-nose, HS-SPME-GC-MS and HS-GC-IMS. *Food Res. Int.* **2020**, *138*, 109717. [CrossRef] [PubMed]
22. Gil, M.M.; Miller, F.A.; Brandao, T.R.; Silva, C.L. On the use of the Gompertz model to predict microbial thermal inactivation under isothermal and non-isothermal conditions. *Food Eng. Rev.* **2011**, *3*, 17–25. [CrossRef]
23. Zuluaga, C.; Martínez, A.; Fernández, J.; López-Baldó, J.; Quiles, A.; Rodrigo, D. Effect of high pressure processing on carotenoid and phenolic compounds, antioxidant capacity, and microbial counts of bee-pollen paste and bee-pollen-based beverage. *Innov. Food Sci. Emerg. Technol.* **2016**, *37*, 10–17. [CrossRef]
24. Sun, L.-C.; Sridhar, K.; Tsai, P.-J.; Chou, C.-S. Effect of traditional thermal and high-pressure processing (HPP) methods on the color stability and antioxidant capacities of Djulis (*Chenopodium formosanum* Koidz.). *LWT* **2019**, *109*, 342–349. [CrossRef]
25. Queiroz, C.; Lopes, M.L.M.; Da Silva, A.J.R.; Fialho, E.; Valente-Mesquita, V.L. Effect of high hydrostatic pressure and storage in fresh-cut cashew apple: Changes in phenolic profile and polyphenol oxidase activity. *J. Food Process. Preserv.* **2021**, *45*, e15857 [CrossRef]
26. Carullo, D.; Barbosa-Cánovas, G.; Ferrari, G. Changes of structural and techno-functional properties of high hydrostatic pressure (HHP) treated whey protein isolate over refrigerated storage. *LWT* **2021**, *137*, 110436. [CrossRef]
27. Zhang, Y.; Zielinska, M.; Vidyarthi, S.K.; Zhao, J.-H.; Pei, Y.-P.; Li, G.; Zheng, Z.-A.; Wu, M.; Gao, Z.-J.; Xiao, H.-W. Pulsed pressure pickling enhances acetic acid transfer, thiosulfinates degradation, color and ultrastructure changes of "Laba" garlic. *Innov. Food Sci. Emerg. Technol.* **2020**, *65*, 102438. [CrossRef]
28. Huang, L.; Qu, L.; Jia, S.; Ding, S.; Zhao, J.; Li, F. The interaction of allicin with bovine serum albumin and its influence on the structure of protein. *Process Biochem.* **2022**, *112*, 139–144. [CrossRef]
29. Li, H.; Zhu, K.; Zhou, H.; Peng, W. Effects of high hydrostatic pressure treatment on allergenicity and structural properties of soybean protein isolate for infant formula. *Food Chem.* **2012**, *132*, 808–814. [CrossRef]
30. Rade-Kukic, K.; Schmitt, C.; Rawel, H.M. Formation of conjugates between β-lactoglobulin and allyl isothiocyanate: Effect on protein heat aggregation, foaming and emulsifying properties. *Food Hydrocoll.* **2011**, *25*, 694–706. [CrossRef]
31. Ferioli, F.; Giambanelli, E.; D'Antuono, L.F. Comparison of Two Extraction Techniques (SDE vs. SPME) for the Determination of Garlic and Elephant Garlic Volatile Compounds. *Food Anal. Methods* **2022**, *15*, 1867–1879. [CrossRef]
32. Molina-Calle, M.; Priego-Capote, F.; de Castro, M.D.L. Headspace−GC−MS volatile profile of black garlic vs fresh garlic: Evolution along fermentation and behavior under heating. *LWT* **2017**, *80*, 98–105. [CrossRef]
33. Ferioli, F.; Giambanelli, E.; D'Alessandro, V.; D'Antuono, L.F. Comparison of two extraction methods (high pressure extraction vs. maceration) for the total and relative amount of hydrophilic and lipophilic organosulfur compounds in garlic cloves and stems. An application to the Italian ecotype "Aglio Rosso di Sulmona"(Sulmona Red Garlic). *Food Chem.* **2020**, *312*, 126086.
34. Mengers, H.G.; Schier, C.; Zimmermann, M.; Gruhlke, M.C.; Block, E.; Blank, L.M.; Slusarenko, A.J. Seeing the smell of garlic: Detection of gas phase volatiles from crushed garlic (*Allium sativum*), onion (*Allium cepa*), ramsons (*Allium ursinum*) and human garlic breath using SESI-Orbitrap MS. *Food Chem.* **2022**, *397*, 133804. [CrossRef] [PubMed]
35. Momin, K.; Thomas, S. GC-MS analysis of antioxidant compounds present in different extracts of an endemic plant *Dillenia scabrella* (dilleniaceae) leaves and barks. *Int. J. Pharm. Sci. Res* **2020**, *11*, 2262–2273.
36. Auersvald, M.; Kejla, L.; Eschenbacher, A.; Thi, H.D.; Van Geem, K.M.; Šimáček, P. Detailed characterization of sulfur compounds in fast pyrolysis bio-oils using GC × GC-SCD and GC–MS. *J. Anal. Appl. Pyrolysis* **2021**, *159*, 105288. [CrossRef]
37. Zhao, R.; Zhang, B.; Sun, J.; Zheng, Z.; Qiao, X. Evaluation of degradation of pigments formed during garlic discoloration in different pH. *Food Res. Int.* **2021**, *140*, 109957. [CrossRef] [PubMed]

Disclaimer/Publisher's Note: The statements, opinions and data contained in all publications are solely those of the individual author(s) and contributor(s) and not of MDPI and/or the editor(s). MDPI and/or the editor(s) disclaim responsibility for any injury to people or property resulting from any ideas, methods, instructions or products referred to in the content.

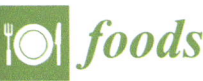

Article

Effects of Novel Preparation Technology on Flavor of Vegetable-Soy Sauce Compound Condiment

Tiantian Tang [1,2], Min Zhang [1,3,*] and Bhesh Bhandari [4]

[1] State Key Laboratory of Food Science and Technology, Jiangnan University, Wuxi 214122, China
[2] International Joint Laboratory on Food Safety, Jiangnan University, Wuxi 214122, China
[3] Jiangsu Province International Joint Laboratory on Fresh Food Smart Processing and Quality Monitoring, Jiangnan University, Wuxi 214122, China
[4] School of Agriculture and Food Sciences, University of Queensland, Brisbane, QLD 4072, Australia
* Correspondence: min@jiangnan.edu.cn; Tel./Fax: +86-510-85877225

Abstract: Vegetables contain important bioactive substances which have unique tastes and aromas and provide beneficial effects to human health. In this study, multiflavor blended soy sauce was prepared with the juice of eight kinds of vegetables, dried shrimp boiled stock, and six kinds of commercial soy sauce as raw materials, and thermal ultrasound was used as the sterilization method. The effects of adding different formulas of vegetable and seafood stock on the basic physical and chemical parameters, nutrition, antioxidant activity, flavor, and taste of soy sauce were investigated. The results showed that the basic physicochemical indices such as pH, total acid, color, soluble solids, and amino acid nitrogen of the product with a ratio of soy sauce to vegetable-seafood stock of 1:0.5 (v/v) could meet the production standards of soy sauce, and its flavor, taste, and sensory scores were relatively good, with the highest likeability (overall acceptability). The mixed soy sauce with a ratio of 1:2 (v/v) had higher vegetable and seafood flavors, and different vegetable flavors (celery, carrot, and onion) were more obvious, but its nutritional index was relatively low. Multiflavor vegetable-soy sauce can be used for quick cooking by chefs of catering enterprises, and may be used as a seasoning bag for prefabricated dishes and convenient foods, attracting increasing attention from manufacturers and consumers.

Keywords: vegetables; soy sauce; seafood; flavor; condiments

1. Introduction

Soy sauce is a condiment made from soybean, wheat, or corn and other grains using solid-state fermentation (koji) and brine fermentation (moromi). It has a strong umami taste and a very unique aroma [1] and is often used in Eastern and Western cuisines for dipping or stir frying, such as sushi, sashimi, fried noodles, salad, and various meat dishes. It can enhance the overall saltiness of various dishes, giving color and aroma to food, and is becoming more and more popular worldwide [2,3]. Flavor is a crucial attribute of soy sauce and is gradually becoming a key factor determining consumer acceptance and preference. It has been reported that nearly 300 different volatile compounds have been identified in soy sauce [4,5]. The formation of aroma compounds in traditional soy sauce is generally related to its key processing stages, including the cooking of raw materials, koji culture, moromi fermentation, and pasteurization.

In recent years, a variety of flavors of soy sauce have been developed, such as steamed fish soy sauce, seafood soy sauce, shiitake mushroom soy sauce, oak mushroom soy sauce, *Hericium erinaceus* fermented soy sauce, iron-fortified soy sauce, etc. It is worth noting that some vegetable soy sauce is attracting the attention of various condiment manufacturers and consumers. Although no relevant research articles have been reported so far, some patents have been published. Seong and Woong [6] proposed a kind of *Allium hookeri* soy sauce, in which the addition of *Allium hookeri* improved the storage performance and antioxidant effect of the soy sauce. Gong [7] reported a kind of fruit and vegetable health-care soy sauce. The preselected fruits and vegetables were washed, chopped, mixed with various spices, and boiled with water, followed by mixing with fermented soy sauce raw juice for thermal treatment to obtain the fruit and vegetable health soy sauce. Ok [8] added beef broth, fruit juice (brewed from apples and jujubes), and vegetable juice (brewed from garlic, kelp, onion, ginseng, and ginger) into soy sauce to produce a soy sauce mixture. Soo et al. [9] reported a unique-flavor soy sauce containing vegetables such as mustard, broccoli, cabbage, and Chinese cabbage. Ma [10] provided a processing method of *Toona sinensis* soy sauce. Ground *Toona sinensis* was added to soy to make a slurry, which was soaked in a closed container for more than 2 h, and finally, the soy sauce with a strong *Toona sinensis* flavor was filtered out. In addition, there are herb soy sauce [11], mustard soy sauce [12], *Rosmarinus officinalis* health-care soy sauce [13], and other soy sauce related products that have been patented. US condiment brand OhSaucy has launched a vegetable soy sauce, which can be used as an alternative to traditional soy sauce. Its main ingredients are brewing soy sauce, kelp concentrate, anchovy concentrate, fructo-oligosaccharides, mixed-vegetable concentrate, apple concentrate, pear concentrate, yeast extract, and water. On the basis of brewing soy sauce, seafood and the concentrated juice of vegetables and fruits are added, which not only reduces the salinity to the maximum, conforming to the healthy lifestyle of salt reduction, but also greatly improves the taste after cooking.

Soy sauce is an essential condiment for catering enterprises and chefs. Different soy sauces may have different tastes, and chefs may waste time using various soy sauces in the cooking process. In addition, the excessive use of soy sauce will make the color of the dishes dark brown or more salty, losing the original fragrance of the dishes. Therefore, according to the real demand of catering enterprises, this study aims to prepare a kind of multiflavor vegetable-soy sauce compound condiment suitable for fast cooking or convenient fast food. At the same time, the influence of adding vegetable juice on the nutritional ingredients and flavor of soy sauce is explored.

2. Materials and Methods

2.1. Materials and Reagents

Seafood soy sauce (Haitian), jinbiao soy sauce (Haitian), steamed fish soy sauce (Lee Kum Kee), spicy fresh dew (Knorr), fresh shellfish sauce (Totole), Maggi fresh (Nestle), celery, carrot, onion, green onion, red pepper, ginger, garlic, coriander, dried shrimps, dried shitake mushrooms, and rock sugar were purchased from local supermarkets in Wuxi, China. Food-grade ascorbic acid and potassium sorbate were purchased from Henan Wanbang Industrial Co., Ltd. (Zhengzhou, China). The juicer was purchased from Midea Group Co., Ltd. (Foshan, China).

Methanol (chromatographically pure) and acetonitrile (chromatographically pure) were purchased from Tedia Co., Ltd. (Fairfield, Ohio, USA). Tetrahydrofuran, triethylamine, hydrochloric acid, crystalline sodium acetate, and trichloroacetic acid were of analytical grade, and water was Millipore ultrapure water. Seventeen amino acid standards, including alanine (Ala), arginine (Arg), glycine (Gly), glutamic acid (Glu), aspartic acid (Asp), methionine (Met), serine (Ser), histidine (His), leucine (Leu), phenylalanine (Phe), isoleucine (Iso), cysteine (Cys), tyrosine (Tyr), lysine (Lys), threonine (Thr), valine (Val), and proline (Pro), were purchased from Sigma-Aldrich (Shanghai) Trading Co., Ltd. (Shanghai, China).

2.2. Preparation of Vegetable-Soy Sauce Compound Condiment

Seafood soy sauce, jinbiao soy sauce, steamed fish soy sauce, spicy fresh dew, fresh shellfish sauce, and Maggi fresh were mixed according to the volume ratio of 12:4:1:1:1:1 (v/v), and used as soy sauce mixed juice for later use. The celery, carrot, onion, green onion, red pepper, ginger, garlic, and coriander were mixed and squeezed according to the weight ratio of 15:1:5:1:1:1:1:1, 5:15:1:1:1:1:1:1, and 1:5:15:1:1:1:1:1 (w/w), respectively. After that, the mixed-vegetable juice was filtered through a 150-mesh sieve. A centrifuge (TG16-WS, Hunan Xiangyi Laboratory Instrument Development Co., Ltd., Changsha, China) was used to collect supernatant at 9000 rpm for 10 min. The three mixed-vegetable juices were, respectively, recorded as celery-flavored, carrot-flavored, and onion-flavored vegetable juices according to the highest added amount of vegetables. Amounts of 0.05% (w/w) ascorbic acid and 0.05% (w/w) potassium sorbate were added by weight of the vegetable juice. Dried shrimps (50 g), dried shiitake mushrooms (25 g), rock sugar (15 g), and distilled water (500 mL) were mixed and boiled for 10 min (about 200 mL of water remained). Above boiled juice was then diluted to 500 mL with distilled water. The juices were filtered through a 150-mesh sieve and centrifuged (9000 rpm, 15 min), and the supernatant was taken as seafood stock for later use. The vegetable juices with the three flavors were mixed with the seafood stock in a ratio of 1:1 (v/v) to obtain the mixed vegetable-seafood juice.

The soy sauce mixed juice and mixed vegetable-seafood liquid were mixed in a ratio of 1:0.5 and 1:2 (v/v), and centrifuged (9000 rpm, 10 min), and the supernatant was treated with thermal ultrasound at 100 kHz, 70 °C for 20 min. According to the ratio of soy sauce and 3 kinds of mixed vegetables and seafood stock (v/v), the final product was recorded as 1:0.5 (celery), 1:0.5 (carrot), 1:0.5 (onion), 1:2 (celery), 1:2 (carrot), and 1:2 (onion), and marked as CE1, CA1, ON1, CE2, CA2, and ON2, respectively. The samples mixed with soy sauce and distilled water at ratios of 1:0 (no addition), 1:0.5, and 1:2 (v/v) were used as blank controls and denoted as S, W1, and W2, respectively.

2.3. Analysis of Basic Physical and Chemical Parameters for Vegetable-Soy Sauce Compound Condiment

The colors of S, W1, CE1, CA1, ON1, W2, CE2, CA2, and ON2 soy sauce samples were determined using a colorimeter (CR-400, Konica Minolta Co., Osaka, Japan). Colors were represented by CIE a^*, b^*, and L^* values, which represent redness/greenness, yellowness/blueness, and brightness, respectively. The pH of each soy sauce sample was determined using a pH meter (pHS-3C acidity meter; Shanghai Precision Science Instrument Co., Ltd., Shanghai, China). The total soluble solids (TSS) content was determined by a hand-held refractometer (Aipli Co., Hangzhou, China), expressed as °Brix. The total acid content of soy sauce was determined with alkaline titration. A 20 mL appropriately diluted sample was titrated to pH 8.2 with 0.1 N NaOH, and the result was reported as lactic acid content (g/100 mL). Salt content (NaCl, g/100 mL) was assessed by volumetric titration with $AgNO_3$ using the Mohr's method [14]. The salt content (dried at 105 °C to constant weight) was subtracted from the total solid content to give a non-salt soluble solid (g/100 mL). The amino acid nitrogen (AAN) in soy sauce was measured using the colorimetric method according to Chinese national standard GB 5009.235-2016. In sodium acetate-acetic acid buffer pH 4.8, amino acid nitrogen reacted with acetylacetone and formaldehyde to generate yellow 3,5-diacetic acid-2,6-dimethyl-1,4-dihydropyridine amino acid derivative. The absorbance was determined at a wavelength of 400 nm and quantified compared to the standard series.

2.4. Determination of Free Amino Acids

The determination of free amino acid content was slightly modified according to the method of Wu et al. [15] and Zheng et al. [16]. Sample pretreatment: 12.5 mL of 10% trichloroacetic acid (10 g/100 mL) was added to 1 mL of soy sauce (its weight was accurately recorded) and allowed to stand for 1 h. After that, the volume was fixed to 25 mL with distilled water. After mixing, the sample solution (1 mL) was transferred to a 1.5 mL centrifuge tube and centrifuged (15,000 rpm, 30 min). The supernatant was filtered with a 0.22 µm aqueous membrane and placed in a liquid-phase sample bottle.

HPLC analysis: Agilentl 100 HPLC system (Agilent Technologies Co. Ltd. (Palo Alto, CA, USA), including VWD detector (G1314A), autosampler (G1313A), quaternary pump (G1311A), and online degasser (G1322A). Mobile Phase A (pH 7.2): triethylamine, tetrahydrofuran, and 27.6 mmo/L sodium acetate (volume ratio 0.11:2.5:500). Mobile Phase B (pH 7.2): acetonitrile, methanol, and 80.9 mmol/L sodium acetate (volume ratio 2:2:1). Agilent Hypersil ODS column (5 µm, 4.0 mm × 250 mm). Gradient elution was performed with the following procedure: 0.0 min, 8% B; 17.0 min, 50% B; 20.1 min, 100% B; and 24.0 min, 0% B.

The column temperature was 40 °C, and the mobile phase flow rate was 1.0 mL/min. The ultraviolet detector detection wavelength was 338 nm, and the proline detection wavelength was 262 nm. The external standard method was used for the quantification of amino acid content.

2.5. Determination of Total Phenolic and Flavonoid Content and Antioxidant Capacity

The total phenolic content of soy sauce was measured according to the Folin-Ciocalteu method reported by Li et al. [17]. Briefly, a 150-fold dilution of soy sauce (1 mL) was mixed with Folin phenol (1 mL) and reacted for 3 min, followed by the addition of 3 mL of sodium carbonate (75 g/L) and incubation in the dark for 90 min at room temperature. The absorbance was measured at 760 nm using a spectrophotometer (UV2600, TECHCOMP, China). The measurement results are based on the calibration curve of gallic acid, expressed as milligrams of gallic acid equivalent (GAE) per milliliter of soy sauce (mg GAE/mL). The total flavonoid was measured with the colorimetric method [18]. Briefly, 1 mL of soy sauce sample was added to 4 mL of distilled water and 0.3 mL of sodium nitrite solution (5%, w/v). After 5 min, 0.3 mL of aluminum chloride (10%, w/v) was added. After 6 min, 2 mL of NaOH (1 mol/L) was added and the volume was adjusted to 10 mL with distilled water. The absorbance was measured at 510 nm using a spectrophotometer. The results were calculated based on the standard curve of rutin, expressed as milligrams of rutin equivalent (RE) per milligram of soy sauce (mg RE/mL).

The DPPH radical scavenging activity of soy sauce was determined using the method reported by Shi et al. [19]. The diluted soy sauce sample was mixed with the DPPH solution and reacted at room temperature in the dark for 30 min, and the absorbance measurement wavelength was 517 nm. The scavenging activity of ABTS radicals was determined according to the method described by Qiu et al. [20]. ABTS radical reserve solution was prepared by mixing ABTS aqueous solution with potassium persulfate solution in equal amounts and leaving it to stand in the dark at room temperature for 12 h. The diluted soy sauce sample was mixed with ABTS radical reserve solution, and then reacted in the dark at room temperature for 15 min, and the absorbance was measured at a wavelength of 734 nm.

2.6. Electronic Nose Analysis

The flavor of each soy sauce product was analyzed with an electronic nose (iNose, Isenso, Ruifen Trading Co., Shanghai, China). Table 1 shows the responsive compounds corresponding to the 18 sensor array systems of the electronic nose. Soy sauce (4 mL) was placed in a glass bottle specifically designed for electronic nose testing and allowed to stand for 2 h under a seal to enrich the sufficient flavor compounds, following the method of Zhang et al. [21] with slight modifications. The sensor was cleaned and calibrated with an air flow rate of 1 L·min^{-1} for more than 50 min before the start of the experiment. Each sample had the same measurement time of 60 s, sensor wash time of 120 s, and air flow rate of 1 L min^{-1}. At the end of the experiment, the sensor was cleaned for more than 30 min.

Table 1. Response substances and substance categories corresponding to the sensor [22].

Sensor	Response Substance	Substance Category
S1	Alkanes and smog	Propane, natural gas, and smog
S2	Alcohols, aldehydes, and short-chain alkanes	Alcohol, smog, isobutane, and formaldehyde
S3	Ozone	—
S4	Sulfides	Hydrogen sulfide
S5	Organic amines	Ammonia, methylamine, and ethanolamine
S6	Organic gases, phenylketones, aldehydes, and aromatic compounds	Toluene, acetone, ethanol, hydrogen, and other organic vapors
S7	Short-chain alkanes	Methane, natural gas, and methane
S8	Short-chain alkanes	Propane and liquefied gas
S9	Aromatic compounds and aldehydes	Toluene, formaldehyde, benzene, alcohol, and acetone
S10	Hydrogen-containing gases	Hydrogen

Table 1. Cont.

Sensor	Response Substance	Substance Category
S11	Alkanes and olefin	Liquefied gas, alkane, and alkene
S12	Short-chain alkanes	Liquefied gas and methane
S13	Combustible gases	Methane
S14	Flammable gas	Flammable gas and smoke
S15	Alkane and organic gas	Smoke, isobutane, organic acid esters, and aliphatic hydrocarbons
S16	Sulfides	Sulfur compounds
S17	Nitrides	Nitrogen oxides
S18	Ketone and alcohol	Acetone, ethanol, and organic solvent

2.7. Electronic Tongue Analysis

According to the description of Zheng et al. [23] and Lao et al. [24], the taste of soy sauce was tested using a commercial electronic tongue instrument (Insent, taste sensing system SA402B, Intelligent Sensor Technology, Inc., Kanagawa, Japan). The electronic tongue was capable of measuring eight basic sensory qualities including sourness, saltiness, bitterness, bitter aftertaste (aftertaste-B), astringency, astringent aftertaste (aftertaste-A), richness, and umami. The taste reference solution was configured to contain 2.2365 g of KCl and 0.045 g of tartaric acid in 1000 mL of distilled water, and the sensor response of this reference solution was zero. The soy sauce was diluted 30 times to meet the requirements of determination. The measurements were started when the biofilm sensor (taste sensor) was stable, and after a single measurement, the sensor was cleaned to measure the next sample.

2.8. Sensory Evaluation

Sensory evaluation was conducted within 5 h after soy sauce production in the Research Center for Food Resources and Comprehensive Utilization of Jiangnan University. The sensory evaluation group consisted of 20 well-trained individuals in the 20–40 age group from Jiangnan University. All panel members were asked to avoid stimulating food, alcohol, and tobacco use for 8 h prior to the assessment and rinsed their mouth to clean their sense of taste before each sample was evaluated. The sensory analysis of color, appearance, soy sauce flavor, vegetable flavor, seafood flavor, and likeability (overall acceptability) of S, W1, CE1, CA1, ON1, W2, CE2, CA2, and ON2 soy sauces was performed by these team members. According to Table 2, the score for each evaluated attribute ranged from 1 (very disliked) to 9 (very liked).

Table 2. Sensory scoring parameters.

Attribute	Descriptive Terms	Full Score of 9 (Minimum of 1 is Extremely Poor or Disliked)
Colour	Thick, black, reddish brown or tawny, shiny, and bright.	• Glossy and bright color (6–9). • Incorrect color (1–5).
Appearance	Concentration, viscosity, clarity, the presence of precipitation, and the presence of suspended solids.	• Thin and moderately thick, clear and transparent, no precipitation, no suspended matter, and uniform liquid (6–9). • Thin and not moderate, with suspended sediment (1–5).
Soy sauce flavor	Rich sauce flavor, mellow flavor, ester flavor, koji flavor, caramel flavor, amino acid flavor, ammonia gas, and musty flavor.	• Soy sauce with strong flavor such as sauce flavor, mellow flavor, and ester flavor (6–9). • Soy sauce has low flavor, burnt smell, musty smell, and ammonia gas (1–5).
Vegetable flavor	The delicate fragrance and pungent taste of vegetables.	• Strong vegetable fragrance (5–9). • Vegetable taste is low and it has a pungent spiciness (1–5).

Table 2. Cont.

Attribute	Descriptive Terms	Full Score of 9 (Minimum of 1 is Extremely Poor or Disliked)
Seafood flavor	Rich or light seafood flavor and fishy smell.	• Has a good seafood flavor (6–9). • Seafood taste is low and it is fishy (1–5).
Likeability	——	• Prefer (7–9), average (4–6), and dislike (1–3).

2.9. Statistical Analysis

Electronic nose and electronic tongue experiments were repeated 5 times. Other experiments were repeated 3–6 times. GraphPad Prism 9.0 (GraphPad Software Inc., San Diego, CA, USA), Origin 2018 (OriginLab, Northampton, MA, USA), and SPSS 26.0 (IBM, Chicago, IL, USA) were used for plotting and data analysis. At the 95% confidence level, significant differences between the means were determined using a one-way analysis of variance (ANOVA). Different letters were used to indicate the significant difference of data ($p < 0.05$), and experimental result data were expressed as mean ± SD.

3. Results and Discussion

3.1. General Physicochemical Property Analysis

Table 3 shows the results of determination of general physicochemical properties of vegetable juice-soy sauce compound condiment. The color directly affects the appearance quality of soy sauce and consumers' purchase intention [25]. The red/dark brown color of soy sauce is the result of the Maillard reaction of reducing sugars and amino acids produced by the enzymatic hydrolysis of carbohydrates and proteins during fermentation [26]. According to Table 3, the difference in brightness (L^*) of the soy sauce with different formulations was not significant. Compared to W1 and W2, the soy sauce with the addition of vegetable-seafood stock had a higher redness value (a^*) and yellowness value (b^*), which might be due to the yellowish color of carrots and boiled shrimp skin. In addition, compared to pure soy sauce S, the overall color of the compound soy sauce product became lighter due to the dilution effect. It was previously reported that either too-low or too-high L^* values did not affect soy sauce appearance, while high a^* and b^* values were important contributors to high-quality soy sauce [27]. Light-colored soy sauce was generally more popular than traditional soy sauce [28]. In the development of new soy sauce products, controlling the color of soy sauce is beneficial to improving customer acceptance.

The pH plays a vital role in the process of moromi fermentation. Microbial fermentation, substance hydrolysis, microbial cell autolysis, and the release of organic acids, free fatty acids, and amino acids can all lead to decreases in pH [29]. Typically, Japanese soy sauce has a pH between 4.6 and 4.9 [27,28]. Syifaa et al. [30] measured a pH range of 4.01–4.88 for common soy sauces in Southeast Asia. Commercially available soy sauce in Brazil had a pH between 4.00 and 5.27 [31]. The pH of the radish-, apple-, and pear-fermented soy sauce products ranged from 4.85 to 5.47 [32]. In this study, the pH values of all soy sauce products were in the range of 5.10–5.24; the pH value of pure soy sauce S was the lowest at 5.10. The larger the ratio of vegetable to seafood juice was, the higher the pH value was. The total acid content of soy sauce increased continuously during the fermentation process due to the production of organic acids. The highest total acid content of pure soy sauce S was 1.51 g/100 mL (calculated based on lactic acid), and with the addition of vegetable-seafood juice, the total acid content decreased due to the dilution effect. The 1:2 formula soy sauce samples (W2, CE2, CA2, and ON2) had the lowest total acid content, and there was no significant difference between the samples. Hoang et al. [33] recommended that the total acid content in soy sauce products should not exceed 2.0 g/100 mL and be less than 1.4 g/100 mL. The Chinese Soy Sauce Hygiene Standard GB 2717-2003 stipulated that the total acid content in soy sauce should be less than 2.5 g/100 mL (calculated based on lactic acid).

Table 3. Basic physicochemical parameters of different soy sauce.

Samples	L*	a*	b*	pH	Total Acid (Lactic Acid, g/100 mL)	TSS (°Brix)	Sodium Chloride (g/100 mL)	Non-Salt Soluble Solid (g/100 mL)	Amino Acid Nitrogen (g/100 mL)
S	34.29 ± 0.88 [a]	−0.14 ± 0.07 [ab]	−0.24 ± 0.06 [e]	5.10 ± 0.03 [e]	1.51 ± 0.02 [a]	39.50 ± 0.05 [a]	18.33 ± 0.55 [a]	19.17 ± 0.20 [a]	0.79 ± 0.04 [a]
W1	24.39 ± 1.23 [bc]	−0.28 ± 0.2 [abc]	0.50 ± 0.16 [cd]	5.11 ± 0.02 [de]	0.92 ± 0.02 [c]	27.88 ± 0.54 [d]	12.87 ± 0.96 [b]	11.43 ± 0.45 [d]	0.49 ± 0.02 [d]
CE1	25.33 ± 1.04 [b]	−0.35 ± 0.11 [bc]	0.72 ± 0.26 [d]	5.12 ± 0.01 [d]	1.04 ± 0.05 [b]	28.25 ± 1.03 [cd]	13.65 ± 0.55 [b]	11.63 ± 0.13 [cd]	0.59 ± 0.03 [b]
CA1	25.44 ± 1.38 [b]	−0.29 ± 0.28 [abc]	1.10 ± 0.36 [bc]	5.11 ± 0.01 [de]	1.06 ± 0.02 [b]	29.38 ± 0.96 [bc]	13.26 ± 0.55 [b]	12.32 ± 0.33 [bc]	0.56 ± 0.01 [c]
ON1	24.43 ± 1.56 [bc]	−0.26 ± 0.12 [ab]	1.00 ± 0.26 [bcd]	5.11 ± 0.01 [de]	1.01 ± 0.02 [bc]	29.75 ± 0.25 [b]	13.26 ± 0.55 [b]	12.64 ± 0.25 [b]	0.54 ± 0.01 [c]
W2	25.69 ± 1.56 [b]	−0.49 ± 0.28 [c]	0.67 ± 0.17 [d]	5.16 ± 0.01 [c]	0.52 ± 0.02 [d]	17.75 ± 0.83 [f]	8.78 ± 0.59 [c]	3.08 ± 0.05 [g]	0.25 ± 0.01 [e]
CE2	22.81 ± 1.99 [c]	−0.27 ± 0.09 [abc]	1.61 ± 0.46 [a]	5.22 ± 0.01 [b]	0.54 ± 0.05 [d]	20.25 ± 0.25 [e]	8.97 ± 0.55 [c]	5.81 ± 0.02 [f]	0.25 ± 0.01 [e]
CA2	25.72 ± 1.34 [b]	−0.17 ± 0.13 [ab]	1.90 ± 0.25 [a]	5.24 ± 0.03 [a]	0.56 ± 0.02 [d]	20.75 ± 0.56 [e]	8.97 ± 0.55 [c]	6.51 ± 0.13 [ef]	0.24 ± 0.02 [ef]
ON2	26.23 ± 2.1 [b]	−0.10 ± 0.14 [a]	1.23 ± 0.12 [b]	5.22 ± 0.02 [b]	0.50 ± 0.05 [d]	20.75 ± 0.56 [e]	8.58 ± 0.55 [c]	6.65 ± 0.13 [e]	0.22 ± 0.01 [f]

Notes: Means with different letters in the same column are statistically significant at $p < 0.05$.

The TSS content of pure soy sauce S was the highest (39.50 °Brix), and the 1:0.5 soy sauce (27.88–29.75 °Brix) contained more soluble solids than the 1:2 soy sauce (17.75–20.75 °Brix) Compared to W1 and W2, the content of TSS increased through the addition of vegetable and seafood juice. In general, soy sauce has a higher concentration of sodium chloride to prevent microbial spoilage. The sodium chloride and non-salt-soluble solid contents of pure soy sauce S were up to 18.33 g/100 mL and 19.17 g/100 mL, respectively. The sodium chloride and non-salt-soluble solid contents of 1:0.5 soy sauce juice ranged from 12.87 to 13.65 and 11.43 to 12.64 g/100 mL, and that of 1:2 ranged from 8.78 to 8.97 and 3.08 to 6.65 g/100 mL. The soy sauce with added vegetable-seafood juice had a higher sodium chloride content than W1 and W2, which might be due to the salt in the dried shrimp being boiled in the seafood stock. Previous studies have shown that the TSS content of soy sauce is generally in the range of 24.8–57.9 g/100 mL, and the salt content is in the range of 11.09–22.18 g/100 mL [34]. Li et al. [35] measured soy sauce, and it contained 38.6 g/100 mL TSS and 18.9 g/100 mL non-salt soluble solids. Amino acid nitrogen content is considered as the main parameter to evaluate the quality of soy sauce products [36]. According to the current Chinese standard, the amino acid nitrogen content of fermented soy sauce should be higher than 0.4 g/100 mL (GB 2717-2018). The amino acid nitrogen content in that blended soy sauce was generally less than 0.4 g/100 mL [37]. The amino acid nitrogen content of pure soy sauce S was 0.79 g/100 mL, and that of W1, CE1, CA1, and ON1 were 0.49, 0.59, 0.56, and 0.54 g/100 mL, respectively. However, the amino acid nitrogen content of 1:2 soy sauce products was lower than 0.4 g/100 mL. In summary, most of the physicochemical parameters of pure soy sauce decreased after the addition of vegetable juice due to the dilution effect, and the soy sauce juice with the formula of 1:0.5 basically met the general quality standards for the production of soy sauce.

3.2. Free Amino Acids (FAAs)

During the fermentation of soy sauce, the action of protease and glutaminase leads to the hydrolysis of proteins and the formation of FAAs [38]. Free amino acids are considered important contributors to the unique taste of soy sauce. A quantitative analysis of 17 common FAAs in blended soy sauce samples was conducted in this study (Table 4). It was found that Glu, Asp, Leu, Pro, and Val were the main amino acids in soy sauce, especially glutamic acid, which accounted for more than 50% of the total FAA content and was considered to be an important contributor to the flavor of soy sauce. The umami amino acids represented by Glu and Asp accounted for about 60% of the total FAA content. Glu is an essential umami substance, and other amino acids can promote umami through synergistic effects [28]. The proportion of sweet (16.73–18.71%) and bitter (20.46–22.64%) amino acids in the total FAA content was not significantly different among different soy sauce samples and was generally lower than the umami (59.12–61.97%) amino acid content. These results were basically consistent with the report by Kong et al. [39], where the content of umami amino acids in Chinese commercial soy sauce accounted for 28.83–97.18% of the total FAAs, with an average of 62.42%, and Glu, Leu, Ala, and Pro were the main free amino acids. By contrast, the soy sauce used in this research was mainly seafood soy sauce with high umami, and the proportion of umami amino acids was significantly higher than that of soy-brewed soy sauce. It was reported that the umami amino acids (Glu and Asp) in soy sauce made from soybean accounted for more than 23.94% of the total FAA content [38]. Similarly, Lin et al. [40] measured the umami amino acids of soy sauce made from soybeans, finding that they accounted for 6.06–25.20% of the total FAAs.

Table 4. Free amino acid content of soy sauce with different formulations.

Taste	FAAs (g/100 mL)	S	W1	CE1	CA1	ON1	W2	CE2	CA2	ON2
Umami	Asp	0.50 ± 0.03 [a]	0.36 ± 0.01 [cd]	0.40 ± 0.01 [b]	0.38 ± 0.01 [bc]	0.34 ± 0.00 [d]	0.17 ± 0.01 [e]	0.18 ± 0.01 [e]	0.18 ± 0.00 [e]	0.18 ± 0.01 [e]
Umami	Glu	4.34 ± 0.03 [a]	3.10 ± 0.09 [c]	3.46 ± 0.09 [b]	3.40 ± 0.07 [b]	3.02 ± 0.03 [c]	1.52 ± 0.12 [d]	1.60 ± 0.05 [d]	1.57 ± 0.02 [d]	1.57 ± 0.04 [d]
	Relative	61.58%	61.57%	61.66%	61.97%	61.76%	61.23%	59.73%	59.52%	59.12%
Sweet	Ser	0.10 ± 0.01 [a]	0.06 ± 0.00 [c]	0.07 ± 0.00 [b]	0.09 ± 0.00 [a]	0.07 ± 0.00 [b]	0.04 ± 0.01 [d]	0.04 ± 0.00 [d]	0.04 ± 0.00 [d]	0.04 ± 0.00 [d]
Sweet/Bitter	Lys	0.29 ± 0.02 [a]	0.20 ± 0.01 [c]	0.22 ± 0.00 [b]	0.23 ± 0.01 [b]	0.20 ± 0.00 [c]	0.10 ± 0.01 [d]	0.11 ± 0.00 [d]	0.11 ± 0.00 [d]	0.11 ± 0.00 [d]
Sweet/Bitter	Pro	0.32 ± 0.03 [a]	0.24 ± 0.01 [b]	0.25 ± 0.00 [b]	0.15 ± 0.03 [c]	0.14 ± 0.01 [c]	0.08 ± 0.02 [d]	0.09 ± 0.01 [d]	0.10 ± 0.01 [d]	0.10 ± 0.00 [d]
Sweet	Gly	0.20 ± 0.01 [a]	0.14 ± 0.00 [c]	0.16 ± 0.00 [b]	0.17 ± 0.00 [b]	0.15 ± 0.00 [c]	0.08 ± 0.00 [d]	0.10 ± 0.00 [d]	0.10 ± 0.00 [d]	0.10 ± 0.01 [d]
Sweet	Thr	0.22 ± 0.01 [a]	0.16 ± 0.00 [c]	0.18 ± 0.00 [b]	0.17 ± 0.00 [b]	0.15 ± 0.00 [c]	0.08 ± 0.01 [d]	0.09 ± 0.00 [d]	0.09 ± 0.00 [d]	0.08 ± 0.01 [d]
Sweet	Ala	0.28 ± 0.02 [a]	0.20 ± 0.01 [c]	0.23 ± 0.01 [b]	0.23 ± 0.00 [b]	0.20 ± 0.00 [c]	0.10 ± 0.01 [d]	0.11 ± 0.00 [d]	0.11 ± 0.00 [d]	0.11 ± 0.00 [d]
	Relative	17.94%	17.79%	17.73%	17.05%	16.73%	17.39%	18.12%	18.71%	18.24%
Bitter	Tyr	0.08 ± 0.01 [a]	0.06 ± 0.00 [b]	0.07 ± 0.00 [b]	0.07 ± 0.00 [b]	0.06 ± 0.00 [b]	0.03 ± 0.00 [c]	0.04 ± 0.00 [c]	0.04 ± 0.00 [c]	0.04 ± 0.00 [c]
Bitter	Val	0.31 ± 0.02 [a]	0.22 ± 0.01 [c]	0.25 ± 0.01 [b]	0.25 ± 0.00 [b]	0.22 ± 0.00 [c]	0.11 ± 0.01 [d]	0.12 ± 0.00 [d]	0.12 ± 0.00 [d]	0.12 ± 0.01 [d]
Bitter	Met	0.07 ± 0.01 [a]	0.05 ± 0.00 [c]	0.06 ± 0.00 [b]	0.06 ± 0.00 [b]	0.05 ± 0.00 [c]	0.02 ± 0.00 [e]	0.03 ± 0.00 [d]	0.03 ± 0.00 [d]	0.03 ± 0.00 [d]
Bitter	Phe	0.24 ± 0.02 [a]	0.17 ± 0.01 [c]	0.19 ± 0.00 [b]	0.19 ± 0.01 [bc]	0.17 ± 0.00 [c]	0.09 ± 0.01 [d]	0.09 ± 0.00 [d]	0.09 ± 0.00 [d]	0.09 ± 0.00 [d]
Bitter	Ile	0.27 ± 0.02 [a]	0.19 ± 0.01 [c]	0.21 ± 0.00 [b]	0.21 ± 0.00 [b]	0.19 ± 0.00 [c]	0.10 ± 0.01 [d]	0.10 ± 0.00 [d]	0.10 ± 0.00 [d]	0.10 ± 0.00 [d]
Bitter	Leu	0.42 ± 0.03 [a]	0.30 ± 0.01 [c]	0.33 ± 0.01 [b]	0.33 ± 0.01 [b]	0.29 ± 0.00 [c]	0.15 ± 0.01 [d]	0.16 ± 0.01 [d]	0.16 ± 0.00 [d]	0.16 ± 0.01 [d]
Bitter	His	0.10 ± 0.01 [a]	0.07 ± 0.00 [bc]	0.08 ± 0.00 [b]	0.07 ± 0.00 [bc]	0.06 ± 0.00 [c]	0.04 ± 0.00 [d]	0.04 ± 0.00 [d]	0.04 ± 0.01 [d]	0.04 ± 0.00 [d]
Bitter	Arg	0.12 ± 0.01 [a]	0.09 ± 0.00 [c]	0.11 ± 0.00 [b]	0.11 ± 0.00 [b]	0.11 ± 0.00 [b]	0.05 ± 0.00 [f]	0.08 ± 0.00 [de]	0.08 ± 0.00 [e]	0.09 ± 0.00 [cd]
	Relative	20.48%	20.46%	20.77%	21.15%	21.14%	21.38%	22.15%	22.45%	22.64%
Tasteless	Cys	0.01 ± 0.01 [a]	0.01 ± 0.00 [a]	0.01 ± 0.00 [ab]	0.01 ± 0.00 [ab]	0.01 ± 0.00 [ab]	0.01 ± 0.01 [ab]	0.00 ± 0.00 [b]	0.00 ± 0.00 [b]	0.01 ± 0.00 [ab]
	Relative	0.13%	0.18%	0.16%	0.16%	0.18%	0.36%	0%	0%	0.34%
	Total Amino Acids	7.86 ± 0.55 [a]	5.62 ± 0.17 [cd]	6.26 ± 0.14 [b]	6.10 ± 0.07 [bc]	5.44 ± 0.04 [d]	2.76 ± 0.22 [e]	2.98 ± 0.05 [e]	2.94 ± 0.03 [e]	2.96 ± 0.10 [e]

Notes: Means with different letters in the same column are statistically significant at $p < 0.05$.

As expected, S had the highest content of FAAs (7.86 g/100 mL), followed by CE1 (6.26 g/100 mL), CA1 (6.10 g/100 mL), W1 (5.62 g/100 mL), and ON1 (5.44 g/100 mL), and the 1:2 soy sauce formulation generally had low FAA content (about 3.00 g/100 mL). The total FAA content of CE1 and CA1 was 11.39% and 8.54% higher than that of W1, respectively, and the Glu content was 11.61% and 9.68% higher than that of W1, respectively. This may be due to the addition of seafood juice containing a certain amount of free amino acids. Glu, Gly, and Ala are considered to be the main flavor amino acids in oyster juice [41]. The most abundant amino acids in shrimp cooking juice are, in sequence, Glu, Gly, Pro, Asp, and Arg [42]. Gly, Ala, Glu, and Arg account for about 40% of the total FAAs in oyster cooker effluent [43]. In addition, vegetable juice also contains a certain amount of free FAAs. For example, the total FAA concentration of broccoli juice is 256.66 mg/100 mL, and Arg accounts for 21% [44]. Therefore, adding vegetable-seafood juice is helpful to increase the content of FAAs in soy sauce, but at a ratio of 1:0.5, it will not exceed the content of FAAs in pure soy sauce due to the dilution effect.

3.3. Total Phenolic, Flavonoid and Antioxidant Activity

The total phenolic and total flavonoid contents of pure soy sauce S reached 2.58 mg GAE/mL and 1.53 mg RE/mL, respectively (Figure 1A). The total phenolic content was similar to the result previously reported by Gao et al. [45] and higher than that of citrus-peel-fermented soy sauce [46]. Phenols and flavonoids are secondary metabolites abundantly present in fruits and vegetables, which significantly promote human health. The total phenolic and flavonoid contents of the soy sauce with the formula of 1:0.5 and 1:2 with added vegetable juice were higher than those of the control group (W1 and W2) and lower than S. The total phenolic contents of CA1 and ON1 were 14.85% and 14.36% higher than that of W1, respectively, and the flavonoid contents of CE1, CA1, and ON1 were 13.68%, 11.11%, and 12.82% higher than that of W1, respectively. Previous studies have shown a close positive correlation between the content of phenolic compounds and antioxidant activity [47,48].

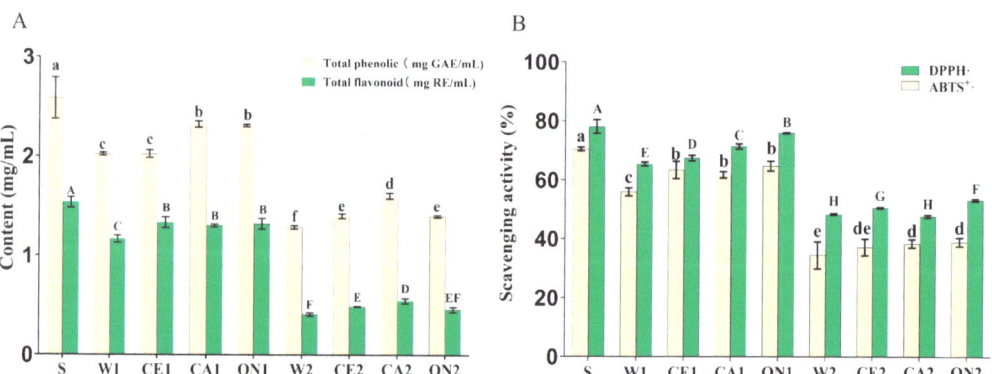

Figure 1. Total phenolics, flavonoids (**A**), and antioxidant capacity (**B**) of soy sauce. Different letters represent significant differences between groups ($p < 0.05$).

Figure 1B shows the antioxidant activity of the soy sauce products. S had the highest antioxidant activity, with the scavenging abilities of ABTS and DPPH radicals of 70.40% and 78.04%, respectively. Basically consistent with the change trend in total phenolic and flavonoid content, the free radical scavenging ability of the 1:0.5 and 1:2 formula soy sauce with added vegetable juice was higher than that of the control group (W1 and W2) and lower than that of S. The total phenolic contents of CE1, CA1, and ON1 were 13.22%, 10.38%, and 15.63% higher than those of W1, respectively, and the flavonoid contents were 13.68%, 11.11%, and 12.82% higher than those of W1, respectively. CE1, CA1, and ON1 had better antioxidant activity because they contained celery, carrots, and onions, etc., and their potential role as an antioxidant has been well documented in the literature [49,50]. In addition, many reports indicated that amino acids have strong antioxidant activity [45,51], which may be one reason for the better antioxidant properties of vegetable-seafood soy sauce. Fan et al. [52] reported that aromatic amino acids and histidine are considered effective radical scavengers because they can easily provide protons to electron-deficient radicals while maintaining their stability through resonance structures. Amino acids can act as a synergistic antioxidant as a natural component of food materials [53].

3.4. Electronic Nose Analysis

Electronic noses are sensitive to the overall smell of food, and slight changes in the presence of volatile compounds can cause differences in the sensor response [54]. Electronic noses are a common tool for analyzing the flavor changes in soy sauce [55,56]. Figure 2A shows the radar map of the odor distribution of the soy sauce with different formulations. The sensors with relatively strong responses to soy sauce samples were S1, S4, S5, S6, S9, S11, S12, S14, S16, S17, and S18, which were, respectively, sensitive to alkanes, sulfides, organic amines, aromatic compounds, aldehydes, alkenes, short-chain alkanes, flammable gases, sulfides, nitrides, and alcohols. The sensor response values of the S, W1, and W2 groups decreased successively, indicating that the overall flavor of the soy sauce became weaker with the increase in dilution degree. The sensor response value of soy sauce with added vegetable-seafood juice was larger, and the soy sauce flavor response value of the 1:2 formula was higher than that of the 1:0.5 formula, which indicated that the addition of vegetable-seafood juice enhanced the overall flavor of the soy sauce.

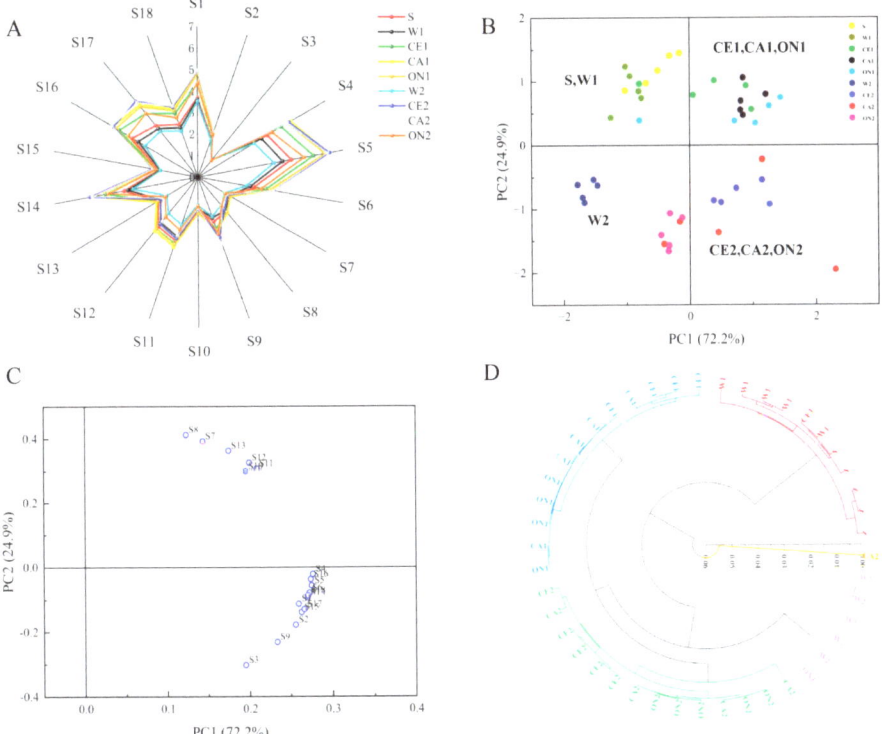

Figure 2. Radar plot (**A**), PCA score plot (**B**), loading plot (**C**), and HCA analysis plot (**D**) of soy sauce based on e-nose response data.

A principal component analysis (PCA) was performed on the response signals of the 18 sensors for each sample (Figure 2B). The contribution rates of the first and second principal components were 72.2% and 24.9%, respectively, and the total contribution rate was 97.1%, which covered almost all the variable information, indicating that the principal components could reflect all the characteristics of the volatile odor of different soy sauce samples. CE1, CA1, and ON1 samples were mainly distributed in the first quadrant with relatively close distances, and the differences between the samples were small. CE2, CA2, and ON2 were mainly distributed in the third and fourth quadrants, with little difference among the samples. S and W1 were in the second quadrant, while W2 was far away from other samples. This indicated that the samples of the soy sauce group (S, W1, and W2), the 1:0.5 soy sauce, and the 1:2 soy sauce were distributed in their independent regions, which were clearly distinguished by the PCA, and the flavor differences among the three groups were larger. However, the difference in flavor was small among different vegetables (celery, carrot, and onion). In the loading diagram (Figure 2C), the coordinates of each sensor can accurately reflect its contribution to the volatile odor of the sample. The farther from the origin, the greater the sensor's contribution to the principal component, and vice versa. Among the eighteen sensors, the sensors that contributed more to the first principal component were S4, S16, S5, and S6, and the one that contributed the most to the second principal component was S8. This indicated that sulfide, organic amine, aromatic compounds, and short-chain alkane played the main roles in the differentiation of soy sauce with different formulations.

A hierarchical cluster analysis (HCA) was performed on the response values of 18 sensors to visually and objectively clarify the flavor differences between the samples. The earlier the samples were gathered into the same group, the closer they became. As shown in Figure 2D, the soy sauce samples were mainly classified into four groups. S and W1 were clustered into one group; W2 was clustered into one group individually; CE1, CA1, and ON1 were clustered into one group; and CE2, CA2, and ON2 were clustered into one group. The HCA results were consistent with the PCA results. Compared to the control W1, the addition of vegetable-seafood juice could change the flavor of soy sauce and significantly improve the aroma quality, but the flavor differences between the celery, carrot, and onion soy sauce samples were small.

3.5. Electronic Tongue Analysis

The electronic tongue uses artificial lipid membrane sensor technology to quantitatively analyze the six basic tastes of soy sauce: sourness, saltiness, astringency, aftertaste-A (astringency aftertaste), bitterness, aftertaste-B (bitterness aftertaste), richness, and umami [57]. Before determining the taste of the soy sauce, the taste of the distilled water used for preparing the soy sauce was first measured. The results showed that the saltiness, sourness, bitterness, aftertaste-B, astringency, aftertaste-A, umami, and richness of the distilled water were −20.11, −17.83, 16.13, −0.73, −4.43, −0.39, −5.30, and 0.35, respectively. Figure 3A shows the saltiness and sourness of soy sauce. Pure soy sauce S had the most salty taste, followed by the soy sauce with a formula of 1:0.5. The salty taste of CE1, CA1, and ON1 was higher than that of W1, which might be due to the salty taste of boiled seafood sauce. The sourness of the sauce was caused by lactic acid and other organic acids produced by lactic acid bacteria fermentation [58]. The sourness of the soy sauce did not change significantly after adding vegetable-seafood juice, and the sourness of all the samples was lower than that of the distilled water. The bitterness and umami of soy sauce are related to the amino acids produced during the fermentation process. After the soy sauce was diluted (W1 and W2), its bitterness significantly increased (Figure 3B), mainly due to the presence of a certain bitterness in distilled water [59]. The bitter aftertaste of all the soy sauce samples was lower than that of the distilled water. The variation trend in the astringency and astringency aftertaste of the soy sauce was basically the same. That is, the astringency and astringency aftertaste of the soy sauce increased significantly after adding vegetable and seafood juice, and the order was celery > carrot > onion-flavored soy sauce (Figure 3C). The umami taste of the soy sauce decreased after dilution. Compared to the control groups W1 and W2, the umami of the vegetable-seafood soy sauce was significantly increased, but still lower than that of the pure soy sauce (Figure 3D). The richness of CE2 was the highest, which may be due to the obvious taste of celery.

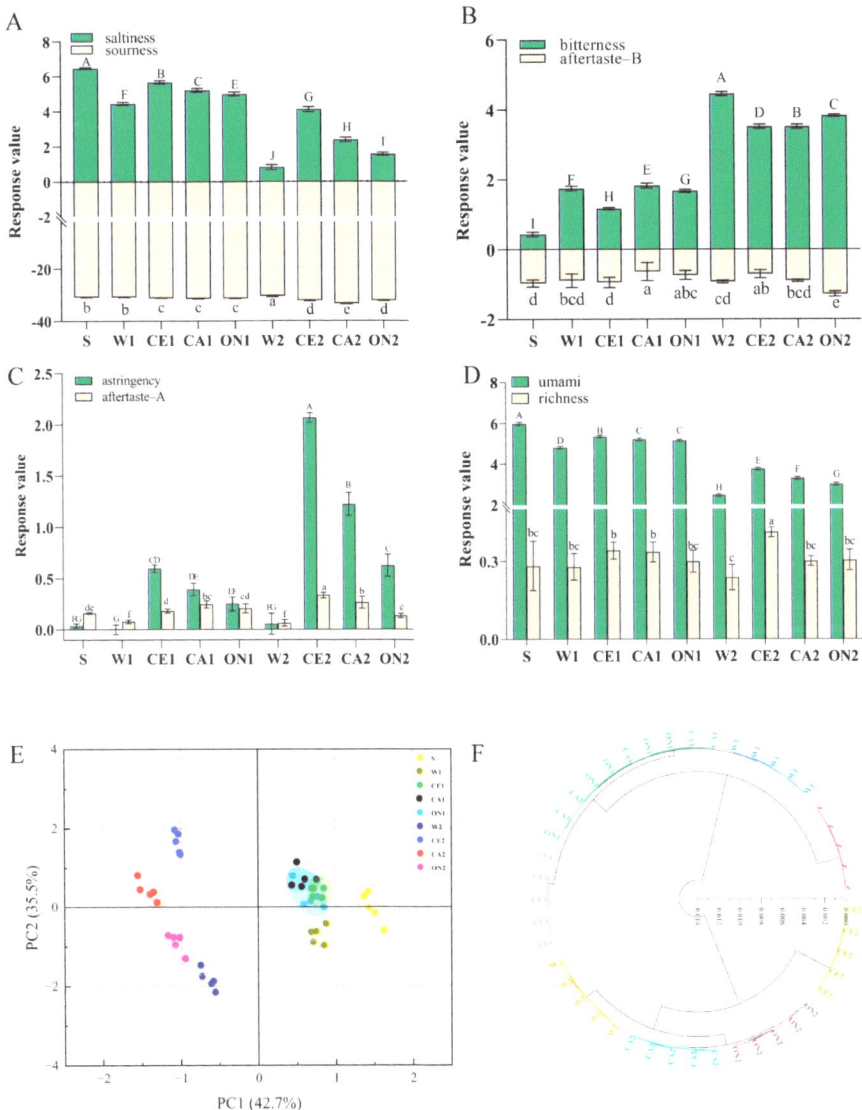

Figure 3. Saltiness and sourness (**A**), bitterness and bitterness aftertaste (**B**), astringency and astringency aftertaste (**C**), umami and richness (**D**) of different soy sauces; PCA score plot (**E**) and HCA analysis plot (**F**) of soy sauce taste based on electronic tongue response data. Different letters represent significant differences between groups ($p < 0.05$).

Figure 3E shows the PCA scores of different soy sauce seasonings based on the electronic tongue response data. PC1 and PC2 accounted for 42.7% and 35.5% of the total variance, respectively, for a total contribution of 78.2%. The scores showed that the soy sauce groups (S, W1, and W2) could be distinguished to a certain extent. CE1, CA1, and

ON1 were close to each other, indicating that their tastes were similar. Soy sauce samples that were 1:2 formulated (W2, CE2, CA2, and ON2) showed good overall discrimination and large taste difference. HCA was performed on the response data of the electronic tongue. As shown in Figure 3F, the soy sauce condiments with different formulations were mainly divided into eight categories. S, W1, CE1, W2, CE2, CA2, and ON2 could be clustered into one group alone, indicating that there were significant differences in taste among different samples. CA1 and ON1 were gathered into one group, indicating that the tastes were similar. This result was basically consistent with that of the PCA. The taste of the soy sauce after adding vegetable-seafood juice was different from that of the pure soy sauce or diluted soy sauce, and there were some differences in the taste of the soy sauce from different vegetables (celery, carrot, and onion).

3.6. Sensory Evaluation

Twenty panel members conducted a sensory evaluation on the color, appearance, soy sauce flavor, vegetable flavor, seafood flavor, and likeability (overall acceptability) of the soy sauce products. As shown in Figure 4, S and W1 had the highest color and appearance scores, followed by the 1:0.5 vegetable soy sauce (CE1, CA1, and ON1), with both color and appearance scores greater than 7. This indicated that the color and appearance of soy sauce would decrease with the addition of vegetable-seafood juice, and the 1:0.5 formula had little influence on the soy sauce. For the flavor of the soy sauce, S, W1, and W2 scored the highest, followed by the 1:0.5 vegetable formula soy sauce. CE2, CA2, and ON2 had the highest scores for vegetable and seafood flavor, while S, W1, and W2 had the lowest scores. This showed that the more vegetable and seafood juice added, the lower the flavor of soy sauce and the higher the flavor of vegetables and seafood would be, and this flavor difference could be identified by human senses. In terms of the popularity of soy sauce products, the 1:0.5 vegetable-seafood soy sauce (CE1, CA1, and ON1) had the highest score, indicating that consumers might have a high acceptance rate of mixed-vegetable soy sauce.

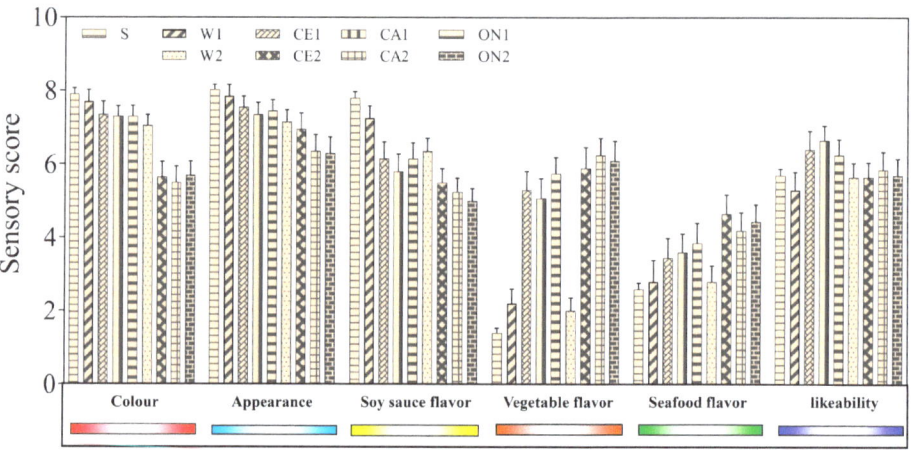

Figure 4. Sensory evaluation results of soy sauce with different formulations.

4. Conclusions

In this study, according to the catering enterprises and the real demand, a variety of flavors of mixed-vegetable seafood soy sauce were developed, and the influence of different formula proportions on the physical and chemical parameters, nutrition, flavor, and taste of soy sauce was studied. The results showed that the product with the ratio of soy sauce to vegetable-seafood juice of 1:0.5 (v/v) had relatively good flavor, mouthfeel, and sensory scores, but the flavors of different vegetables (celery, carrot, and onion) were difficult to distinguish. It is suggested that manufacturers or catering enterprises should control the ratio of vegetables to soy sauce within 1:0.5 and strive to develop more soy sauce with multiple flavors to meet the needs of consumers or chefs.

Author Contributions: Methodology, T.T.; Formal analysis, T.T.; Investigation, B.B.; Resources, M.Z.; Writing—original draft, T.T.; Writing—review & editing, M.Z. and B.B.; Supervision, M.Z. All authors have read and agreed to the published version of the manuscript.

Funding: We acknowledge financial support from the National Key R&D Program of China (No. 2018YFD0700303), Jiangsu Province Key Laboratory Project of Advanced Food Manufacturing Equipment and Technology (No. FMZ202003), and the National First-Class Discipline Program of Food Science and Technology (No. JUFSTR20180205), all of which enabled us to carry out this study.

Institutional Review Board Statement: Not applicable.

Informed Consent Statement: Not applicable.

Data Availability Statement: Data are available on request to the authors.

Conflicts of Interest: The authors declare no conflict of interest.

References

1. Devanthi, P.V.P.; Gkatzionis, K. Soy sauce fermentation: Microorganisms, aroma formation, and process modification. *Food Res. Int.* **2019**, *120*, 364–374. [CrossRef]
2. Pujchakarn, T.; Suwonsichon, S.; Suwonsichon, T. Development of a sensory lexicon for a specific subcategory of soy sauce: Seasoning soy sauce. *J. Sens. Stud.* **2016**, *31*, 443–452. [CrossRef]
3. Diez-Simon, C.; Eichelsheim, C.; Mumm, R.; Hall, R.D. Chemical and Sensory Characteristics of Soy Sauce: A Review. *J. Agric. Food Chem.* **2020**, *68*, 11612–11630. [CrossRef]
4. Feng, Y.; Cui, C.; Zhao, H.; Gao, X.; Zhao, M.; Sun, W. Effect of koji fermentation on generation of volatile compounds in soy sauce production. *Int. J. Food Sci. Technol.* **2013**, *48*, 609–619. [CrossRef]
5. Steinhaus, P.; Schieberle, P. Characterization of the Key Aroma Compounds in Soy Sauce Using Approaches of Molecular Sensory Science. *J. Agric. Food Chem.* **2007**, *15*, 6262–6269. [CrossRef] [PubMed]
6. Seong, P.T.; Woong, K.D. Method for Producing Allium Hookeri Soy Sauce and Allium Hookeri Soy Sauce Using Thereof. Republic of Korea Patent KR101877875B1, 12 July 2018.
7. Gong, Z. Method for Preparing Fruit and Vegetable Health-Care Soy Sauce and Fruit and Vegetable Health-Care Soy Sauce. China Patent CN102132860A, 27 July 2011.
8. Ok, Y.S. Manufacturing Method of Soy Sauce. Republic of Korea Patent KR101423194B1, 28 July 2014.
9. Soo, C.B.; Suck, C.K.; Kyung, L.M. Making Process of Soy Sauce Comprising Antimicrobial Substance and Soy Sauce Comprising Antimicrobial Substance. Republic of Korea Patent KR100874785B1, 18 December 2008.
10. Ma, D. Toona Sinensis Soy Sauce Processing Method. China Patent CN105533635A, 14 May 2016.
11. Bok, L.S. Herb Soy Sauce and Producing Method Thereof. Republic of Korea Patent KR100647878B1, 23 November 2016.
12. Chen, H. Manufacturing Process and Preparation Method of Mustard Soy Sauce. China Patent CN112890163A, 4 June 2021.
13. Wang, L. Rosmarinus Officinalis Health-Care Soy Sauce and Preparation Method Thereof. China Patent CN109418922A, 5 March 2019.
14. Gao, X.; Zhang, J.; Liu, E.; Yang, M.; Chen, S.; Hu, F.; Ma, H.; Liu, Z.; Yu, X. Enhancing the taste of raw soy sauce using low intensity ultrasound treatment during moromi fermentation. *Food Chem.* **2019**, *298*, 124928. [CrossRef]
15. Wu, J.; Zhang, M.; Zhang, L.; Liu, Y. Effect of ultrasound combined with sodium bicarbonate pretreatment on the taste and flavor of chicken broth. *J. Food Process Eng.* **2022**, e14072. [CrossRef]
16. Zheng, Z.; Zhang, M.; Fan, H.; Liu, Y. Effect of microwave combined with ultrasonic pretreatment on flavor and antioxidant activity of hydrolysates based on enzymatic hydrolysis of bovine bone. *Food Biosci.* **2021**, *44*, 101399. [CrossRef]
17. Li, L.; Zhang, M.; Zhou, L. A promising pulse-spouted microwave freeze drying method used for Chinese yam cubes dehydration: Quality, energy consumption, and uniformity. *Dry. Technol.* **2021**, *39*, 148–161. [CrossRef]
18. Chitrakar, B.; Zhang, M.; Zhang, X.; Bhandari, B. Valorization of asparagus-leaf by-product through nutritionally enriched chips to evaluate the effect of powder particle size on functional properties and rutin contents. *Dry. Technol.* **2023**, *41*, 34–45. [CrossRef]
19. Shi, H.; Zhang, M.; Bhandari, B.; Wang, Y.; Yi, S. Effects of superfine grinding on the properties and qualities of *Cordyceps militaris* and its spent substrate. *J. Food Process. Preserv.* **2019**, *43*, e14169. [CrossRef]
20. Qiu, L.; Zhang, M.; Adhikari, B.; Chang, L. Microencapsulation of rose essential oil in mung bean protein isolate-apricot peel pectin complex coacervates and characterization of microcapsules. *Food Hydrocoll.* **2022**, *124*, 107366. [CrossRef]
21. Zhang, X.J.; Zhang, M.; Law, C.L.; Guo, Z. High-voltage electrostatic field-assisted modified atmosphere packaging for long-term storage of pakchoi and avoidance of off-flavors. *Innov. Food Sci. Emerg. Technol.* **2022**, *79*, 103032. [CrossRef]
22. Tang, T.; Zhang, M.; Mujumdar, A.S.; Teng, X. 3D printed white radish/potato gel with microcapsules: Color/flavor change induced by microwave-infrared heating. *Food Res. Int.* **2022**, *158*, 111496. [CrossRef] [PubMed]

23. Zheng, Z.; Zhang, M.; Liu, W.; Liu, Y. Effect of beef tallow, phospholipid and microwave combined ultrasonic pretreatment on Maillard reaction of bovine bone enzymatic hydrolysate. *Food Chem.* **2022**, *377*, 131902. [CrossRef] [PubMed]
24. Lao, Y.; Zhang, M.; Li, Z.; Bhandari, B. A novel combination of enzymatic hydrolysis and fermentation: Effects on the flavor and nutritional quality of fermented *Cordyceps militaris* beverage. *LWT* **2020**, *120*, 108934. [CrossRef]
25. Wongthahan, P.; Sae-Eaw, A.; Prinyawiwatkul, W. Sensory lexicon and relationships among brown colour, saltiness perception and sensory liking evaluated by regular users and culinary chefs: A case of soy sauces. *Int. J. Food Sci. Technol.* **2020**, *55*, 2841–2850. [CrossRef]
26. Ito, K.; Matsuyama, A. Koji Molds for Japanese Soy Sauce Brewing: Characteristics and Key Enzymes. *J. Fungi* **2021**, *7*, 658. [CrossRef] [PubMed]
27. Wang, S.; Zhang, H.; Liu, X.; Tamura, T.; Kyouno, N.; Chen, J.Y. Relationship between Chemical Characteristics and Sensory Evaluation of Koikuchi Soy Sauce. *Anal. Lett.* **2018**, *51*, 2192–2204. [CrossRef]
28. Miyagi, A.; Suzuki, T.; Nabetani, H.; Nakajima, M. Color control of Japanese soy sauce (shoyu) using membrane technology. *Food Bioprod. Process.* **2013**, *91*, 507–514. [CrossRef]
29. Kim, J.-S.; Lee, Y.-S. A study of chemical characteristics of soy sauce and mixed soy sauce: Chemical characteristics of soy sauce. *Eur. Food Res. Technol.* **2007**, *227*, 933–944. [CrossRef]
30. Syifaa, A.S.; Jinap, S.; Sanny, M.; Khatib, A. Chemical profiling of different types of soy sauce and the relationship with its sensory attributes. *J. Food Qual.* **2016**, *39*, 714–725. [CrossRef]
31. Guidi, L.R.; Gloria, M.B. Bioactive amines in soy sauce: Validation of method, occurrence and potential health effects. *Food Chem.* **2012**, *133*, 323–328. [CrossRef]
32. Bahuguna, A.; Jo, I.G.; Lee, J.S.; Kim, M. Effects of Radishes, Apples, and Pears on the Lactic Acid Bacteria and Nutritional and Functional Qualities of Flavored Soy Sauce. *Foods* **2020**, *9*, 1562. [CrossRef]
33. Hoang, N.X.; Ferng, S.; Ting, C.-H.; Huang, W.-H.; Chiou, R.Y.-Y.; Hsu, C.-K. Optimizing the initial moromi fermentation conditions to improve the quality of soy sauce. *LWT* **2016**, *74*, 242–250. [CrossRef]
34. Li, Y.; Zhao, H.; Zhao, M.; Cui, C. Relationships between antioxidant activity and quality indices of soy sauce: An application of multivariate analysis. *Int. J. Food Sci. Technol.* **2009**, *45*, 133–139. [CrossRef]
35. Li, Y.; Zhao, M.; Parkin, K.L. beta-carboline derivatives and diphenols from soy sauce are in vitro quinone reductase (QR) inducers. *J. Agric. Food Chem.* **2011**, *59*, 2332–2340. [CrossRef] [PubMed]
36. Liu, X.; Qian, M.; Shen, Y.; Qin, X.; Huang, H.; Yang, H.; He, Y.; Bai, W. An high-throughput sequencing approach to the preliminary analysis of bacterial communities associated with changes in amino acid nitrogen, organic acid and reducing sugar contents during soy sauce fermentation. *Food Chem.* **2021**, *349*, 129131. [CrossRef]
37. Luo, T.; Xie, Y.; Dong, Y.; Liu, A.; Dong, Y. Quality assessment of soy sauce using underivatized amino acids by capillary electrophoresis. *Int. J. Food Prop.* **2018**, *20*, S3052–S3061. [CrossRef]
38. Zhou, W.; Sun-Waterhouse, D.; Xiong, J.; Cui, C.; Wang, W.; Dong, K. Desired soy sauce characteristics and autolysis of *Aspergillus oryzae* induced by low temperature conditions during initial moromi fermentation. *J. Food Sci. Technol.* **2019**, *56*, 2888–2898. [CrossRef]
39. Kong, Y.; Zhang, L.-L.; Zhang, Y.-Y.; Sun, B.-G.; Sun, Y.; Zhao, J.; Chen, H.-T. Evaluation of non-volatile taste components in commercial soy sauces. *Int. J. Food Prop.* **2018**, *21*, 1854–1866. [CrossRef]
40. Lin, W.; Song, J.; Hu, W.; Miao, J.; Gao, X. Relationship between Extracellular Cellulase, Pectinase and Xylanase Activity of Isolated *Aspergillus oryzae* Strains Grown on Koji and the Umami-Tasting Amino Acid Content of Soy Sauce. *Food Biotechnol.* **2016**, *30*, 278–291. [CrossRef]
41. Chen, Y.Y.; Chen, S.S.; Qiu, W.Q.; Li, Q.L. Identification of Different Varieties of Oyster Juice Based on the Comparison of Free Amino Acids. *Adv. Mater. Res.* **2013**, *781–784*, 1534–1539. [CrossRef]
42. Pérez-Santín, E.; Calvo, M.M.; López-Caballero, M.E.; Montero, P.; Gómez-Guillén, M.C. Compositional properties and bioactive potential of waste material from shrimp cooking juice. *LWT—Food Sci. Technol.* **2013**, *54*, 87–94. [CrossRef]
43. Kim, D.S.; Baek, H.H.; Ahn, C.B.; Byun, D.S.; Jung, K.J.; Lee, H.G.; Cadwallader, K.R.; Kim, H.R. Development and characterization of a flavoring agent from oyster cooker effluent. *J. Agric. Food Chem.* **2000**, *48*, 4839–4843. [CrossRef]
44. Sánchez-Vega, R.; Garde-Cerdán, T.; Rodríguez-Roque, M.J.; Elez-Martínez, P.; Martín-Belloso, O. High-intensity pulsed electric fields or thermal treatment of broccoli juice: The effects of processing on minerals and free amino acids. *Eur. Food Res. Technol.* **2020**, *246*, 539–548. [CrossRef]
45. Gao, X.; Liu, E.; Zhang, J.; Yang, M.; Chen, S.; Liu, Z.; Ma, H.; Hu, F. Effects of sonication during moromi fermentation on antioxidant activities of compounds in raw soy sauce. *LWT* **2019**, *116*, 108605. [CrossRef]
46. Peng, M.; Liu, J.; Liu, Z.; Fu, B.; Hu, Y.; Zhou, M.; Fu, C.; Gao, B.; Wang, C.; Li, D.; et al. Effect of citrus peel on phenolic compounds, organic acids and antioxidant activity of soy sauce. *LWT* **2018**, *90*, 627–635. [CrossRef]
47. Velioglu, Y.S.; Mazza, G.; Gao, L.; Oomah, B.D. Antioxidant Activity and Total Phenolics in Selected Fruits, Vegetables, and Grain Products. *J. Agric. Food Chem.* **1998**, *46*, 4113–4117. [CrossRef]
48. Piao, Y.Z.; Eun, J.B. Physicochemical characteristics and isoflavones content during manufacture of short-time fermented soybean product (cheonggukjang). *J. Food Sci. Technol.* **2020**, *57*, 2190–2197. [CrossRef]
49. Chu, Y.F.; Sun, J.I.E.; Wu, X.; Liu, R.H. Antioxidant and antiproliferative activities of common vegetables. *J. Agric. Food Chem.* **2002**, *50*, 6910–6916. [CrossRef] [PubMed]

50. Song, W.; Derito, C.M.; Liu, M.K.; He, X.; Dong, M.; Liu, R.H. Cellular antioxidant activity of common vegetables. *J. Agric. Food Chem.* **2010**, *58*, 6621–6629. [CrossRef] [PubMed]
51. Xu, N.; Chen, G.; Liu, H. Antioxidative Categorization of Twenty Amino Acids Based on Experimental Evaluation. *Molecules* **2017**, *22*, 2066. [CrossRef] [PubMed]
52. Fan, J.; Zhang, Y.; Chang, X.; Saito, M.; Li, Z. Changes in the radical scavenging activity of bacterial-type douchi, a traditional fermented soybean product, during the primary fermentation process. *Biosci. Biotechnol. Biochem.* **2009**, *73*, 2749–2753. [CrossRef]
53. Marcuse, R. Antioxidative Effect of Amino-Acids. *Nature* **1960**, *186*, 886–887. [CrossRef]
54. Du, H.; Chen, Q.; Liu, Q.; Wang, Y.; Kong, B. Evaluation of flavor characteristics of bacon smoked with different woodchips by HS-SPME-GC-MS combined with an electronic tongue and electronic nose. *Meat Sci.* **2021**, *182*, 108626. [CrossRef]
55. Gao, L.; Liu, T.; An, X.; Zhang, J.; Ma, X.; Cui, J. Analysis of volatile flavor compounds influencing Chinese-type soy sauces using GC-MS combined with HS-SPME and discrimination with electronic nose. *J. Food Sci. Technol.* **2017**, *54*, 130–143. [CrossRef]
56. Zhu, L.; Yan, Y.; Gu, D.-C.; Lu, Y.; Gan, J.-H.; Tao, N.-P.; Wang, X.-C.; Xu, C.-H. Rapid Quality Discrimination and Amino Nitrogen Quantitative Evaluation of Soy Sauces by Tri-Step IR and E-nose. *Food Anal. Methods* **2018**, *11*, 3201–3210. [CrossRef]
57. Zhao, G.; Feng, Y.; Hadiatullah, H.; Zheng, F.; Yao, Y. Chemical Characteristics of Three Kinds of Japanese Soy Sauce Based on Electronic Senses and GC-MS Analyses. *Front. Microbiol.* **2020**, *11*, 579808. [CrossRef] [PubMed]
58. Luan, C.; Zhang, M.; Devahastin, S.; Liu, Y. Effect of two-step fermentation with lactic acid bacteria and Saccharomyces cerevisiae on key chemical properties, molecular structure and flavor characteristics of horseradish sauce. *LWT* **2021**, *147*, 111637. [CrossRef]
59. McBurney, D.H.; Shick, T.R. Taste and water taste of twenty-six compounds for man. *Percept. Psychophys.* **1971**, *10*, 249–252. [CrossRef]

Disclaimer/Publisher's Note: The statements, opinions and data contained in all publications are solely those of the individual author(s) and contributor(s) and not of MDPI and/or the editor(s). MDPI and/or the editor(s) disclaim responsibility for any injury to people or property resulting from any ideas, methods, instructions or products referred to in the content.

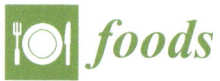

Article

Characteristics and Antioxidant Activity of Walnut Oil Using Various Pretreatment and Processing Technologies

Pan Gao [1,2,*], Yunpeng Ding [1], Zhe Chen [2], Zhangtao Zhou [1], Wu Zhong [1,2], Chuanrong Hu [1], Dongping He [1,2] and Xingguo Wang [1,3]

[1] Key Laboratory for Deep Processing of Major Grain and Oil (Wuhan Polytechnic University) of Ministry of Education in China, College of Food Science and Engineering, Wuhan Polytechnic University, 68 Xuefu South Road, Changqing Garden, Wuhan 430023, China; dyp99112@163.com (Y.D.); 18162571387@163.com (Z.Z.); zhongwu@whpu.edu.cn (W.Z.); hcr305@163.com (C.H.); hedp123456@163.com (D.H.); wangxg1002@gmail.com (X.W.)

[2] Key Laboratory of Edible Oil Quality and Safety for State Market Regulation, Wuhan Institute for Food and Cosmetic Control, 1137 Jinshan Avenue, Wuhan 430012, China; whpuchenzhe@163.com

[3] National Engineering Research Center for Functional Food, School of Food Science and Technology, Jiangnan University, 1800 Lihu Road, Wuxi 214122, China

* Correspondence: gaopan@whpu.edu.cn; Tel./Fax: +86-027-8391-0015

Citation: Gao, P.; Ding, Y.; Chen, Z.; Zhou, Z.; Zhong, W.; Hu, C.; He, D.; Wang, X. Characteristics and Antioxidant Activity of Walnut Oil Using Various Pretreatment and Processing Technologies. *Foods* **2022**, *11*, 1698. https://doi.org/10.3390/foods11121698

Academic Editors: Antonio José Pérez-López and Luis Noguera-Artiaga

Received: 23 May 2022
Accepted: 7 June 2022
Published: 9 June 2022

Publisher's Note: MDPI stays neutral with regard to jurisdictional claims in published maps and institutional affiliations.

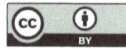

Copyright: © 2022 by the authors. Licensee MDPI, Basel, Switzerland. This article is an open access article distributed under the terms and conditions of the Creative Commons Attribution (CC BY) license (https://creativecommons.org/licenses/by/4.0/).

Abstract: This study was the first time the effects of pretreatment technology (microwave roasting, MR; oven roasting, OR; steaming roasting, SR) and processing technology (screw pressing, SP; aqueous enzymatic extraction, AEE; subcritical butane extraction, SBE) on the quality (physicochemical properties, phytochemical content, and antioxidant ability) of walnut oil were systematically compared. The results showed that the roasting pretreatment would reduce the lipid yield of walnut oil and SBE (59.53–61.19%) was the processing method with the highest yield. SR-AEE oil provided higher acid value (2.49 mg/g) and peroxide value (4.16 mmol/kg), while MR-SP oil had the highest content of polyunsaturated fatty acid (73.69%), total tocopherol (419.85 mg/kg) and total phenolic compounds (TPC, 13.12 mg/kg). The DPPH-polar and ABTS free radicals' scavenging abilities were accorded with SBE > AEE > SP. SBE is the recommended process for improving the extraction yield and antioxidant ability of walnut oil. Hierarchical cluster analysis showed that processing technology had a greater impact on walnut oil than pretreatment technology. In addition, multiple linear regression revealed C18:0, δ-tocopherol and TPC had positive effects on the antioxidant ability of walnut oil, while C18:1n-9, C18:3n-3 and γ-tocopherol were negatively correlated with antioxidant activity. Thus, this a promising implication for walnut oil production.

Keywords: walnut oil; pretreatment; processing; subcritical butane extraction; steaming roasting

1. Introduction

Walnuts (*Juglans regia* L.) are widely cultivated and important oilseed crops in China [1]. Chinese walnut production is 1.78 million tons and its output is 4795.9 kilotons, which accounts for half of the world's walnut production (2020, FAO stat). Walnuts have been eaten in China for thousands of years, influenced by the traditional concept of "shape compensation", as the kinds of nuts that have benefits for brain health [2]. This speculation has also been demonstrated in walnut oil; a recent date showed that walnut oil could reduce memory impairment in mice [3] because walnut oil has anti-inflammatory properties [4]. In recent years, the research on walnut oil has become popular because walnut oil is a kind of edible oil with high nutritional value. Walnut oil nutrition research mainly focuses on the role of walnut oil in intestinal diseases, which is widely used in traditional medicine around the world and is prescribed as beneficial food oil in agroindustry [5]. Walnut oil is a prominent functional food candidate for inflammatory bowel disease treatment [6] and ulcerative colitis treatment [7] because it has good antiaging activity in vivo [8] and can increase antioxidant capacity [9]. The anti-inflammatory action is more dominant in the cases of ameliorating inflammatory bowel disease and ulcerative colitis. Moreover, for the above-mentioned health outcome of preventing memory impairment, antiaging and antioxidative potentials would serve more beneficial roles. The antioxidant capacity of walnut oil is closely related to its processing technology [10]. Therefore, the reports related to walnut oil processing have attracted extensive attention.

Walnut oil processing traditionally focuses on organic solvent extraction [11,12], and it has high volatility, toxicity and flammability [13], which usually involve immense environmental pollution, human health risks and high operating costs [14]. Thus, growing attention has been attracted to developing an environmentally friendly method of extracting walnut oil in recent years. Screw pressing (SP) can produce high-quality oils, be environmentally friendly and require less energy than organic solvent extraction [15]. However, its main disadvantage is that it generates low extraction yields, which limits its industrial use [16]. Aqueous enzymatic extraction (AEE) is a promising methodology since it is ecofriendly and provides healthful nutrition [17]. In addition, the oil obtained is of better quality because it does not present organic solvents or antinutritional compounds (3,4-benzypyrene and other polycyclic aromatic compounds) and the walnut meal is also of superior quality for human and animal consumption [13]. The subcritical butane extraction (SBE) method is another environmentally friendly process method, which is also proven to reduce the degradation of the bioactive components, resulting in a final extracted product that is free of toxic residual solvents [18]. However, AEE and SBE have several disadvantages, such as high costs and low lipid yield [19]. Our previous study [20] proved that roasting pretreatment could improve the lipid yield and bioactive components of walnut oil. Therefore, to improve oil extraction yields or nutrition value, suitable roasting pretreatment methods should be used.

The research on the roasting pretreatment methods of walnut oil focuses on roasting conditions [21–23]. In addition, the effects of walnut oil produced by microwaves and soaking on antioxidant and antiproliferative activity have been compared [24]. Microwave roasting (MR) pretreatment has been proven to improve the oil extraction yield of yellow horn seed kernels [25] and camellia oleifera seed [26]. There are significant differences between MR and oven roasting (OR): the volatile compounds of camellia seed oil prepared by MR and OR are different [27] and the bioactive composition of orange seed oil pretreated by these two methods have differences [28]. In addition, steaming roasting (SR) is also the conventional processing pretreatment of flaxseed oil [29] and camellia seed oil [30]. The advantages of this pretreatment are preventing oil oxidation with an oxygen-free environment and enhancing thermal degradation by increasing heat transfer [31]. Notably, the study of steaming technology to pretreat walnuts and its effect on the nutritional components of walnut oil are scarce.

There are many small walnut oil production enterprises in China and pretreatment and processing methods are various. Therefore, it is very important to systematically compare the effects of roasting pretreatment and processing methods on the quality of walnut oil. In the present study, walnut oil produced using different pretreatment and processing methods was analyzed, including the lipid yield, physicochemical properties, fatty acid composition, phytochemical content, and antioxidant capacity. To guide the production of walnut oil with high nutritional value and better antioxidant capacity, the effects of pretreatment and processing methods on the quality of walnut oil were compared by hierarchical cluster analysis (HCA). Moreover, the main functional substances responsible for the antioxidant capacity of walnut oil were screened by multiple linear regression (MLR). It can be clarified that the impact of pretreatment and processing technologies on the chemical composition of walnut oil obtained the best processing technology of walnut oil and promoted the development of the related industry.

2. Materials and Methods

2.1. Materials

The walnuts were collected from the walnut planting base of Hubei Guicuiyuan Technology Co., Ltd. (Xiangyang, China). The walnut variety is Qingxiang, which was harvested during the 2020–2021 season. The mean value of annual precipitation is about 24.0 to 34.0 mm, air temperature ranges between 10.2 and 12.3 °C, the number of frost-free days is 200 to 230 and the sunshine duration is 2683.5 to 3167.1 h. The walnuts after harvest were transported to the laboratory, dried in an oven at 40 °C for 72 h to make their moisture content less than 8% and processed to walnut oil immediately. Walnut shells were broken by hand, and the kernels were separated from the shells before processing.

2.2. Chemicals and Standards

Standards of 37-fatty acid methyl esters, 2,2-Diphenyl-1-picrylhydrazyl (DPPH), 2,4,6-Tris (2-pyridyl)-S-triazine (TPTZ), 2,2′-Azino-bis (3-ethylbenzothiazoline-6-sulfonic acid) diammonium salt (ABTS) and 6-hydroxy-2,5,7,8-tetramethylchroman-2-carboxylic acid (Trolox) were purchased from Sigma-Aldrich Chemical Co. Ltd. (Shanghai, China). Standards of tocopherols (α-, β-, γ- and δ-tocopherol, purity > 95%), 5α-cholestane, campesterol, stigmasterol and β-sitosterol were provided by Aladdin Chemical Co. Ltd. (Shanghai, China). Cellulase (EC 3.2.1.1, ≥ 400 U/mg) and pectinase (EC 3.2.1.15, ≥ 500 U/mg) were purchased from Pangbo Biological Engineering Co., Ltd. (Nanning, China). Other solvents were obtained from Macklin Reagent Co., Ltd. (Wuhan, Hubei, China).

2.3. Oil Extraction

2.3.1. Roasting Pretreatment

MR: Walnut kernels (500 g) were treated by a microwave-assisted extraction apparatus (Media, Guangzhou, China) for 10 min by applying a 1 min-pause mode, 1 min-run mode action with the condition of microwave power 540 W at a frequency of 2450 MHz.

OR: Walnut kernels (500 g) were subjected to roasting in an oven (GZX-9080, Boxun, China) under 160 °C for 10 min.

SR: Walnut kernels (500 g) were put into a steam generator (FY50, Sanshen, China) under 160 °C for 10 min at 0.54 MPa.

2.3.2. Processing

SP: The walnut samples were pressed at room temperature using a ZJ-707 screw press (Wenfeng, Dongguan, China) to afford the oil, and 10% walnut shell was used as filler. The oil was centrifuged at 4000× g for 20 min at 4 °C.

AEE: The method was according to Cheng et al. [32] with some modifications. The samples were ground into a fine powder and commixed with distilled water at a ratio of 1:5 (w/v); the slurry was heated to 50 °C, held for 30 min and then cooled to the enzymatic digestion temperature. The cellulase and pectinase ratio 1:1 (w/w) was added and the mixture was agitated for 30 min at 40 °C. Enzymatic hydrolysis proceeded for a further 10 min at 90 °C under constant horizontal shaking in a Maxi Mix III rotary shaker (Thomas Scientific, Shanghai, China). The suspension was then centrifuged at 4000× g for 20 min at 4 °C.

SBE: The method was according to our previously published paper [10]. The samples were ground into a fine powder and extracted by subcritical extraction equipment (Zhengzhou, Henan, China) at 45 °C for 60 min in 0.5 MPa with a butane-to-kernel ratio of 7:1 (v/w). The oil was centrifuged at 4000× g for 20 min at 4 °C.

2.4. Physicochemical Properties

The acid value (AV) and peroxide value (PV) were determined according to the Cd 3d-63 and Cd 8b-90 official recommended by AOCS. The oil yield was recorded by the mass of oil extracted and the weight of the walnut kernel at room temperature (25 °C). The continuous bubbling of air at a flow rate of 20 L/h through oil samples (3.0 g) held at

120 °C was used to measure the oxidation stability index (OSI) with a Rancimat 892 model (Metrohm, Switzerland), which was expressed in hours.

2.5. Fatty Acid Composition

The fatty acid composition was carried out by the Agilent 7890A gas chromatography (GC) system (Agilent, CA, USA) by Gao et al. [20] with some modifications. The oil of 0.20 mg was methylated under alkaline conditions and analyzed by a DB-5 capillary column (30 m × 0.25 mm, 0.25 µm, Agilent, CA, USA). The GC adopted a programmed temperature rising mode, with an initial temperature of 60 °C for 3 min and then a temperature of 170 °C at a rate of 5 °C/min for 5 min and a temperature of 220 °C at a rate of 2 °C/min for 10 min. The carrier gas was helium (99.999%) with a flow rate of 1.0 mL/min, the inlet temperature was 250 °C, the injection volume was 1 µL, and the split ratio was 100:1. The fatty acid methyl ester peaks were identified by comparison to the retention times of known standards, and the percentage of each peak area to the sum of all peak areas was quantified.

2.6. Phytochemicals Content

The determination of phytosterols, tocopherols and squalene in pretreatment was as described by Liu et al. [33]. The mobile phase for HPLC-DAD (Ultimate 3000, Thermo Fisher, Waltham, MA, USA) analysis used methanol. The samples were injected onto a C18 Column (5 µm, 150 mm × 2.1 mm; ZORBAX Eclipse Plus, Agilent, CA, USA). The flow rate was 0.7 mL/min with a 10 µL injection volume and maintained the column at 30 °C. The quantification of the analytes by DAD and the wavelengths were 210 nm. The phytochemicals were identified by comparison with authentic standard retention times, and the results were expressed in mg/kg.

A solid phase extraction column (Sepax Technologies, Inc., Newark, DE, USA) and a Folin–Ciocalteu reagent method were used to analyze the content of total phenolic compounds (TPC), which was according to our previous report [9]. According to the gallic acid standard, the TPC content in each walnut oil sample was calculated, and the results were expressed in mg/kg.

2.7. Free Radical Scavenging Capacity

The 2.5 g of walnut oil was added to 5 mL of methanol and shaken 3 min in the dark. The supernatant was separated as the polar extract, and the remainder was retained as the nonpolar extract. Approximately 0.12 g of the walnut oil sample was used as a whole oil for the DPPH assay. Details of the employed methods can be found in our previous paper [10].

2.8. Statistical Analysis

All samples were analyzed in triplicate, and the results were expressed as means ± standard deviations (SDs). Statistical analysis was carried out using SPSS 23.0 (IBM, Armonk, NY, USA). For all evaluated parameters (Duncan's multiple-range tests), ANOVA test results were considered to be statistically different at a level of 5%. Prior to regression analysis, to remove the influence of independent variable units, all independent variables were standardized (converted to z-scores). Hierarchical cluster analysis (HCA) was assessed based on the squared Euclidean distance, and centroid clustering was used to group the samples. Multiple linear regression (MLR) was conducted using a stepwise method.

3. Results and Discussion

3.1. Lipid Yield

Table 1 lists the lipid yields of walnut oils. The results showed that the lipid yield of walnut oil processing decreased in the order of SBE (59.53–61.19%) > AEE (50.64–53.65%) > SP (40.73–46.31%). This may be because SBE has the lowest loss of lipids in a sealed environment. The highest oil content was that of OR-SBE oil, which was 14.88% higher than that of the control (46.31%). However, the effect of pretreatment on the yield had no obvious regularity. The pretreatment decreased the lipid yield of SP oil; the average yield of SP oil samples with pretreatment was 41.60%, which was 4.71% less than that of the control. It proved that pretreatment had a negative effect on the processing of walnut oil by SP. The lipid yield of AEE oil in our study was lower than that of the report (75.4%) [34], which might be because the reaction conditions of AEE were not optimized. The lipid yield of AEE oil would improve by properly optimizing the experimental conditions.

Table 1. The physiochemical indexes and fatty acid compositions (%) of walnut oils.

	SP	MR-SP	OR-SP	SR-SP	MR-AEE	OR-AEE	SR-AEE	MR-SBE	OR-SBE	SR-SBE
Lipid yield (%)	46.31±0.55 f *	40.73 ± 0.41 h	40.79 ± 0.17 h	43.29 ± 0.71 g	53.65 ± 0.33 c	52.73 ± 0.31 d	50.64 ± 0.39 e	60.75 ± 0.30 a	61.19 ± 0.25 a	59.53 ± 0.44 b
Acid value (mg/g)	0.45 ± 0.10 cd	0.57 ± 0.00 c	0.14 ± 0.02 f	0.33 ± 0.01 de	1.12 ± 0.03 b	1.14 ± 0.01 b	2.49 ± 0.16 a	0.26 ± 0.01 ef	0.23 ± 0.00 ef	0.23 ± 0.00 ef
Peroxide value (mmol/kg)	5.56 ± 0.07 a	3.38 ± 0.34 c	2.63 ± 0.24 de	2.45 ± 0.02 e	3.37 ± 0.08 c	2.52 ± 0.18 de	4.16 ± 0.11 b	2.33 ± 0.02 e	2.61 ± 0.05 de	2.81 ± 0.04 d
					Fatty acid (%)					
C16:0	6.41 ± 0.02 a	6.14 ± 0.00 f	6.18 ± 0.02 e	6.19 ± 0.00 de	6.21 ± 0.00 d	6.21 ± 0.01 d	6.25 ± 0.00 c	6.23 ± 0.02 c	6.21 ± 0.01 d	6.30 ± 0.01 b
C18:0	2.75 ± 0.00 abc	2.62 ± 0.01 e	2.70 ± 0.01 d	2.70 ± 0.02 d	2.77 ± 0.02 a	2.76 ± 0.01 ab	2.74 ± 0.00 bc	2.76 ± 0.01 abc	2.74 ± 0.01 c	2.75 ± 0.01 abc
C18:1n-9	18.51 ± 0.03 b	17.36 ± 0.04 i	17.70 ± 0.02 g	18.03 ± 0.02 f	18.84 ± 0.02 a	18.53 ± 0.02 b	18.35 ± 0.02 c	18.10 ± 0.02 e	18.15 ± 0.01 d	17.51 ± 0.02 h
C18:2n-6	62.10 ± 0.01 h	64.95 ± 0.06 a	63.21 ± 0.02 c	62.94 ± 0.01 d	61.73 ± 0.02 j	61.98 ± 0.03 i	62.31 ± 0.02 g	62.55 ± 0.02 f	62.64 ± 0.01 e	63.89 ± 0.02 b
C18:3n-3	10.04 ± 0.02 de	8.75 ± 0.01 h	10.01 ± 0.01 e	9.95 ± 0.01 f	10.26 ± 0.02 b	10.33 ± 0.05 a	10.17 ± 0.03 c	10.17 ± 0.01 c	10.08 ± 0.02 d	9.36 ± 0.02 g
C20:1	0.18 ± 0.00 a	0.19 ± 0.00 a	0.19 ± 0.01 a	0.19 ± 0.00 a	0.19 ± 0.01 a	0.19 ± 0.01 a	0.19 ± 0.00 a	0.19 ± 0.01 a	0.18 ± 0.01 a	0.19 ± 0.00 a
SFA #	9.16 ± 0.02 a	8.76 ± 0.01 f	8.89 ± 0.01 e	8.89 ± 0.02 e	8.98 ± 0.02 c	8.97 ± 0.02 cd	8.99 ± 0.00 c	8.99 ± 0.02 c	8.94 ± 0.01 d	9.05 ± 0.01 b
MUFA	18.69 ± 0.03 b	17.55 ± 0.04 i	17.89 ± 0.01 g	18.22 ± 0.02 f	19.03 ± 0.02 a	18.71 ± 0.02 b	18.54 ± 0.02 c	18.29 ± 0.03 e	18.34 ± 0.02 de	17.70 ± 0.02 h
PUFA	72.15 ± 0.01 g	73.69 ± 0.05 a	73.22 ± 0.02 b	72.89 ± 0.00 c	71.99 ± 0.03 h	72.32 ± 0.03 f	72.47 ± 0.02 e	72.72 ± 0.03 d	72.72 ± 0.02 d	73.25 ± 0.01 b

* Values are means ± standard deviations. The superscript letters indicate the statistical differences in rows at significance level of 5%. # SFA: C14:0 + C16:0 + C18:0, MUFA: C16:1 + C18:1 + C20:1, PUFA: C18:2 + C18:3.

3.2. Physicochemical Properties

The physicochemical properties of walnut oils are shown in Table 1. The AV of oils ranged from 0.14 to 2.49 mg KOH/g, which was lower than the standard of walnut oil in China (≤3 mg KOH/g). The AV of AEE walnut oil was the highest, with an average value of 1.58 mg KOH/g, which was much higher than that of SP (0.35 mg KOH/g) and SBE (0.24 mg KOH/g). Similar to AV results, the PV of SR-AEE oil was also higher (4.16 mmol/kg) than that of other samples. This might be because the triglycerides were broken down into free fatty acids under the action of enzymes, which would produce more free fatty acids, resulting in higher AV and PV [35]. The PV of the control (5.56 mmol/kg) was higher than that of others, which proved that the pretreatment processing could significantly reduce the PV of oils.

3.3. Fatty Acid Composition

Table 1 also shows the fatty acid composition and content of walnut oils. The result was obtained that the pretreatment and processing methods could not change the composition of fatty acid. The main fatty acids of walnut oil were palmitic acid (C16:0, 6.14–6.41%), stearic acid (C18:0, 2.62–2.77%), oleic acid (C18:1n-9, 17.36–18.84%), linoleic acid (C18:2n-6, 61.73–64.95%) and linolenic acid (C18:3n-3, 8.75–10.33%). The C18:1n-9 of AEE oils (average value 18.57%) was higher than that of SP and SBE oils (average values 17.70% and 17.92%, respectively), while the C18:2n-6 content (average value 62.00%) was lower than that of the other two (average values 63.70% and 63.03%, respectively). The result accorded with the rule that C18:1n-9 and C18:2n-6 transformed each other in the process of walnut oil ripening, and their sum was equal (Gao et al., 2021). The C18:2n-6 was the main component of PUFA, MR-SP had the highest C18:2n-6 content (64.95%), and, although the C18:3n-3 content of MR-SP (8.75%) was significantly lower than that of other samples, its PUFA content (73.69%) was the highest among all walnut oils.

3.4. Phytochemicals Content

Table 2 lists the phytochemicals present in walnut oil produced by different pretreatment and processing methods, which included three forms of tocopherol (α, γ and δ), phytosterols, squalene and TPC. The α, γ, δ and total tocopherol contents of all samples were significantly higher than those of the control, which proved that pretreatment and processing could improve the content of tocopherol in walnut oil. For walnut oil with the same processing method, the content of α-tocopherol was MR (17.76–18.84 mg/kg) > OR (16.94–18.62 mg/kg) > SR (13.73–17.56 mg/kg) in descending order according to the pretreatment method, and the content of SR was significantly lower than that of the other two groups. γ-Tocopherol was the major tocopherol in walnut oil, and MR-SP had the highest content (359.90 mg/kg) of all walnut oils, which was 96.42 mg/kg higher than OR-SP. Therefore, its total tocopherol content (419.85 mg/kg) was also the highest, which was 27.41% higher than that of OR-SP. There were significant differences in the δ-tocopherol contents of walnut oils in different processing methods, and the contents were: SBE (45.88–46.71 mg/kg) > AEE (42.97–44.70 mg/kg) > SP (38.36–42.19 mg/kg). Tocopherol is very sensitive and might decompose in an environment subjected to heat and solvents [20].

Table 2. The phytochemicals content (mg/kg) of walnut oils.

	α-Tocopherol	γ-Tocopherol	δ-Tocopherol	Total Tocopherol	Phytosterols	Squalene	TPC
SP	5.64 ± 0.22 [g] *	244.67 ± 14.49 [f]	35.64 ± 0.21 [g]	285.95 ± 14.40 [e]	1474.18 ± 6.31 [d]	8.39 ± 0.01 [g]	6.48 ± 0.02 [e]
MR-SP	17.76 ± 0.11 [b]	359.90 ± 15.02 [a]	42.19 ± 0.09 [e]	419.85 ± 15.01 [a]	1462.65 ± 3.34 [e]	9.60 ± 0.01 [c]	13.12 ± 0.05 [a]
OR-SP	16.94 ± 0.35 [f]	263.48 ± 7.12 [e]	38.36 ± 0.43 [h]	304.78 ± 7.14 [d]	1361.36 ± 4.62 [g]	9.91 ± 0.01 [a]	12.27 ± 0.12 [ab]
SR-SP	13.73 ± 0.17 [e]	313.36 ± 3.00 [cd]	39.64 ± 0.27 [f]	366.73 ± 3.10 [bc]	1367.10 ± 1.31 [g]	8.86 ± 0.01 [f]	10.59 ± 0.14 [c]
MR-AEE	17.76 ± 0.02 [b]	316.42 ± 3.50 [c]	44.61 ± 0.43 [c]	378.79 ± 3.42 [b]	1394.32 ± 3.30 [g]	8.12 ± 0.02 [i]	9.64 ± 0.10 [d]
OR-AEE	17.41 ± 0.09 [c]	296.60 ± 3.31 [d]	44.70 ± 0.09 [c]	358.71 ± 3.29 [c]	1416.75 ± 1.91 [f]	8.24 ± 0.03 [h]	8.13 ± 0.07 [c]
SR-AEE	15.60 ± 0.13 [d]	318.93 ± 6.40 [cd]	42.97 ± 0.60 [d]	377.50 ± 6.31 [b]	1557.00 ± 9.21 [b]	7.65 ± 0.02 [j]	10.45 ± 0.16 [ab]
MR-SBE	18.84 ± 0.04 [a]	305.25 ± 3.19 [cd]	45.88 ± 0.30 [b]	369.97 ± 2.99 [bc]	1560.01 ± 8.19 [b]	9.77 ± 0.03 [b]	10.30 ± 0.11 [ab]
OR-SBE	18.62 ± 0.10 [a]	305.68 ± 3.86 [c]	46.71 ± 0.59 [a]	371.00 ± 4.24 [bc]	1489.75 ± 4.32 [c]	9.10 ± 0.02 [e]	12.16 ± 0.10 [ab]
SR-SBE	17.56 ± 0.17 [bc]	340.23 ± 3.81 [b]	46.17 ± 0.44 [b]	403.96 ± 4.09 [a]	1610.05 ± 7.69 [a]	9.50 ± 0.02 [d]	11.22 ± 0.05 [b]

* Values are means ± standard deviations. The superscript letters indicate the statistical differences in lines at significance level of 5%.

Table 2 also presents the phytosterols, squalene and TPC contents of walnut oil samples. The pretreatment method would reduce the phytosterols content of SP oils, which was significantly lower than that of the control (1474.18 mg/kg). The SR-SBE oil had the highest content, 248.69 mg/kg higher than that of the lowest OR-SP oil. This might be because phytosterols undergo oxidation, isomerization, dehydroxylation, hydrolysis, dehydrogenation and other intermolecular transformation reactions during processing, resulting in significant differences in their contents. In addition, the content of squalene in walnut oil was low (7.65–9.91 mg/kg), while pretreatment methods could significantly increase the content in SP samples. The average squalene content of AEE oils (8.00 mg/kg) was lower than that of the other two; the average contents of SP and SBE were both 9.46 mg/kg. In addition, the results of TPC were similar to those of squalene, pretreatment technology had little influence on the TPC content of walnut oil, and the content had a decreasing order of SP > SBE > AEE > control. MR-SP oil had the highest content (13.12 mg/kg), which was 6.64 mg/kg higher than that of the control.

3.5. Antioxidant Activity

The OSI could be used to predict the shelf life of oil, and the free radical scavenging capacity could evaluate the antioxidant activity of oil from a physiological point of view.

The OSIs and free radical scavenging capacities of walnut oils are shown in Table 3. The OSIs of different walnut oil samples were significantly higher than that of the control (1.80 h), and MR-SP oil had the best oxidative stability (2.63 h). According to the detection rules of the oxidation stabilizer, the oxidation rate was doubled every 10 degrees. Therefore, the results here are better than those of our previous paper [10].

Table 3. Oxidation stability indexes (h) and free radical scavenging capacities (μmol TE /kg) of walnut oils.

	OSI	DPPH-Oil	DPPH-Nonpolar	DPPH-Polar	ABTS	FRAP
SP	1.80 ± 0.05 [e] *	132.93 ± 4.63 [de]	91.64 ± 3.97 [cd]	105.40 ± 10.56 [e]	233.54 ± 3.72 [def]	85.50 ± 5.01 [bc]
MR-SP	2.63 ± 0.08 [a]	171.70 ± 12.20 [abc]	73.26 ± 1.30 [f]	30.69 ± 2.48 [f]	206.70 ± 3.06 [g]	105.61 ± 5.13 [a]
OR-SP	2.53 ± 0.06 [ab]	193.19 ± 4.05 [a]	76.83 ± 3.02 [ef]	43.40 ± 4.92 [f]	227.08 ± 1.22 [f]	67.22 ± 5.95 [e]
SR-SP	2.34 ± 0.05 [c]	157.76 ± 17.96 [bc]	72.59 ± 7.79 [f]	44.70 ± 6.31 [f]	231.06 ± 5.76 [ef]	84.79 ± 3.54 [bc]
MR-AEE	2.14 ± 0.06 [d]	153.92 ± 7.77 [cd]	108.36 ± 3.59 [a]	248.76 ± 9.54 [c]	241.50 ± 3.06 [d]	50.49 ± 5.60 [f]
OR-AEE	2.32 ± 0.02 [c]	128.07 ± 9.33 [e]	101.96 ± 5.86 [ab]	245.03 ± 24.71 [c]	260.39 ± 0.70 [c]	50.25 ± 4.88 [f]
SR-AEE	2.51 ± 0.03 [ab]	147.11 ± 13.64 [de]	94.88 ± 9.22 [bcd]	163.04 ± 18.90 [d]	239.51 ± 9.30 [de]	69.49 ± 7.05 [de]
MR-SBE	2.52 ± 0.04 [ab]	158.22 ± 11.38 [bc]	107.01 ± 4.23 [ab]	373.14 ± 20.78 [a]	269.34 ± 4.28 [b]	80.97 ± 3.94 [bcd]
OR-SBE	2.51 ± 0.08 [ab]	180.54 ± 7.76 [ab]	87.15 ± 10.40 [de]	341.24 ± 21.02 [a]	275.80 ± 2.54 [ab]	91.81 ± 7.28 [b]
SR-SBE	2.48 ± 0.03 [b]	181.67 ± 7.78 [ab]	109.46 ± 2.85 [a]	287.59 ± 20.48 [b]	280.28 ± 1.86 [a]	77.85 ± 1.54 [cde]

* Values are means ± standard deviations. The superscript letters indicate the statistical differences in lines at significance level of 5%.

The DPPH free radical scavenging capacity of the samples was assessed by whole oil, nonpolar and polar extract parts. Except for that of OR-AEE oil (128.07 μmol TE/kg), the DPPH-oil free radical scavenging capacity of all walnut oils was better than that of the control. The DPPH-oil free radical scavenging capacities with different processing methods were significantly different, and AEE oils featured lower capacities than that of others. In contrast, pretreatment methods would reduce the DPPH-nonpolar extract free radical scavenging capacity of SP oils. The free radical scavenging capacities of SP samples (72.59–76.83 μmol TE/kg) were significantly lower than that of the control (91.64 μmol TE/kg). The pretreatment method of DPPH-polar free radical scavenging capacity in SP oils also showed a negative influence, which increased in the order of SP (30.69–44.70 μmol TE/kg) < control (105.40 μmol TE/kg) < AEE (163.04–248.76 μmol TE/kg) < SBE (287.59–373.14 μmol TE/kg). MR-SBE oil with the strongest DPPH-polar free radical scavenging capacity was 12 times higher than that of MR-SP oil, which had the worst effect.

The trend of walnut oil ABTS free radical scavenging capacity was consistent with the DPPH-polar results, which decreased in the order of SBE (269.34–280.28 μmol TE/kg) > AEE (239.51–260.39 μmol TE/kg) > control (233.54 μmol TE/kg) > SP (206.70–231.06 μmol TE/kg). This might be because both DPPH-polar and ABTS assess the ability to quench free radicals by hydrogen donation, which is according to hydrogen atom transfer methods [20]. Generally, the scavenging reaction between radicals and antioxidants present in the oil starts with the transfer of the most labile H atom from the scavenger molecule to the free radical [36]. The FRAP free radical scavenging capacity of AEE oil was lower than that of others, and the OR-AEE oil was the lowest (50.25 μmol TE/kg). MR-SP oil had the highest capacity (105.61 μmol TE/kg) of FRAP, which was 23.52% higher than that of the control and 55.36 μmol TE/kg higher than that of OR-AEE oil.

3.6. HCA Analysis

HCA was used to evaluate the similarities among walnut oils. These results are presented as a dendrogram in Figure 1, which is utilized to convey a hierarchy based on the similarities among different pretreatment and process samples. When the 25-distance threshold was selected, the tree structure of the cluster analysis was divided into two main parts, and walnut oil from SP and other process methods could be clearly distinguished. The results revealed that the processing method significantly affected the chemical components and antioxidant capacity of walnut oil. AEE technology used biological enzyme preparation to destroy or dissolve the cell wall and oil complex after mechanical crushing, and then the oil was extracted by the characteristics of the immiscibility of oil and water [37], while SBE technology used butane as an extraction solvent, according to the principle of similarity and intervisibility [38]. Although the principles of AEE and SBE were different, both of them belonged to extraction technology, which was much different with the SP method. Therefore, we could conclude that processing method had the greatest influence on the characterizations and antioxidant capacity of walnut oil. In addition, the walnut oils obtained with MR and OR pretreatment were more similar in composition and character. This might be because although the heat conduction rates of MR and OR are different, their principles are similar. In heating or roasting, thermal energy reached the surface of walnut kernels by radiation or convection heating, which was then transferred gradually to the bulk of the kernel via conduction [39]. Thus, the contents of phytochemicals and their antioxidant properties were affected in walnut oil.

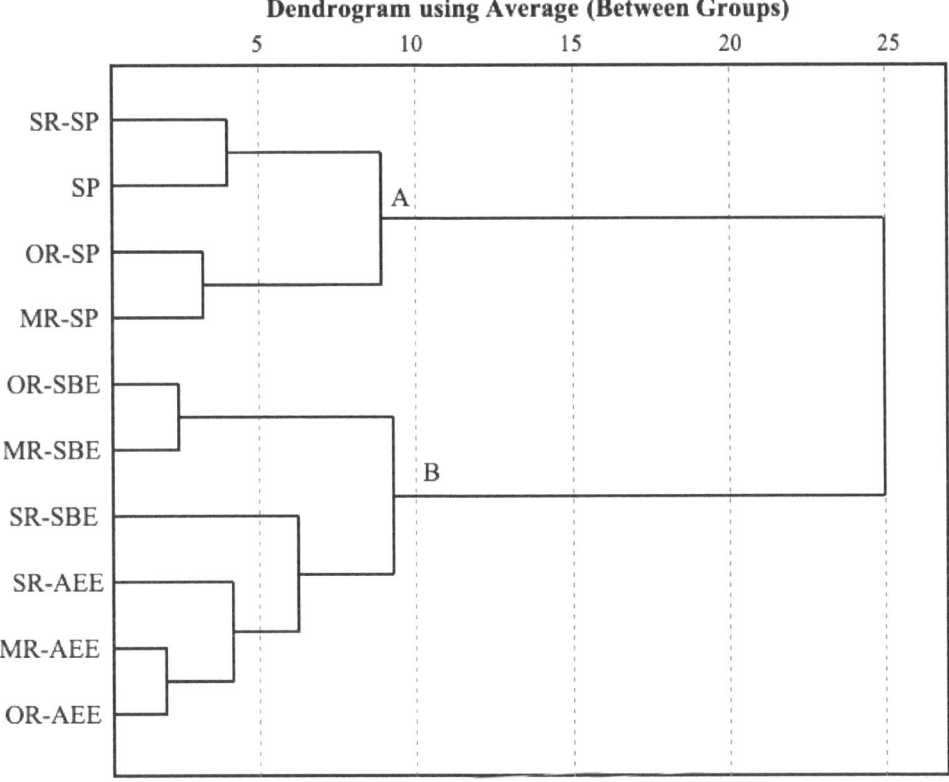

Figure 1. Hierarchical cluster analysis of walnut oils.

3.7. MLR Analysis

As some chemical components of walnut oil might exhibit antioxidant activity, MLR was used to shed light on a certain correlation and mutual restriction between overall antioxidant capacity and that of single or multiple chemical components (Table 4). The OSI and DPPH-oil models showed 0.727 and 0.711 of adjusted R^2, with the partial correlation coefficients of the predicted equation equaling 0.870 and 0.862 for TPC, respectively. The obtained results indicated that the antioxidant activity of whole oil was related only to TPC. OSI and DPPH-oil were two different types of indicators expressing the antioxidant capacity of walnut oil. Our previous research (Gao et al., 2018; Gao et al., 2021) reported that the antioxidant capacity of walnut oil was related to TPC, which was demonstrated again.

Table 4. Equations, variables and regression coefficients in the prediction of antioxidant capacity by multiple linear regression.

Dependent Variable	Adjusted R^2	Variable	Standardized Coefficient	Significance (Two Tails p)	Equation
OSI	0.727	TPC	0.870	0.001	Y = 0.870 (TPC)
DPPH-oil	0.711	TPC	0.862	0.001	Y = 0.862 (TPC)
DPPH-nonpolar	0.772	C18:0	1.344	0.001	Y = 1.344 (C18:0) − 0.689 (C18:3)
		C18:3	−0.689	0.032	
DPPH-polar	0.910	δ-tocopherol	1.260	0.000	Y = 1.260 (δ-tocopherol) − 0.699 (γ-tocopherol)
		γ-tocopherol	−0.699	0.001	
ABTS	0.954	C18:0	0.647	0.007	Y = 0.647 (C18:0) − 0.657 (C18:1) + 0.942 (δ-tocopherol) − 0.601 (γ-tocopherol)
		C18:1	−0.657	0.002	
		δ-tocopherol	0.942	0.002	
		γ-tocopherol	−0.601	0.016	
FRAP	0.395	C18:3	−0.680	0.030	Y = −0.680 (C18:3)

The nonpolar extracts in walnut oil were mainly triglycerides and free fatty acids; thus, C18:0 and C18:3n-3 were the significantly independent variables of DPPH-nonpolar assay. In addition, the model constructed using the results of the ABTS assay showed the highest regression coefficient (R^2 = 0.954) and C18:0, C18:1n-9, δ-tocopherol and γ-tocopherol contents were correlated as Y = 0.647 (C18:0) − 0.657 (C18:1n-9) + 0.942 (δ-tocopherol) − 0.601 (γ-tocopherol). Furthermore, γ-tocopherol exhibited a significant negative contribution to DPPH-polar, while δ-tocopherol (R = 1.260) played an important positive role. Moreover, C18:3n-3 (R = 0.395) influenced the FRAP radical scavenging activity of the samples.

C18:3n-3 was the highest unsaturated fatty acid in walnut oil, and the double bond contained in C18:3n-3 was the main reason for lipid oxidation because the double bond was easy to open and became a free radical receptor under light, heat or other oxidation conditions, which intensified the oxidation reaction; thus, C18:0 could inhibit oxidation. The phenolic hydroxyl groups in tocopherol structure were the main sources of its antioxidant activity, but the methyl substitution of hydroxyl groups at different positions would affect the antioxidant activity and steric hindrance of tocopherol monomers. Therefore, γ-tocopherol and δ-tocopherol showed opposite antioxidant effects in walnut oil.

4. Conclusions

This study investigated the effects of different pretreatment and processing on the chemical properties and quality characteristics of walnut oil. The oil yield of SBE oils (59.53–61.19%) was higher than that of other processing technologies, which also had better DPPH-polar (287.59–373.14 μmol TE/kg) and ABTS (269.34–280.28 μmol TE/kg) free radical scavenging ability. Owing to higher oil yield and better antioxidant activity, SBE processing is recommended for extracting oil from walnuts for various applications in industry. The SR-AEE process resulted in higher acid value (2.49 mg/g) and peroxide value (4.16 mmol/kg), while the MR-SP process would increase the content of PUFA (73.69%), total tocopherol (419.85 mg/kg) and total phenolic compounds (TPC, 13.12 mg/kg). HCA results showed that processing technology formed the main factor affecting the chemical characterizations of walnut oil. Moreover, MLR confirmed that C18:0, C18:1n-9, C18:3n-3, γ- tocopherol, δ-tocopherol and TPC were strongly correlated with the antioxidant capacity of walnut oil.

Author Contributions: Conceptualization, P.G.; methodology, Z.C. and W.Z.; validation, Z.Z. and P.G.; data curation, Y.D.; writing—original draft preparation, P.G.; writing—review and editing, P.G.; supervision, D.H. and X.W.; project administration, C.H. All authors have read and agreed to the published version of the manuscript.

Funding: This work was supported by the National Natural Science Foundation of China Youth Science Foundation Project under Grant 32001735 and the Major Science and Technology Special Project of Yunnan Province "Major Special Projects of Bio-Breeding Industry and Deep Processing of Agricultural Products" (202102AE090055).

Institutional Review Board Statement: Not applicable.

Informed Consent Statement: Not applicable.

Data Availability Statement: No new data were created or analyzed in this study. Data sharing is not applicable to this article.

Acknowledgments: The authors thank the National Natural Science Foundation of China and Key Laboratory of Edible Oil Quality and Safety for State Market Regulation financial support for this research project.

Conflicts of Interest: The authors declare no conflict of interest.

References

1. Garcia-Mendoza, M.D.P.; Espinosa-Pardo, F.A.; Savoire, R.; Etchegoyen, C.; Harscoat-Schiavo, C.; Subra-Paternault, P. Recovery and antioxidant activity of phenolic compounds extracted from walnut press-cake using various methods and conditions. *Ind. Crop. Prod.* **2021**, *167*, 113546. [CrossRef]
2. Zhao, F.; Liu, C.; Fang, L.; Lu, H.; Wang, J.; Gao, Y.; Gabbianelli, R.; Min, W. Walnut-Derived Peptide Activates PINK1 via the NRF2/KEAP1/HO-1 Pathway, Promotes Mitophagy, and Alleviates Learning and Memory Impairments in a Mice Model. *J. Agric. Food Chem.* **2021**, *69*, 2758–2772. [CrossRef] [PubMed]
3. Liao, J.; Nai, Y.; Feng, L.; Chen, Y.; Li, M.; Xu, H. Walnut Oil Prevents Scopolamine-Induced Memory Dysfunction in a Mouse Model. *Molecules* **2020**, *25*, 1630. [CrossRef] [PubMed]
4. Bartoszek, A.; Makaro, A.; Bartoszek, A.; Kordek, R.; Fichna, J.; Salaga, M. Walnut Oil Alleviates Intestinal Inflammation and Restores Intestinal Barrier Function in Mice. *Nutrients* **2020**, *12*, 1302. [CrossRef] [PubMed]
5. Miao, F.; Shan, C.; Shah, S.A.H.; Akhtar, R.W.; Wang, X.; Ning, D. Effect of walnut (*Juglans sigillata*) oil on intestinal antioxidant, anti-inflammatory, immunity, and gut microbiota modulation in mice. *J. Food Biochem.* **2020**, *45*, e13567. [CrossRef] [PubMed]
6. Miao, F.; Shan, C.; Ning, D. Walnut oil alleviates LPS-induced intestinal epithelial cells injury by inhibiting TLR4/MyD88/NF-κB pathway activation. *J. Food Biochem.* **2021**, *45*, e13955. [CrossRef]
7. Miao, F.; Shan, C.; Ma, T.; Geng, S.; Ning, D. Walnut oil alleviates DSS–induced colitis in mice by inhibiting NLRP3 inflammasome activation and regulating gut microbiota. *Microb. Pathog.* **2021**, *154*, 104866. [CrossRef]
8. Tian, W.; Wu, B.; Sun, L.; Zhuang, Y. Protective effect against d-gal-induced aging mice and components of polypeptides and polyphenols in defatted walnut kernel during simulated gastrointestinal digestion. *J. Food Sci.* **2021**, *86*, 2736–2752. [CrossRef]
9. Gencoglu, H.; Orhan, C.; Tuzcu, M.; Sahin, N.; Juturu, V.; Sahin, K. Effects of walnut oil on metabolic profile and transcription factors in rats fed high-carbohydrate/fat diets. *J. Food Biochem.* **2020**, *44*, e13235. [CrossRef]
10. Gao, P.; Liu, R.; Jin, Q.; Wang, X. Effects of processing methods on the chemical composition and antioxidant capacity of walnut (*Juglans regia* L.) oil. *LWT* **2021**, *135*, 109958. [CrossRef]
11. Juhaimi, F.; Özcan, M.M.; Ghafoor, K.; Babiker, E.E.; Hussain, S. Comparison of cold-pressing and soxhlet extraction systems for bioactive compounds, antioxidant properties, polyphenols, fatty acids and tocopherols in eight nut oils. *J. Food Sci. Technol.* **2018**, *55*, 3163–3173. [CrossRef] [PubMed]
12. Gharibzahedi, S.M.T.; Mousavi, M.; Hamedi, M.; Rezaei, K.; Khodaiyan, F. Evaluation of physicochemical properties and antioxidant activities of Persian walnut oil obtained by several extraction methods. *Ind. Crop. Prod.* **2013**, *45*, 133–140. [CrossRef]
13. Aquino, D.S.; Fanhani, A.; Stevanato, N.; Da Silva, C. Sunflower oil from enzymatic aqueous extraction process: Maximization of free oil yield and oil characterization. *J. Food Process Eng.* **2019**, *42*, e13169. [CrossRef]
14. Liu, Z.; Gui, M.; Xu, T.; Zhang, L.; Kong, L.; Qin, L.; Zou, Z. Efficient aqueous enzymatic-ultrasonication extraction of oil from Sapindus mukorossi seed kernels. *Ind. Crop. Prod.* **2019**, *134*, 124–133. [CrossRef]
15. Rabadán, A.; Pardo, J.E.; Gómez, R.; Álvarez-Ortí, M. Influence of temperature in the extraction of nut oils by means of screw pressing. *LWT* **2018**, *93*, 354–361. [CrossRef]
16. Díaz-Suárez, P.; Rosales-Quintero, A.; Fernandez-Lafuente, R.; Pola-Sánchez, E.; Hernández-Cruz, M.C.; Ovando-Chacón, S.L.; Rodrigues, R.C.; Tacias-Pascacio, V.G. Aqueous enzymatic extraction of *Ricinus communis* seeds oil using *Viscozyme L*. *Ind. Crop. Prod.* **2021**, *170*, 113811. [CrossRef]
17. Liu, J.J.; Gasmalla, M.A.A.; Li, P.; Yang, R. Enzyme-assisted extraction processing from oilseeds: Principle, processing and application. *Innov. Food Sci. Emerg. Technol.* **2016**, *35*, 184–193. [CrossRef]
18. Uoonlue, N.; Muangrat, R. Effect of different solvents on subcritical solvent extraction of oil from Assam tea seeds (*Camellia sinensis* var. *assamica*): Optimization of oil extraction and physicochemical analysis. *J. Food Process Eng.* **2019**, *42*, e12960. [CrossRef]
19. Song, Y.; Zhang, W.; Wu, J.; Admassu, H.; Liu, J.; Zhao, W.; Yang, R. Ethanol-Assisted Aqueous Enzymatic Extraction of Peony Seed Oil. *J. Am. Oil Chem. Soc.* **2019**, *96*, 595–606. [CrossRef]

20. Gao, P.; Liu, R.; Jin, Q.; Wang, X. Comparison of Different Processing Methods of Iron Walnut Oils (*Juglans sigillata*): Lipid Yield, Lipid Compositions, Minor Components, and Antioxidant Capacity. *Eur. J. Lipid Sci. Technol.* **2018**, *120*, 1800151. [CrossRef]
21. Niu, B.; Olajide, T.; Liu, H.; Pasdar, H.; Weng, X. Effects of different baking techniques on the quality of walnut and its oil. *Grasas y Aceites* **2021**, *72*, e406. [CrossRef]
22. Ghafoor, K.; Al Juhaimi, F.; Geçgel, Ü.; EBabiker, E.; Özcan, M.M. Influence of Roasting on Oil Content, Bioactive Components of Different Walnut Kernel. *J. Oleo Sci.* **2020**, *69*, 423–428. [CrossRef] [PubMed]
23. Chang, S.K.; Alasalvar, C.; Bolling, B.; Shahidi, F. Nuts and their co-products: The impact of processing (roasting) on phenolics, bioavailability, and health benefits—A comprehensive review. *J. Funct. Foods* **2016**, *26*, 88–122. [CrossRef]
24. Anjum, S.; Gani, A.; Ahmad, M.; Shah, A.; Masoodi, F.A.; Shah, Y.; Gani, A. Antioxidant and Antiproliferative Activity of Walnut Extract (*Juglans regia* L.) Processed by Different Methods and Identification of Compounds Using GC/MS and LC/MS Technique. *J. Food Process. Preserv.* **2017**, *41*, e12756. [CrossRef]
25. Li, J.; Zu, Y.G.; Luo, M.; Gu, C.B.; Zhao, C.; Efferth, T.; Fu, Y.J. Aqueous enzymatic process assisted by microwave extraction of oil from yellow horn (*Xanthoceras sorbifolia* Bunge.) seed kernels and its quality evaluation. *Food Chem.* **2013**, *138*, 2152–2158. [CrossRef]
26. Zhang, W.G. Aqueous Extraction and Nutraceuticals Content of Oil Using Industrial Enzymes from Microwave Puffing-pretreated Camellia oleifera Seed Powder. *Food Sci. Technol. Res.* **2016**, *22*, 31–38. [CrossRef]
27. Suri, K.; Singh, B.; Kaur, A.; Yadav, M.P.; Singh, N. Influence of microwave roasting on chemical composition, oxidative stability and fatty acid composition of flaxseed (*Linum usitatissimum* L.) oil. *Food Chem.* **2020**, *326*, 126974. [CrossRef]
28. Güneşer, B.A.; Yilmaz, E. Comparing the effects of conventional and microwave roasting methods for bioactive composition and the sensory quality of cold-pressed orange seed oil. *J. Food Sci. Technol.* **2018**, *56*, 634–642. [CrossRef]
29. Yu, G.; Guo, T.; Huang, Q.; Shi, X.; Zhou, X. Preparation of high-quality concentrated fragrance flaxseed oil by steam explosion pretreatment technology. *Food Sci. Nutr.* **2020**, *8*, 2112–2123. [CrossRef]
30. He, J.; Wu, X.; Zhou, Y.; Chen, J. Effects of different preheat treatments on volatile compounds of camellia (*Camellia oleifera* Abel.) seed oil and formation mechanism of key aroma compounds. *J. Food Biochem.* **2021**, *45*, e13649. [CrossRef]
31. Idrus, N.F.M.; Zzaman, W.; Yang, T.A.; Easa, A.M.; Sharifudin, M.S.; Noorakmar, B.W.; Jahurul, M.H.A. Effect of superheated-steam roasting on physicochemical properties of peanut (*Arachis hypogea*) oil. *Food Sci. Biotechnol.* **2017**, *26*, 911–920. [CrossRef] [PubMed]
32. Cheng, M.H.; Rosentrater, K.A.; Sekhon, J.; Wang, T.; Jung, S.; Johnson, L.A. Economic Feasibility of Soybean Oil Production by Enzyme-Assisted Aqueous Extraction Processing. *Food Bioprocess Technol.* **2019**, *12*, 539–550. [CrossRef]
33. Liu, S.; Hu, H.; Yu, Y.; Zhao, J.; Liu, L.; Zhao, S.; Xie, J.; Li, C.; Shen, M. Simultaneous Determination of Tocopherols, Phytosterols, and Squalene in Vegetable Oils by High Performance Liquid Chromatography-Tandem Mass Spectrometry. *Food Anal. Methods* **2021**, *14*, 1567–1576. [CrossRef]
34. González-Gómez, D.; Ayuso-Yuste, M.C.; Blanco-Roque, C.; Bernalte-García, M.J. Optimization of enzyme-assisted aqueous method for the extraction of oil from walnuts using response surface methodology. *J. Food Process. Preserv.* **2019**, *43*, e14218. [CrossRef]
35. Soo, P.; Ali, Y.; Lai, O.; Kuan, C.; Tang, T.; Lee, Y.; Phuah, E. Enzymatic and Mechanical Extraction of Virgin Coconut Oil. *Eur. J. Lipid Sci. Technol.* **2020**, *122*, 1900220. [CrossRef]
36. Brozničć, D.; Jurešić, G.; Milin, Č. Involvement of α-, γ- and δ-tocopherol isomers from pumpkin (*Cucurbita pepo* L.) seed oil or oil mixtures in the biphasic DPPH disappearance kinetics. *Food Technol. Biotechnol.* **2016**, *54*, 200–210. [CrossRef]
37. Nguyen, H.C.; Vuong, D.P.; Nguyen, N.T.T.; Nguyen, N.P.; Su, C.H.; Wang, F.-M.; Juan, H.Y. Aqueous enzymatic extraction of polyunsaturated fatty acid–rich sacha inchi (*Plukenetia volubilis* L.) seed oil: An eco-friendly approach. *LWT* **2020**, *133*, 109992. [CrossRef]
38. Teixeira, G.L.; Ghazani, S.M.; Corazza, M.L.; Marangoni, A.G.; Ribani, R.H. Assessment of subcritical propane, supercritical CO_2 and Soxhlet extraction of oil from sapucaia (*Lecythis pisonis*) nuts. *J. Supercrit. Fluids* **2018**, *133*, 122–132. [CrossRef]
39. Mazaheri, Y.; Torbati, M.; Azadmard-Damirchi, S.; Savage, G.P. Effect of roasting and microwave pre-treatments of *Nigella sativa* L. seeds on lipase activity and the quality of the oil. *Food Chem.* **2019**, *274*, 480–486. [CrossRef]

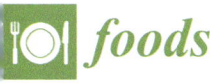

Article

Effect of Pulsed Light on Quality of Shelled Walnuts

Vicente Manuel Gómez-López [1], Luis Noguera-Artiaga [2], Fernando Figueroa-Morales [3], Francisco Girón [3], Ángel Antonio Carbonell-Barrachina [2], José Antonio Gabaldón [3] and Antonio Jose Pérez-López [3,*]

[1] Catedra Alimentos para la Salud, Campus de los Jerónimos, Universidad Católica San Antonio de Murcia (UCAM), 30107 Murcia, Spain; vmgomez@ucam.edu
[2] Research Group "Food Quality and Safety", Centro de Investigación e Innovación Agroalimentaria y Agroambiental (CIAGRO-UMH), Miguel Hernández University of Elche (UMH), Carretera de Beniel km 3.2, 03312 Orihuela, Spain; lnoguera@umh.es (L.N.-A.); angel.carbonell@umh.es (Á.A.C.-B.)
[3] Department of Food Technology and Nutrition, Catholic University of San Antonio, Campus de los Jerónimos s/n, Guadalupe, 30107 Murcia, Spain; ffigueroa@ucam.edu (F.F.-M.); fgiron@ucam.edu (F.G.); jagabaldon@ucam.edu (J.A.G)
* Correspondence: ajperez@ucam.edu; Tel.: + 34-968-278-622

Abstract: Shelled walnuts are considered a microbiologically low-risk food but have been linked to some outbreaks, and a treatment aiming to decrease this risk is desirable. Pulsed light (PL) may be an alternative, providing it does not seriously impair their quality. This work assessed the impact of PL on some quality attributes of walnuts. To do this, measurements of rancidity, volatiles, total phenols, antioxidant activity, and descriptive sensory analysis were carried out on untreated and PL (43 J/cm^2)-treated kernels. PL had no statistically significant ($p > 0.05$) effects on TBARS, peroxide value, total phenols, and antioxidant activity but significantly increased the concentration of volatiles related to green/herbaceous odors and decreased compounds related to fruity and citrus odors. The descriptors nut overall, walnut odor and flavor, and aftertaste were given statistically significantly ($p < 0.05$) higher scores, while descriptors woody odor and sweet received lower scores; 16 other traits such as all those related to color, texture, and rancidity were unaffected. No significant ($p > 0.05$) effects on total phenols and antioxidant activity in general were observed during the course of PL treatment. It can be concluded that PL technology may be used in shelled walnuts with only mild effects on their quality; a storage study must be carried out in order to determine the effect of PL treatment on its shelf-life.

Keywords: pulsed light; walnut; UV light; non-thermal; rancidity; sensory; volatiles; food quality; nut

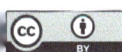

1. Introduction

Pulsed light (PL) is a non-thermal processing technology based on the application of repetitive flashes of a non-coherent, broad-spectrum, high-intensity light. It has been developed in the context of the technologies aimed to increase the safety of foods avoiding the deleterious effect of heating. Its spectrum is composed of infrared, visible light, and UV light. The UV-C sub-band accounts for much of its microbicide action. Its application is limited to the decontamination of surfaces and UV-transparent liquids because of its low penetration power [1]. The capability of PL to yield fast effects is one of its main features. It is more efficient than low- and medium-pressure mercury lamps on a per time and fluence basis, and it is more ecologically friendly than them because lamps are filled with an inert (xenon) gas rather than mercury [2]. Fluence (J/cm^2) is the unit used to characterize PL treatments; it is the measure of the amount of energy impinging a target surface per amount of target surface [3].

The efficacy of PL to inactivate microorganisms on food surfaces has been successfully tested in a wide variety of foods, including nuts such as almond kernels [4] and shelled walnuts [5].

Walnuts (*Juglans regia* L.) are considered a low-risk food from the microbiological point of view due to their low water activity; however, several outbreaks caused by their consumption have been reported. In 2011, an outbreak linked to the consumption of shelled walnuts contaminated by *Escherichia coli* O157:H7 was reported in Canada. Some affected people were hospitalized, and a few developed hemolytic uremic syndrome [6]. *Salmonella* has been detected in walnuts [7–10] and in a pre-packed mixture of nuts that included walnuts [11]. A total of 11 out of 20 walnut recalls due to food pathogen concerns registered in the USA between 2010 and 2015 were linked to *Salmonella* [12]. This pathogen has been shown to be capable of long-term survival on the surface of walnut kernels [8]. Santillana-Farakos et al. (2019) [13], based on a quantitative risk assessment of human salmonellosis from consumption of walnuts in the United States, have predicted that a minimum 3-log *Salmonella* reduction treatment would result in less than one case of salmonellosis per year linked to the consumption of walnuts. It has recently been shown that PL can achieve that level of *Salmonella* inactivation in shelled walnuts [5] when applying 41.2 J/cm^2. However, this finding would not have a practical application if PL deteriorates the quality of nuts. Walnuts are very rich in lipids; they are rich in polyunsaturated fatty acids with a high linoleic acid content and particularly high ω3:ω6 ratio, which is the highest of all the tree nuts [14]. It is well known that the exposure to UV light in foods with high amounts of unsaturated fatty acids in the presence of oxygen promotes rancidity; therefore, a detailed analysis of the potentially harmful effects of PL applied to shelled walnuts at a fluence level required to reach 3-log *Salmonella* reduction is deserved. Izmirlioglu et al. (2020) [5] reported that PL has no significant effect on the color nor malondialdehyde levels (rancidity indicator) of shelled walnuts; however, the fluences applied to the samples used in these determinations were far below the fluence they used to achieve the 3-log *Salmonella* reduction. Furthermore, walnuts have a wide arrange of volatile compounds that affect their quality perception and stability, and the potential generation of new volatile compounds after walnut processing by novel technologies should be assessed.

Walnuts exhibit interesting nutritional properties due to their high content of linoleic acid and phenolic compounds, which have antioxidant activity [15,16]. The preservation of their antioxidant capacity is desirable not only because it is related to health properties but also because it helps to prevent fatty acid oxidation [17].

Therefore, in order to assess the actual potential application of PL to achieve 3-log *Salmonella* reduction in shelled walnuts without significantly harming their quality, a comprehensive evaluation of the effect of the required fluence (41.2 J/cm^2) on the quality of this product is deserved. Research with this aim was undertaken, which included measurements of lipid oxidation, volatile compounds, and descriptive sensory analysis together with determinations of health-related compounds such as total phenols as well as antioxidant capacity.

2. Materials and Methods

2.1. Walnut Source and Composition

Walnuts (*Juglans regia* L. var. Chandler) were provided by a local supplier from Orihuela (Alicante, Spain) and stored at 8 °C until used. Walnut shells were mechanically broken and kernels extracted and halved.

Moisture was determined by drying the samples to constant weight at 95–100 °C (AOAC method 925.40, 2005) [18]. Ashes were quantified by means of sample incineration in a muffle furnace as described by AOAC [19]. The protein content in walnuts was calculated by multiplying the total nitrogen content obtained by the Kjeldahl method [20] by a conversion factor of 5.30 [21]. The quantitative determination of the total oil of the samples was carried out by extraction in Soxtec equipment (Avanti 2055) according to AOAC [22]. Carbohydrates were calculated by difference.

2.2. Walnut Treatment

PL was applied to shelled walnuts by using a commercial system (XeMaticA-Basic-1 L, Steribeam, Germany), whose characteristics can be found in Pérez-López et al. (2020) [23]. Eight halves of walnuts were placed in two rows along the longitudinal axis of the lamp below it. The position of halves was changed clockwise in order to maximize a homogeneous exposition to the lamp. Once the pre-set number of pulses was delivered, samples were turned upside down, and the same number of pulses was applied on the other side. Treatments were carried out in triplicate, and samples were analyzed immediately post treatment or their oil immediately extracted, depending on the intended analysis.

Light pulses were generated at 2.5 kV, which gives place to a characteristic emission spectrum that has previously been reported [24]. Each light pulse delivered a fluence at the walnut surface of 2.14 J/cm^2. Samples were treated with 0, 5, 10, 15, or 20 pulses, which correspond respectively to fluences of 0, 10.7, 21.4, 32.1, and 42.8 J/cm^2.

2.3. Lipid Oxidation

In order to extract the oil, the shell was removed from the samples manually until obtaining 25 g of walnut. This quantity was mixed with 250 mL of hexane (1:10 w/v) (Scharlau, Sentmenat, Spain) and homogenized in Ultraturrax T-18 basic for 3 min. The lipid fraction was taken to a rotary evaporator, distilling under vacuum until the removal of the hexane. The hexane-free oil was dried over sodium sulfate (Merck Darmstadt, Germany) and filtered (Whatman # 4 filter paper). The samples were stored in the dark at $-80\,°C$ until further analysis (up to 24 h).

2.3.1. Thiobarbituric Acid Reactive Substances (TBARS)

For the determination of TBARS, 5 mL of oil and 5 mL of thiobarbituric acid solution (Sigma, Steinheim, Germany) were mixed and heated for pink color development at 80 °C for 40 min in a water bath. Once finished, samples were cooled to room temperature (~22 °C; 1 h), and the absorbance (532 nm) was measured with a Varian Cary 50 Bio spectrophotometer (Varian, Palo Alto, CA, USA). The concentration of TBARS in samples was obtained from a standard curve of malondialdehyde (Sigma, Steinheim, Germany) and expressed as mg of malondialdehyde per liter of oil [25].

2.3.2. Peroxide Value

The method developed by Buege and Aust (1978) [26], with slight modifications, was used to the determination of the peroxide value (mmol O_2/g of walnut oil). A total of 5 g of walnut oil and 30 mL of acetic acid solution (50% acetic acid (Normapur, NWR), 50% chloroform (Normapur, NWR)) were homogenized in a 250 mL test flask.

After vortexing, the samples were incubated in hot water (50 °C) for 30 min. Then, samples were filtered using Whatman # 4 filter paper. The filtrate was received in 0.5 mL of KI (Scharlau, Sentmenat, Spain) (50%), kept in darkness for 2 min, three drops of 1% starch (Panreac-Apllichem, Barcelona, Spain) were added (as an indicator), and the mixture was titrated with $Na_2S_2O_3 \cdot 5H_2O$ (Scharlau, Sentmenat, Spain) (0.01M) added dropwise until reaching the end point.

The peroxide value, expressed in milliequivalents of active oxygen per kg of oil, was calculated using the following formula: PV = volume of sodium thiosulphate × 0.1 N × 1000/mass of oil.

2.4. Volatile Compounds

The volatile composition of the walnut samples untreated (control) and subjected to a PL treatment of 42.8 J/cm^2 was determined using headspace solid-phase micro-extraction (HS-SPME) following the method previously described by Noguera-Artiaga et al. (2020) [27]. Prior to the optimization of the method, tests were carried out to determine the amount of sample that offered the best signal results. After that, 2 g of sample, 1 g of NaCl, and 10 g of ultrapure water were weighed and added into a 20 mL vial. The sample was analyzed in a Shimadzu AOC-6000 Plus autosampler (Shimadzu Corporation, Kyoto, Japan), and after 10 min of equilibration time, a 50/30 μm DVB/CAR/PDMS fiber (1 cm) was exposed for 45 min at 40 °C to the sample headspace (throughout the extraction it was kept under constant agitation of 300 rpm). A GC2030 (Shimadzu Scientific Instruments, Inc., Columbia, MD, USA) was used for the separation of compounds, and a mass spectrometer detector (TQ8040 NX triple quadrupole mass spectrometer; Shimadzu Scientific Instruments, Inc., Columbia, MD, USA) was used to the detection. The chromatographic column used was Sapiens X5MS (Teknokroma, Barcelona, Spain), 30 m × 0.25 mm i.d., 0.25 μm film thickness. Only the single quadrupole acquisition mode was used on the TQ8040 NX (Q3 Scan; event time 0.100 s; mass range 40–300 m/z; scan speed 5000 amu/s). The oven temperature program was as follows:

(i) Initial temperature of 40 °C and hold for 5 min;
(ii) Ramp of 2 °C/min up to 140 °C;
(iii) Ramp of 5 °C/min up to 210 °C;
(iv) Ramp of 20 °C/min up to 230 °C, and hold 10 min.

The pressure at the head of the column was 50.4 kPa with a constant linear velocity mode of 36.3 cm/s. The interface temperature was 280 °C. The ion source temperature was 230 °C. The injector temperature was 250 °C. The carrier gas was helium, with a column flow of 1.01 mL/min, and the injector worked in splitless mode and with a purge flow of 6 mL/min.

A commercial alkane standard mixture (Sigma-Aldrich, Steinheim, Germany) was used to obtain the retention indexes, as well as the NIST 17 Mass Spectral and Retention Index Libraries. When it was based only on mass spectral data, the identification was considered tentative. Only compounds with spectra similarity >90% and with a deviation less than 10 units of linear retention similarity were considered as correct hits.

2.5. Descriptive Sensory Analysis

The sensory analysis of shelled walnuts untreated (control) and subjected to a PL treatment of 42.8 J/cm^2 was performed by a panel of 10 highly trained panelists (aged 30 to 62 years; six female) from the Food Quality and Safety research group (Escuela Politécnica Superior de Orihuela, Spain). Each panelist had more than 1000 h of experience with sensory analysis of nuts and other foods. The methodology used for the descriptive sensory analysis was that previously described by Noguera-Artiaga et al. (2019) and Carbonell-Barrachina et al. (2015) [28,29]. The lexicon developed and used for the analysis of the samples is shown in Table 1. A total of 2 appearance descriptors were studied (color and color homogeneity), 6 odor descriptors (nut overall, walnut, roasted, woody, earthy, and rancy), 10 flavor descriptors (nut overall, walnut, roasted, woody, earthy, rancy, sweet, bitter, astringent, and aftertaste), and 5 texture descriptors (hardness, crunchiness, friability, adhesiveness, and oiliness). The scale used ranged from 0 to 10 (0 = without intensity and 10 = high intensity) with increments of 0.5 units. Ten walnuts were served to panelists in odor-free disposable 50 mL biodegradable cups, coded using 3-digit numbers at room temperature (~22 °C). To clean their palates between samples, unsalted crackers and mineral water were provided to panelists. Analyses were run in triplicate ($n = 3$).

Table 1. Appearance, flavor, and texture attributes and definitions used in the study.

Sensory Descriptor	Definition	References and Intensities
Color	Visual evaluation of color intensity of sample	Pantone 17-1052 TCX = 8.5
Color homogeneity	Distribution of the main color in the sample	% of total of sample
Odor and flavor		
Nut overall	The nut-like aromatic that is typical of nuts such as pistachios and almonds.	Nuts Mix "Borges" = 8.0
Walnut	Aromatic reminiscent of walnut	NOW Foods Raw Walnuts = 8.0

Table 1. Cont.

Sensory Descriptor	Definition	References and Intensities
Roasted	Dark-brown odor and flavor notes of products cooked without including bitter or burned notes	Roasted peanuts (Planters) = 5.0
Woody	Aroma associated with woody notes such as those associated with dried fruit shells	Whole peanuts (with shell) = 8.5
Earthy	Aroma related to wet dirt	Pomegranate "Mollar de Elche" = 5.0
Rancy	Aroma related to fat rancidity	Standard of the International Olive Council 5 g L^{-1} = 3.5
Basic tastes		
Sweet	The taste stimulated by substances such as sucrose or stevia	Sucrose solution 2.5 g L^{-1} = 3.5
Bitter	The taste stimulated by substances such as caffeine or quinine	Caffeine solution 1 g L^{-1} = 3.0
Astringent	The puckering or shrinking of the mouth caused by substances such as alum or tannins.	Alum solution 1.5 g L^{-1} = 1.5
Aftertaste	Time that the characteristic flavor of walnut remains in the mouth after swallowing or expectorating the sample.	5 s = 1.0 20 s = 10
Texture		
Hardness	The force required to bite food with molar teeth. Evaluate with the molars and on first bite.	Carrots = 7.5 Land O'Lakes American Cheese = 3.0
Crunchiness	Sound associated with mastication of sample with molars	Cheerios = 7.5
Friability	After chewing, the number of pieces the food breaks into sunke	Carrots fresh = 1.5 Soft brownie Little Debbie = 8.5
Adhesiveness	Amount of product that remains adhered to the teeth after chewing	Mushrooms unpeeled = 2.0 Chocolate MilkyWay bar = 9.5
Oiliness	Oily sensation left in the mouth after chewing the sample	Lay's potato chips = 8.0

2.6. Total Phenolic Compounds and Antioxidant Activity

Sample preparation was carried out following that described by Pérez-Jiménez et al. (2008) [30], with some modifications. Extracts were analyzed the same day of the treatments.

2.6.1. Total Phenolic Compounds

For sample preparation, 5 g of walnuts were homogenized in an Ultraturrax T-18 basic for 2 min, at 24,000 rpm with 20 mL of a 3% methanol (Carlo Erba Reagents, France) + formic acid (Normapur, NWR) solution. The extracts were centrifuged for 10 min at 4000 x g in a Heraeus Biofuge Stratos centrifuge. The supernatant, methanolic extract, was separated from the precipitate and filtered through Whatman # 4 filter paper and collected in opaque flasks. The precipitate was subjected to a new extraction process under identical conditions, and its methanolic extract was joined to that obtained after the first extraction.

The content of total phenolic compounds (TPC) of walnut extracts was determined using the Folin–Ciocalteu method [31]. The reaction mixture contained 1 mL of walnut extracts, 5 mL of the Folin–Ciocalteu reagent (Merck; Darmstadt, Germany, and 20 mL of sodium carbonate (200 mg/L) (Scharlau, Sentmenat, Spain). The final volume was made up to 50 mL with distilled water. After 30 min of reaction, the absorbance at 765 nm was measured in a spectrophotometer Varian Cary 50 Bio (Varian, Palo Alto, CA, USA). The determinations were carried out in triplicate, and TPC content was expressed as g of gallic acid/L by using a calibration curve of pure gallic acid (Sigma-Aldrich, St. Louis, MO, USA).

2.6.2. FRAP Assay

The analysis of antioxidant capacity by the ferric reducing antioxidant power (FRAP) assay was performed according to Benzie and Strain (1996) [32]. The determinations were carried out at 595 nm and 37 °C after 30 min of incubation in a spectrophotometer Molecular Devices LLC (Sunnyvale, CA, USA). Solutions of known Trolox (Sigma, Steinheim, Germany) concentrations are used for calibration. The antioxidant capacity was expressed as µM.

2.6.3. DPPH Assay

The analysis of antioxidant capacity by DPPH radical scavenging was carried out according to Bondet et al. (1997) [33]. Briefly, 5 µL of each sample was added to 1 mL of 2,2-diphenyl-1-picrylhydrazyl (Sigma, Steinheim, Germany) solution (0.094 mM in methanol). Then, after 60 min at 20 °C, the absorbance of samples was determined at 515 nm in a spectrophotometer. The antioxidant capacity was reported as µM equivalents of Trolox.

2.6.4. ABTS Assay

To determine the scavenging capacity of walnuts against the ABTS radical was performed the method previously described by Miller and Rice-Evans (1997) [34]. The blue-green ABTS$^{\bullet+}$ was produced through the reaction between 2,2'-azino-bis(3-ethylbenzothiazoline-6-sulfonic acid (Sigma, Steinheim, Germany) and activated manganese dioxide (Scharlau, Sentmenat, Spain) in water. Then, the solution was kept overnight in darkness before use. To obtain the results, 900 mL of ABTS$^{\bullet+}$ solution was added to the samples, and after 6 min of incubation in the darkness, at room temperature (22 °C), the absorbance was measured at 734 nm. Results were expressed as µM equivalents of Trolox.

2.7. Statistical Analysis

Data were analyzed for normality and homoscedasticity by the Kolmogorov–Smirnov and Levene tests, respectively, and for significant differences by one-way ANOVA and Tukey test, using IBM SPSS Statistics 27. Experiments were repeated three times.

3. Results and Discussion

The proximal composition of the walnuts used in this research was 3.60 ± 0.41 moisture, 16.26 ± 0.70 proteins, 65.73 ± 1.30 oil, 2.77 ± 0.55 ashes, and 11.65 ± 0.12 carbohydrates. These values are in harmony with previous reports [35].

3.1. Lipid Oxidation

It is widely known that the combination of unsaturated fatty acids, oxygen (from air), and UV light gives place to lipid oxidation, which results in rancidity [36]. All these players are present in the treatment of shelled walnuts by PL; therefore, the assessment of the potential sensory changes caused by PL at recommended microbicide fluences is warranted. Oil stability in walnuts is of paramount importance because it is a determinant of their shelf-life; indeed, considerable research has been performed to avoid lipid oxidation in walnuts during storage [37–39].

Table 2 shows the results of measurements of lipid oxidation in walnuts at increasing fluences. Both rancidity indicators, TBARS and peroxide, values were not significantly ($p > 0.05$) changed by PL treatment. Similarly, almonds subjected to a PL treatment (after 1 min water dipping) with the fluence required to achieve a 5-log reduction in *Salmonella* counts did not exhibit a significant increase in lipid oxidation even after 11 days of storage at 39 °C, and no differences in color and appearance were observed [40]. In comparison, the peroxide value of walnut kernels increases at gamma irradiation doses as low as 1.0 kGy [41], and an off-flavor related to oxidative rancidity has been reported for X-ray-treated shelled walnuts [42]. These results point toward a mild character of PL technology for shelled walnut processing. However, because oil stability is a critical attribute of shelled walnuts, more extensive evaluations were undertaken, which are reported next.

3.2. Volatile Compounds

Twenty volatile compounds were found in the volatile composition of walnuts (Table 3). It is necessary to emphasize that the nuts used in this study were not exposed to a roasting treatment. These treatments increase the content of volatile compounds in the nuts, so in this case, the content of volatile compounds found is significantly lower than in other studies.

Table 2. Quality indicators of shelled walnut oil subjected to pulsed light treatment (mean ± standard deviation).

	Fluence (J/cm^2)				
	0	10.7	21.4	32.1	42.8
Rancidity indicators					
TBARS [1] (mg MDA [2]/L oil)	0.27 ± 0.07 a	0.32 ± 0.06 a	0.27 ± 0.08 a	0.31 ± 0.07 a	0.34 ± 0.03 a
PV [3] (mmol O$_2$/g oil)	9.13 ± 0.46 a	9.13 ± 0.64 a	9.27 ± 0.46 a	8.60 ± 0.35 a	8.73 ± 0.23 a
Phenols					
Total phenols (g GAE [4]/l)	0.70 ± 0.17 a	0.69 ± 0.16 a	0.67 ± 0.08 a	0.60 ± 0.07 a	0.67 ± 0.14 a
Antioxidant capacity					
FRAP [5] (µM Fe^{2+} equiv.)	753 ± 55 a	531 ± 43 b	457 ± 21 b	674 ± 15 a	495 ± 13 b
DPPH (µM equiv. Trolox)	469 ± 32 a	464 ± 31 a	466 ± 29 a	469 ± 24 a	462 ± 22 a
ABTS (µM equiv. Trolox)	399 ± 30 a	396 ± 57 a	327 ± 36 a	391 ± 45 a	336 ± 79 a

[1] Thiobarbituric acid reactive substances, [2] malondialdehyde, [3] peroxide value, [4] gallic acid equivalent, [5] ferric reducing antioxidant power. Within rows, values followed by different letters are statistically different ($p < 0.05$).

Table 3. Volatile composition (% relative area) and odor descriptors of walnut organic volatile compounds subjected or not to pulsed light (PL) treatment.

RT (min)	Compound	Odor Description	KI Exp.	KI Lit	ANOVA	Control	PL
7.199	Hexanal	Green, woody, grassy	800	801	***	3.02 b	30.11 a
10.968	1-Hexanol	Herbaceous, green	862	865	***	4.43 b	57.83 a
11.754	Methyl hexanoate	Fruity	915	915	***	45.55 a	0.20 b
16.079	Methyl-2-hexenoate	Fatty	934	933	NS	1.02	0.08
16.775	Benzaldehyde	Bitter almond, cherry, nutty	936	935	NS	1.85	1.11
17.846	1-Heptanol	Musty, leafy, herbal, green, sweet	970	970	NS	0.80	0.48
18.712	Methyl heptenone	Citrus, green	992	994	NS	0.98	1.41
19.803	Ethyl hexanoate	Fruity	1002	1000	**	5.81 a	0.34 b
21.439	β-Cymene	Terpenic	1025	1028	NS	1.82	0.38
21.790	D-Limonene	Citrus, orange, lemon	1029	1031	***	18.20 a	1.80 b
23.982	Sabinene hydrate	Herbal, cooling	1101	1096	NS	0.85	1.04
27.601	Nonanal	Waxy, citrus, green	1115	1105	***	3.10 a	0.95 b
31.633	(E)-Pinocarveol	Herbal, woody, pine	1145	1140	NS	0.93	0.75
34.432	Ethyl octanoate	Waxy, sweet, fruity	1201	1206	NS	0.73	0.20
34.760	Dodecane	-	1206	1200	NS	1.84	0.96
35.007	Decanal	Sweet, waxy, orange	1210	1207	NS	1.84	0.73
35.681	Tridecane	-	1298	1300	NS	0.50	0.24
40.031	Dodecane, 4,6-dimethyl-	-	1327	1325	**	3.06 a	0.84 b
48.395	Tetradecane	-	1401	1400	**	1.55 a	0.44 b
49.082	Isocaryophyllene	Woody, spicy	1459	1461	**	2.22 a	0.13 b

KI exp.: Kovat's index experimental; KI Lit.: Kovats index literature (NIST). Values (mean of 3 replications) followed by the same letter within the same volatile compound were not significantly different ($p > 0.05$), according to Tukey's least significant difference test. NS = not significant at $p > 0.05$; **, ***, significant at $p < 0.01$ and 0.001, respectively.

The compounds found with the highest intensity were 1-hexanol, hexanal, methyl hexanoate, and limonene, although their quantity varied significantly among the treatments studied. These compounds also correspond to those found as the majority in walnut and walnut oil [43,44].

The control sample presented a higher amount of methyl hexanoate and limonene (45.55% and 18.20%, respectively), compounds related to fruity and citrus odors, according to the SAFC Flavors and Fragrances Catalog (SAFC, 2011) [45]. On the contrary, the sample subjected to PL treatment was mainly characterized by the presence of 1-hexanol and hexanal (27.83% and 30.11%, respectively), compounds related to green/herbaceous odors [46]. These four aromatic compounds are present in the volatile composition of this type of nut [37], although their concentration varies depending on the cultivar and agronomic conditions. In this case, the variation in its quantity is directly related to the treatment used. Hexanal has been used as a lipid oxidation marker [39]; however, it has also been identified as the second-most-important volatile compound of the Chandler walnut variety, with concentrations three- and six-fold higher than in the varieties Harley and Lara [43]. On the other side, Crowe et al. (2002) [47] identified hexanal as a walnut oil oxidation product but did not detect it in unoxidized walnuts, while this compound is considered a key important contributor to walnut kernel aroma [46,48]. These contradictory roles assigned to hexanal in Chandler walnut quality deserve to be further evaluated by sensory analysis.

Furthermore, statistically significant differences ($p < 0.05$) were also found in the relative content of ethyl hexanoate, limonene, nonanal, 4,6-dimethyl-dodecane, tetradecane, and isocaryophyllene. In all these compounds, the relative concentration was lower when the PL treatment was applied. These compounds are sensorially related to odors associated with fruity, citrus, and/or spices.

In general, according to the analysis of volatile compounds, the application of PL treatment to walnuts maintains the concentration of volatile compounds related to green nuts.

3.3. Descriptive Sensory Analysis

The descriptive analysis of the walnut samples had statistically significant differences ($p < 0.05$) in only 7 out of the 23 descriptors analyzed (Table 4). The application of light pulses in the walnuts did not have a significant effect on the appearance of the nuts. No differences were found in the color between the control samples and pulses samples (5.5 and 6.0, respectively) or in its color distribution around the inner nut (color homogeneity).

Table 4. Descriptive sensory analysis of walnuts affected by pulsed light (PL) treatment.

Sensory Descriptor	ANOVA	Control	PL
Appearance			
Color	NS	5.5	6.0
Color homogeneity	NS	8.0	8.0
Odor			
Nut overall	**	3.0 b	3.5 a
Walnut	**	3.0 b	3.5 a
Roasted	NS	0.5	0.5
Woody	***	1.5 a	1.0 b
Earthy	NS	0.5	0.5
Rancy	NS	0	0
Flavor			
Nut overall	**	8.0 b	8.5 a
Walnut	***	7.5 b	8.0 a
Roasted	NS	2.2	2.5
Woody	NS	3.5	4.0
Earthy	NS	1.5	1.5
Rancy	NS	0	0
Sweet	**	2.5 a	2.0 b
Bitter	NS	3.5	3.5
Astringent	NS	2.5	2.0
Aftertaste	**	5.0 b	5.5 a
Texture			
Hardness	NS	5.5	5.5
Crunchiness	NS	6.5	6.5
Friability	NS	7.5	7.0
Adhesiveness	NS	6.0	6.5
Oiliness	NS	2.5	2.5

Values (mean of 3 replications) followed by the same letter within the same volatile compound were not significantly different ($p > 0.05$), according to Tukey's least significant difference test. NS = not significant at $p > 0.05$; **, ***, significant at $p < 0.01$ and 0.001, respectively.

Differences were found in the odor of the samples (Table 4). The walnuts that were subjected to PL treatment appeared to have a more intense odor of nut overall (3.5) and walnut (3.5) and a lesser odor of woody (1.0) than the control samples (3.0, 3.0, and 1.5, respectively). The same results were found in the case of the taste analysis of the samples

(Table 4). PL-treated walnuts had a slightly higher intensity of the sensory descriptors of overall walnut (8.5), walnut (8.0), and aftertaste (5.5) than the control samples (8.0, 7.5, and 5.0, respectively). However, the treatment slightly depleted the sweetness of the samples (2.5 control vs. 2.0 pulse). No rancidity was perceived by the panel, which is in harmony with the results shown in Table 2 and reinforces the conclusion about the lack of effect of PL technology on the stability of walnut oil.

Nevertheless, the increased hexanal content in PL-treated walnut kernels deserves further consideration. Previous studies on the oil stability of walnuts [49] and another nut (almond) [50] treated with PL have not included the determination of volatile compounds. However, the volatile composition after PL treatment of other foods less related to walnuts, namely, chicken fillets [51] and Manchego and Gouda cheeses [52], have also revealed an increase in hexanal content together with its lack of relevance to the sensory evaluation, which is in line with our result.

In the case of texture, no statistically significant differences ($p > 0.05$) were found in any of the parameters studied: hardness, crunchiness, friability, adhesiveness, and oiliness (Table 4).

After the sensory analysis of the samples, it can be concluded that the application of PL to walnuts slightly increases their intensity of characteristic odor and flavor without modifying their texture or appearance.

3.4. Total Phenolic Compounds and Antioxidant Activity

Phenolic compounds have been associated with benefits to health and have antioxidant activity. Walnuts have the highest known levels of phenolic antioxidants among all nut species [14]; as an important source of these compounds, their stability under treatment conditions is very important. Table 2 shows the concentration of total phenols and the antioxidant activity, measured by three different methods, of walnuts subjected to PL treatment. No significant ($p > 0.05$) effects on total phenols were observed during the course of PL treatment. As for antioxidant activity, no significant ($p > 0.05$) effects were observed except for a significant ($p < 0.05$) decrease in FRAP values, yet, overall, no effect on antioxidant activity can be concluded.

4. Conclusions

The effect of PL on oil stability, total phenols, antioxidant activity, volatile profile, and descriptive sensory quality of shelled walnuts was assessed under fluence levels relevant to microbiological safety (42.8 J/cm^2). PL had no statistically significant ($p > 0.05$) effects on TBARS, peroxide value, total phenols, and antioxidant activity in general. PL significantly increased ($p < 0.05$) the concentration of volatiles related to green/herbaceous odors and significantly decreased compounds related to fruity and citrus odors. The descriptors nut overall and walnut odor and flavor and aftertaste were given statistically significant ($p < 0.05$) higher scores, while descriptors woody odor and sweet received statistically significant ($p < 0.05$) lower scores, and 16 other traits such as all those related to color and texture including the rancid trait were unaffected. No significant ($p > 0.05$) effects on total phenols and antioxidant activity in general were observed during the course of PL treatment. Therefore, it can be concluded that PL technology may be used in shelled walnuts with mild effects on their quality; a storage study must be carried out in order to determine the effect of PL treatment on the shelf-life of shelled walnuts.

Author Contributions: Conceptualization, V.M.G.-L.; methodology, V.M.G.-L., L.N.-A., A.J.P.-L., Á.A.C.-B., F.G. and F.F.-M.; validation, L.N.-A., A.J.P.-L. and Á.A.C.-B.; formal analysis, V.M.G.-L., L.N.-A., A.J.P.-L. and Á.A.C.-B.; investigation, A.J.P.-L., L.N.-A., F.G. and F.F.-M.; resources, V.M.G.-L.; data curation, L.N.-A.; writing—original draft preparation, V.M.G.-L. and A.J.P.-L.; writing—review and editing, V.M.G.-L., A.J.P.-L. and L.N.-A.; visualization, A.J.P.-L., L.N.-A. and Á.A.C.-B.; supervision, V.M.G.-L., A.J.P.-L. and L.N.-A.; project administration, V.M.G.-L.; funding acquisition, J.A.G. All authors have read and agreed to the published version of the manuscript.

Funding: This research was funded by Universidad Católica de Murcia (UCAM), grant number PMAFI/29/14. The GCMS has been acquired thanks to grant EQC2018-004170-P funded by MCIN/AEI/10.13039/501100011033 and by ERDF A way of making Europe.

Institutional Review Board Statement: Not applicable.

Informed Consent Statement: Not applicable.

Data Availability Statement: Not applicable.

Acknowledgments: The kindness of Ali Demirci (Pennsylvania State University) and his team for providing accurate fluence data for their article "Utilization of pulsed UV light for inactivation of *Salmonella* Enteritidis on shelled walnuts" is highly appreciated.

Conflicts of Interest: The authors declare no conflict of interest. The funders had no role in the design of the study, in the collection, analyses, or interpretation of data, in the writing of the manuscript, or in the decision to publish the results.

References

1. Gómez-López, V.M.; Ragaert, P.; Debevere, J.; Devlieghere, F. Pulsed light for food decontamination: A review. *Trends Food Sci. Technol.* **2007**, *18*, 464–473. [CrossRef]
2. Gómez-López, V.M.; Bhat, R.; Pellicer, J.A. Pulsed light. In *Electromagnetic Technologies in Food Science*; Gómez-López, V.M., Bhat, R., Eds.; Wiley: Oxford, UK, 2022; pp. 200–219. ISBN 978-1-119-75951-5. [CrossRef]
3. Gómez-López, V.M.; Bolton, J.R. An approach to standardize methods for fluence determination in bench-scale pulsed light experiments. *Food Bioprocess Technol.* **2016**, *9*, 1040–1048. [CrossRef]
4. Harguindeguy, M.; Gómez-Camacho, C.E. Pulsed Light (PL) treatments on almond kernels: *Salmonella* Enteritidis inactivation kinetics and infrared thermography insights. *Food Bioprocess Technol.* **2021**, *14*, 2323–2335. [CrossRef] [PubMed]
5. Izmirlioglu, G.; Ouyang, B.; Demirci, A. Utilization of pulsed UV light for inactivation of *Salmonella* Enteritidis on shelled walnuts. *LWT Food Sci. Technol.* **2020**, *134*, 110023. [CrossRef]
6. Rothschild, M. Canada *E. coli* outbreak tied to walnuts. *Food Safety News.* 2011. Available online: https://www.foodsafetynews.com/2011/04/canada-e-coli-outbreak-tied-to-walnuts/ (accessed on 1 March 2022).
7. Riyaz-Ul-Hassan, S.; Verma, V.; Malik, A.; Qazi, G.N. Microbiological quality of walnut kernels and apple juice concentrate. *World J. Microbiol. Biotechnol.* **2003**, *19*, 845–850. [CrossRef]
8. Blessington, T.; Theofel, C.G.; Mitcham, E.J.; Harris, L.J. Survival of foodborne pathogens on inshell walnuts. *Int. J. Food Microbiol.* **2013**, *166*, 341–348. [CrossRef] [PubMed]
9. Davidson, G.R.; Frelka, J.C.; Yang, M.; Jones, T.M.; Harris, L.J. Prevalence of *Escherichia coli* O157:H7 and *Salmonella* on inshell California walnuts. *J. Food Prot.* **2015**, *78*, 1547–1553. [CrossRef]
10. Zhang, G.; Hu, L.; Melka, D.; Wang, H.; Laasri, A.; Brown, E.W.; Strain, E.; Allard, M.; Bunning, V.K.; Musser, S.M.; et al. Prevalence of *Salmonella* in cashews, hazelnuts, macadamia nuts, pecans, pine nuts, and walnuts in the United States. *J. Food Prot.* **2017**, *80*, 459–466. [CrossRef]
11. Little, C.L.; Rawal, N.; de Pinna, E.; McLauchlin, J. Survey of *Salmonella* contamination of edible nut kernels on retail sale in the UK. *Food Microbiol.* **2010**, *27*, 171–174. [CrossRef]
12. Harris, L.J.; Yada, S.; Beuchat, L.R.; Danyluk, M.D. Inactivation of Microorganisms in Nuts and Nut Pastes—Published Treatments. 2021. Available online: https://ucfoodsafety.ucdavis.edu/low-moisture-foods/nuts-and-nut-pastes (accessed on 1 March 2022).
13. Santillana-Farakos, S.M.; Pouillot, R.; Davidson, G.R.; Johnson, R.; Son, I.; Anderson, N.; Van Doren, J.M. A quantitative risk assessment of human salmonellosis from consumption of walnuts in the United States. *J. Food Prot.* **2019**, *82*, 45–57. [CrossRef]
14. Hayes, D.; Angove, M.J.; Tucci, J.; Dennis, C. Walnuts (*Juglans regia*) chemical composition and research in human health. *Crit. Rev. Food Sci. Nutr.* **2015**, *56*, 1231–1241. [CrossRef] [PubMed]
15. Regueiro, J.; Sánchez-González, C.; Vallverdú-Queralt, A.; Simal-Gándara, J.; Lamuela-Raventós, R.; Izquierdo-Pulido, M. Comprehensive identification of walnut polyphenols by liquid chromatography coupled to linear ion trap–Orbitrap mass spectrometry. *Food Chem.* **2014**, *152*, 340–348. [CrossRef] [PubMed]
16. Ojeda-Amador, R.M.; Salvador, M.D.; Gómez-Alonso, S.; Fregapane, G. Characterization of virgin walnut oils and their residual cakes produced from different varieties. *Food Res. Int.* **2018**, *108*, 396–404. [CrossRef] [PubMed]
17. Gharibzahedi, S.M.T.; Mousavi, S.M.; Hamedi, M.; Khodaiyan, F. Determination and characterization of kernel biochemical composition and functional compounds of Persian walnut oil. *J. Food Sci. Technol.* **2014**, *51*, 34–42. [CrossRef] [PubMed]
18. AOAC. Moisture in nuts and nut products. Method 925.40. In *Official Methods of Analysis of AOAC International*, 18th ed.; AOAC: Gaithersburg, MD, USA, 2005.
19. AOAC. *Official Methods of Analysis of AOAC International*, 19th ed.; AOAC: Washington, DC, USA, 2009.
20. FOSS. *The Determination of Nitrogen According to Kjeldahl Using Block Digestion and Steam Distillation*; Foss Application Note AN 300; FOSS: Höganäs, Sweden, 2003.

21. Greenfield, H.; Southgate, H.A.T. *Food Composition Data. Production, Management and Use*, 2nd ed.; Food and Agriculture Organization of the United Nations: Rome, Italy, 2003; Available online: https://www.fao.org/3/y4705e/y4705e.pdf (accessed on 1 March 2022).
22. AOAC. Fat (crude) in nuts and nut products. Method 948.22. In *Official Methods of Analysis of AOAC International*, 18th ed.; AOAC: Gaithersburg, MD, USA, 2005.
23. Pérez-López, A.J.; Rodríguez-López, M.I.; Burló, F.; Carbonell-Barrachina, A.A.; Gabaldón, J.A.; Gómez-López, V.M. Evaluation of pulsed light to inactivate *Brettanomyces bruxellensis* in white wine and assessment of its effects on color and aromatic profile. *Foods* **2020**, *9*, 1903. [CrossRef]
24. Cudemus, E.; Izquier, A.; Medina-Martínez, M.S.; Gómez-López, V.M. Effects of shading and growth phase on the microbial inactivation by pulsed light. *Czech J. Food Sci.* **2013**, *31*, 189–193. [CrossRef]
25. Eliseeva, L.; Gorozhanin, P.; Yurina, O. The study of oxidative processes in walnut fats during storage. *Indian J. Sci. Technol.* **2016**, *9*, 1–6. [CrossRef]
26. Buege, J.A.; Aust, S.D. Microsomal lipid peroxidation. *Methods Enzymol.* **1978**, *52*, 302–310. [CrossRef]
27. Noguera-Artiaga, L.; Sánchez-Bravo, P.; Pérez-López, D.; Szumny, A.; Calín-Sánchez, Á.; Burgos-Hernández, A.; Carbonell-Barrachina, Á.A. Volatile, sensory and functional properties of hydrosos pistachios. *Foods* **2020**, *9*, 158. [CrossRef]
28. Noguera-Artiaga, L.; Salvador, M.D.; Fregapane, G.; Collado-González, J.; Wojdyło, A.; López-Lluch, D.; Carbonell-Barrachina, Á.A. Functional and sensory properties of pistachio nuts as affected by cultivar. *J. Sci. Food Agric.* **2019**, *99*, 6696–6705. [CrossRef]
29. Carbonell-Barrachina, A.A.; Memmi, H.; Noguera-Artiaga, L.; del Carmen Gijón-López, M.; Ciapa, R.; Pérez-López, D. Quality attributes of pistachio nuts as affected by rootstock and deficit irrigation. *J. Sci. Food Agric.* **2015**, *95*, 2866–2873. [CrossRef] [PubMed]
30. Pérez-Jiménez, J.; Arranz, S.; Tabernero, M.; Díaz-Rubio, M.E.; Serrano, J.; Goñi, I.; Saura-Calixto, F. Updated methodology to determine antioxidant capacity in plant foods, oils and beverages: Extraction, measurement and expression of results. *Food Res. Int.* **2008**, *41*, 274–285. [CrossRef]
31. Singleton, V.L.; Rossi, J.A.J. Colorimetry of total phenolics with phosphomolybdic-phosphotungstic acid reagents. *Am. J. Enol. Vitic.* **1965**, *16*, 144–158.
32. Benzie, I.F.; Strain, J.J. The ferric reducing ability of plasma (FRAP) as a measure of antioxidant power: The FRAP assay. *Anal. Biochem.* **1996**, *239*, 70–76. [CrossRef]
33. Bondet, V.; Brand-Williams, W.; Berset, C. Kinetics and mechanisms of antioxidant activity using the DPPH free radical method. *LWT Food Sci. Technol.* **1997**, *30*, 609–615. [CrossRef]
34. Miller, N.J.; Rice-Evans, C.A. Factors influencing the antioxidant activity determined by the ABTS^{+} radical cation assay. *Free Radic. Res.* **1997**, *26*, 195–199. [CrossRef]
35. Al-Bachir, M. Effect of gamma irradiation on fungal load, chemical and sensory characteristics of walnuts (*Juglans regia* L.). *J. Stored Prod. Res.* **2004**, *40*, 355–362. [CrossRef]
36. Ramis-Ramos, G. Antioxidants. Synthetic antioxidants. In *Encyclopedia of Food Sciences and Nutrition*, 2nd ed.; Caballero, B., Ed.; Elsevier: Amsterdam, The Netherlands, 2003; pp. 265–275.
37. Hao, J.; Xu, X.-L.; Jin, F.; Regenstein, J.M.; Wang, F.-J. HS-SPME GC–MS characterization of volatiles in processed walnuts and their oxidative stability. *J. Food Sci. Technol.* **2020**, *57*, 2693–2704. [CrossRef]
38. Grosso, A.L.; Riveros, C.; Asensio, C.M.; Grosso, N.R.; Nepote, V. Improving walnuts' preservation by using walnut phenolic extracts as natural antioxidants through a walnut protein-based edible coating. *J. Food Sci.* **2020**, *85*, 3043–3051. [CrossRef]
39. Mu, H.; Gao, H.; Chen, H.; Fang, X.; Zhou, Y.; Wu, W.; Han, Q. Study on the volatile oxidation compounds and quantitative prediction of oxidation parameters in walnut (*Carya cathayensis* Sarg.) Oil. *Eur. J. Lipid Sci. Technol.* **2019**, *121*, 1800521. [CrossRef]
40. Liu, X.; Fan, X.; Wang, W.; Yao, S.; Chen, H. Wetting raw almonds to enhance pulse light inactivation of *Salmonella* and preserve quality. *Food Control* **2021**, *125*, 107946. [CrossRef]
41. Mexis, S.F.; Kontominas, M.G. Effect of γ-irradiation on the physicochemical and sensory properties of walnuts (*Juglans regia* L.). *Eur Food Res. Technol.* **2009**, *228*, 823–831. [CrossRef]
42. Jeong, S.; Marks, B.P.; Ryser, E.T.; Harte, J.B. The effect of X-ray irradiation on *Salmonella* inactivation and sensory quality of almonds and walnuts as a function of water activity. *Int. J. Food Microbiol.* **2012**, *153*, 365–371. [CrossRef] [PubMed]
43. Kalogiouri, N.P.; Manousi, N.; Rosenberg, E.; Zachariadis, G.A.; Paraskevopoulou, A.; Samanidou, V. Exploring the volatile metabolome of conventional and organic walnut oils by solid-phase microextraction and analysis by GC-MS combined with chemometrics. *Food Chem.* **2021**, *363*, 130331. [CrossRef] [PubMed]
44. Okatan, V.; Gündeşli, M.A.; Kafkas, N.E.; Attar, Ş.H.; Kahramanoğlu, İ.; Usanmaz, S.; Aşkın, M.A. Phenolic Compounds, Antioxidant Activity, Fatty Acids and Volatile Profiles of 18 Different Walnut (*Juglans regia* L.) Cultivars and Genotypes. *Erwerbs-Obstbau* **2022**, 1–14. [CrossRef]
45. SAFC. *Flavors and Fragrances*; SAFC Specialties: Madrid, Spain, 2011.
46. Liu, B.; Chang, Y.; Sui, X.; Wang, R.; Liu, Z.; Sun, J.; Chen, H.; Sun, B.; Zhang, N.; Xia, J. Characterization of Predominant Aroma Components in Raw and Roasted Walnut (*Juglans regia* L.). *Food Anal. Methods* **2022**, *15*, 717–727. [CrossRef]
47. Manousi, N.; Zachariadis, G.A. Determination of Volatile Compounds in nut-based milk alternative beverages by HS-SPME prior to GC-MS analysis. *Molecules* **2019**, *24*, 3091. [CrossRef]

48. Grilo, F.S.; Wang, S.C. Walnut (*Juglans regia* L.) volatile compounds indicate kernel and oil oxidation. *Foods* **2021**, *10*, 329. [CrossRef]
49. Crowe, T.D.; Crowe, T.W.; Johnson, L.A.; White, P.J. Impact of extraction method on yield of lipid oxidation products from oxidized and unoxidized walnuts. *JAOCS* **2002**, *79*, 453–457. [CrossRef]
50. Clark, R.G.; Nursten, H.E. The sensory analysis and identification of volatiles from walnut (*Juglans regia* L.) headspace. *J. Sci. Food Agric.* **1977**, *28*, 69–77. [CrossRef]
51. McLeod, A.; Liland, K.H.; Haugen, J.E.; Sørheim, O.; Myhrer, K.S.; Holck, A.L. Chicken fillets subjected to UV-C and pulsed UV light: Reduction of pathogenic and spoilage bacteria, and changes in sensory quality. *J. Food Saf.* **2018**, *38*, 12421. [CrossRef] [PubMed]
52. Fernández, M.; Hospital, X.F.; Arias, K.; Hierro, E. Application of pulsed light to sliced cheese: Effect on *Listeria* inactivation, sensory quality and volatile profile. *Food Bioprocess Technol.* **2016**, *9*, 1335–1344. [CrossRef]

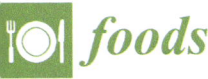

Article

Effect of Salt Reduction on the Quality of Boneless Dry-Cured Ham from Iberian and White Commercially Crossed Pigs

Beatriz Muñoz-Rosique [1], Eva Salazar [2,*], Julio Tapiador [3], Begoña Peinado [4] and Luis Tejada [2]

[1] Departamento de Calidad, Aromaibérica Serrana, S.L. Ctra. Fuente Álamo, km 17,4, 30332 Murcia, Spain; beatriz@aromais.es
[2] Departamento de Tecnología de la Alimentación y Nutrición, UCAM Universidad Católica de Murcia, Campus de los Jerónimos, 30107 Murcia, Spain; ltejada@ucam.edu
[3] Divisa Ibérica Plus S.L, 45519 Novés, Spain; juliotapiador@yahoo.es
[4] Instituto Murciano de Investigación y Desarrollo Agrario y Medioambiental (IMIDA), Equipo de Mejora Genética Animal, 30150 Murcia, Spain; begona.peinado@carm.es
* Correspondence: esalazar@ucam.edu

Abstract: Iberian dry-cured ham has great value in a traditional Spanish diet, although experts have recommended its consumption should be reduced because of its high salt content and link to cardiovascular diseases. Eighteen boneless Iberian hams (RIB), eighteen boneless white commercially crossed pig hams (RWC), and eighteen traditionally salted and processed Iberian hams (TIB) were manufactured to check whether the breed (RIB vs. RWC) or the processing (RIB vs. TIB) affects their physical–chemical and sensory characteristics. Moisture, protein, total nitrogen, nonprotein nitrogen, proteolysis index, NaCl, and ash contents were higher in RWC, contrary to the fat values, which were more than double in RIB. All macrominerals, except Ca, were affected by the processing stage and breed, whereas only the micromineral Zn was higher in RWC. The breed did not affect the free amino acid content; however, the total content was slightly higher in RWC. Regarding the manufacturing process, the deboning of RIB allowed the reduction of salt by over 30%. However, the microbiological stability was not affected, resulting in a safe product. Although deboning and salt reduction significantly affect the hardness, adhesiveness, deformation, and elasticity of dry-cured hams, consumers value all sensory parameters with higher scores in RIB.

Keywords: Iberian dry-cured ham; salt reduction; deboned ham; food labeling; proteolysis

1. Introduction

Iberian dry-cured ham is considered one of the important products of the Spanish meat industry. It is a quality product known worldwide, which has different organoleptic characteristics from other meat products, which make its consumption palatable. It is recognized for its high biological value because of its rich composition of proteins, unsaturated fatty acids, iron, zinc, and vitamin B, among others. In addition, it has a high economic value [1].

Despite having these nutritional characteristics, its consumption has traditionally been limited in at-risk populations, due to its high salt content [2]. High blood levels of sodium cause greater renal perfusion, increasing the excretion of sodium (Na^+) and water. This compensatory mechanism produces normal blood pressure but is progressively depleted, losing self-regulation. Therefore, high sodium intakes predispose hypertension and the appearance of cardiovascular diseases [3].

The increase in sodium consumption and the need to reduce the prevalence of associated diseases has caused the food industry to develop several methods to reduce the sodium added to products [4]. However, salt is an essential ingredient in meat products because it is responsible for the decrease in water activity, delaying and inhibiting microbial growth, and prolonging their useful life. In addition, salt influences the final texture of

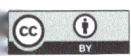

the products and provides a characteristic flavor that differentiates them from others [5]. The reduction of salt in dry-cured ham can have direct and indirect consequences, as the biochemical reactions that occur during the ripening period are affected. Salt influences the behavior of the muscular proteolytic system by acting on enzymes such as cathepsins and calpains. These play a very important role during ripening, since they contribute to the appearance of free amino acids and peptides responsible for developing the aroma, smell, and texture of the dry-cured ham [6]. An excessive hydrolysis of proteins by cathepsin B and B + L have been described as responsible for the softness and adhesiveness in the texture profile and the bitter taste of dry-cured ham [7,8]. Furthermore, the sensory study data of the acceptance of hams and the presence of some amino acid derivatives and small peptides have been correlated as components to distinguish defective and normal hams. [9].

Among the strategies for salt reduction, the most studied has been the total or partial substitution of NaCl with other salts. With dry-cured ham obtained from white pig crosses, Frye et al. [10] described the partial reduction of NaCl, by 50% or less, replaced with KCl is possible while maintaining acceptable physical–chemical and sensory attributes [11]. However, other studies reported that although salted dry-cured hams with partially replaced NaCl for KCl were well evaluated, a bitter taste was detected due to potassium [12,13]. Magnesium salts have also been evaluated, but some observed undesirable flavors appeared in the product and had to use other ingredients to mask those flavors [14]. Furthermore, Seong et al. [15] described the possibility of using natural halophytes in different types of dry-cured hams as salt substitutes, obtaining good physical–chemical results. The possibility of using flavor enhancers as substitutes for salt has also been described in other derived meat products [16]. The use of ultrasound at the time of salting [17] or the use of fresh shaped hams are other technological strategies studied to reduce the salt content. Using fresh shaped hams as a raw material would increase the absorption and the diffusion phenomenon of NaCl because of the greater contact surface, producing dry-cured hams with a reduced salt content [18].

To declare that food has reduced sodium, according to European legislation [19], the reduction must be at least 25% compared to a similar product. This reduction is much more complex in Iberian dry-cured hams because they have a lower level of salt per se than dry-cured hams from white commercially crossed pigs. The higher fat content of Iberian dry-cured ham also makes the reduction of salt in this product more complex because fat complicates the diffusion of salt through the tissues, resulting in a delay in the balance of salt inside the ham in the early stages of ripening [20]; in addition, fat could limit the perception of salinity [21,22]. Furthermore, it has been reported that aroma and flavor decrease with higher fat content [23]. Finally, the possibility that dry-cured ham cured using salt substitutes could require a longer processing time in the early stages should be considered [24].

Despite the limitations stated, there is a scarcity of reports that assess the effect of salt reduction on Iberian dry-cured hams. It is expected that using fresh deboned hams may improve the salt diffusion, reducing the salting time and therefore reducing the salt content of the final product. No study has been found on whether deboning the ham would reduce the salt in the product. Therefore, this work aimed to evaluate the effect of salt reduction on the physicochemical composition, free amino acids, and sensory quality of a reduced salt dry-cured boneless ham from an Iberian pig manufactured using a new process. Furthermore, the effect of breed was analyzed using the same parameters of a commercially crossed white pig, to compare with the Iberian product.

2. Materials and Methods

2.1. Dry-Cured Ham Preparation and Sample Collection

A total of 54 dry-cured hams were used to carry out this study. A batch of Iberian dry-cured hams (RIB) and a batch of dry-cured hams from white commercially crossed pigs (RWC) were produced and supplied by the Spanish meat industry. Fresh raw materials were boned and salted using nitrifying salts and sea salt at a rate of 0.8 days/kg, in a chamber at 3 °C.

After salting, pieces were washed with water, and a traditional curing process was conducted. The resting or postsalting stage started at 3 °C, and the temperature gradually increased to 6 °C. This phase was completed when the hams achieved 18% weight loss. Subsequently, the temperature was increased to 28 °C. The process was concluded when the pieces achieved a loss of 38% of weight. Weight loss was determined by weighing each sample in triplicate in each of the processing stages. The results were expressed as a percentage of weight loss, considering the fresh weight of each piece.

Finally, 18 dry-cured hams were selected from each batch (36 hams). Samples were taken in the following stages: I: Raw muscle; II: Start of post-salting; III: End of postsalting; IV: Drying stage (33% of weight loss); V: Final product (38% of weight loss). To maintain the integrity of the piece throughout processing, samples were taken using a 2 cm diameter stainless steel cylinder, in the area corresponding to the biceps femoris muscle.

Eighteen pieces of Iberian dry-cured hams were manufactured following the traditional curing process as a control product (TIB) (the time of salting stage was 1 day/kg). TIB dry-cured hams were processed with bone.

2.2. Physicochemical and Microbial Analyses

Each sample was analyzed in triplicate for each type of dry-cured ham in each of the physicochemical analyses.

The moisture content was determined by drying 5 g of sample at 105 °C for 24 h following the gravimetric procedure described in the ISO 1442 standard [25]. The method of Folch [26] was followed to obtain the intramuscular fat values of the dry-cured ham samples. The ash content was determined using gravimetry, following the AOAC method 920.153 [27].

For the analysis of dry-cured ham salt content, the Volhard method of the ISO 1841-1 standard [28] was modified, adding 2 mL of nitrobenzene to the sample after mineralization with nitric acid and simultaneous oxidation with potassium permanganate, to eliminate settling phases.

Total nitrogen (TN) and nonprotein nitrogen (NPN) were determined using the Kjeldahl method [29], obtaining the crude protein value by multiplying the TN value by 6.25. The proteolysis index (PI) was calculated as the percentage ratio between NPN and TN [30].

Microbiological counts were conducted on the dry-cured ham, following the protocol of Aaslyng, Vestergaard, and Koch [31] with slight modifications. Briefly, 25 g of each sample was taken in triplicate in the final stage (processing stage V). After serial decimal dilutions in 0.9% saline (Merck 106404, Darmstadt, Germany) enriched with peptone to 0.1% (Merck 1.07214.1000), the samples were seeded in Brain Heart Infusion (BHI) (Oxoid CM1136, Thermo Fisher Scientific, Loughborough, UK)) and All-Purpose Tween (APT) agar (Merck 1.10453.0500) and incubated for 5 days at 20 °C. After incubation, *Listeria monocytogenes* was seeded on Oxford agar (Scharlau Chemie SA, Barcelona, Spain), *Salmonella* on SS-Agar (Sigma, 85640, Buchs (SG), Switzerland), *E. coli* on Levine eosin methylene blue agar (Merck 62087, Darmstadt, Germany), *Staphylococcus* on Baird Parker Agar (Scharlau Chemie S.A., Barcelona, Spain), *Clostridium* on Tryptose Sulphite Cycloserine Agar (TSC) without egg yolk (SGL Lab, Corby, UK), Mesophilic aerobes on PCA (Merck, 1.15363.0500 Darmstadt, Germany), and Enterobacteria on (3M Petrifilm 6421, Madrid, Spain).

Mineral composition of samples was determined following the method of Tejada et al. [32], and the free amino acid content was obtained according to Abellán et al. [33].

2.3. Determination of Instrumental Color and Texture Profile Analysis (TPA)

Instrumental color was determined by colorimetry using a colorimeter (HunterLab, Colorflex) and the CIELab system. The results were expressed through the coordinates L*, a*, and b*, representing the luminosity, the red–green index, and the yellow index, respectively, and the values of the saturation parameter (chroma) and hue angle (h*). The results were calculated as the mean values of three measurements.

Instrumental texture was analyzed using a QTS-25 texturometer (Brookfield CNS Farnell, Borehamwood, Hertfordshire, England) equipped with a 25 kg load cell and a 10 mm diameter probe [34]. The software Texture Pro v. 2.1. was used for data analysis.

The muscle biceps femoris was analyzed. It was cut into $10 \times 10 \times 10$ mm parallelepipeds, using three parallelepipeds per sample. The room was maintained at 20 °C for the analyses.

The test was conducted by applying two consecutive cycles at a constant speed of 30 mm/s and subjecting the sample to a 50% compression in a direction perpendicular to the muscle fibers.

The TPA was performed on hardness, deformation according to hardness, adhesiveness, cohesiveness, recoverable deformation, springiness, gumminess, and chewiness.

2.4. Sensory Analyses (Consumers' Test)

The sensory evaluation of the dry-cured ham samples was conducted by an untrained panel. A total of 47 participants (53.2% men and 46.8% women) came voluntarily without having received prior training or information. The age range of the participants was 18 to 52 years. The study was conducted in one session where the TIB, RIB, and RWC samples were evaluated by the panelists using a questionnaire that included hedonic evaluation of the appearance, color, odor, texture, salty taste, global taste, and global acceptance. Each attribute was scored by assigning a numerical value through a verbal hedonic scale between 1 (I dislike very much) and 5 (I like very much). In addition, a preference study was also conducted.

The samples used for the sensory consumer test were complete slices of a 1 mm thick cross section of the piece, following the method established in the standards UNE-ISO 6658:2019 [35] and UNE-ISO 4121:2006 [36] and were codified with a random three-digit number.

The results were obtained by calculating the average score given to each attribute of the product evaluated by consumers. To determine the preference between the three samples, the percentage values of choice of the consumer panel were obtained in each type of dry-cured ham studied.

2.5. Statistical Analysis

The effect of the processing stage and the effect of breed on physicochemical parameters, salt content, and mineral composition were obtained by a two-way analysis of variance (ANOVA). When the effect of the processing stage or breed was significant ($p < 0.05$), the results were compared using the Fisher LSD test.

To assess if salt reduction and deboning affect the free amino acid content and the sensory quality of Iberian dry-cured ham, a one-way ANOVA was performed. Furthermore, the effect of breed on free amino acid content and sensory quality was studied in salt-reduced dry-cured hams from Iberian and white commercially crossed pigs.

3. Results and Discussion

3.1. Effect of Processing Stage and Breed on Physicochemical Parameters, Salt Content, Microbial Analyses, and Mineral Composition

Table 1 shows the evolution of the physicochemical parameters and salt content of reduced boneless dry-cured ham obtained from commercial crosses of Iberian and white pigs at different processing stages.

The processing stage affected all physicochemical parameters studied in boneless dry-cured ham of different breeds.

The moisture content in the dry-cured RIB ham was significantly reduced ($p \leq 0.001$), mainly between the drying stage and the final product, whereas the intramuscular fat content increased ($p \leq 0.05$), as observed in the protein values. In this parameter, the increase was more marked between the raw muscle and the drying stage, without observing significant differences between the final product (stage V) and the previous processing stages ($p \geq 0.05$); this was observed in both studied breeds. A similar evolution was observed in the NPN, with significantly increased values mainly between the end of postsalting (stage III) and the end of processing (stage V) ($p \leq 0.001$) in RIB and RWC. Consequently, PI also increased significantly during processing ($p \leq 0.001$). The increase in proteolytic activity of dry-cured hams during their ripening stage (stages IV and V) has been related to the rise in temperature that takes place at these manufacturing stages, resulting in a greater activity of proteolytic enzymes [37]. Physicochemical modifications were in line with what is observed in other dry-cured hams throughout processing [38,39].

NaCl and ash concentrations increased significantly, mainly at the start of postsalting stage due to the incorporation of curing salts associated with the manufacturing process ($p \leq 0.001$ in both cases). A marked increase was observed in the NaCl values of both breeds between stages I (raw muscle) and II (start of postsalting), as well as between the end of postsalting and the last two phases of the production process, due to the decrease in moisture, which takes place during the last stages of production. This phenomenon was also observed in the ash concentration of RWC dry-cured ham (Table 1), which reached its maximum values in the last two stages of the production process, whereas the ash values of the RIB dry-cured ham remained stable between the start of the postsalting stage (stage II) and the final product (stage V). Correct diffusion of salt (NaCl) was achieved with the processing method, with the concentration in dry-cured RWC of 3.77% and 2.86% in the RIB final product (processing stage V). Correct diffusion of salt during processing is important because of the role this ingredient plays. It will not only influence the texture, flavor, and aroma of the product, but will also ensure an optimal microbiological quality [40].

Regarding breed, moisture ($p \leq 0.001$), fat ($p \leq 0.001$), protein ($p \leq 0.001$), TN ($p \leq 0.001$), NPN ($p \leq 0.001$), PI ($p \leq 0.05$), NaCl ($p \leq 0.05$), and ash ($p \leq 0.001$) were also affected.

Moisture values and protein content were significantly higher in dry-cured RWC ham ($p \leq 0.001$), in all stages of processing, in contrast to the fat values, in which the RIB dry-cured ham presented more than double the fat content of RWC ($p \leq 0.001$), due to the high adipogenicity of native pig breeds [41]. These differences between breeds in fat and protein content were like those observed by Lorido et al. [23].

NPN values were significantly higher in RWC dry-cured ham ($p \leq 0.001$) throughout the manufacturing process. As expected, the PI was significantly lower in RIB ($p \leq 0.05$), due to the higher calpains and cathepsins activity in the dry-cured hams of commercially crossed white pigs [42]. In contrast, Córdoba et al. [43] described that proteolysis in Iberian hams could be higher than other types of dry-cured hams, such as Parma ham, due to the longer ripening time and the higher temperatures reached during the process. The PI in both breeds was lower than values reported by Schivazzapa and Virgili [44] in reduced salt Italian dry-cured hams obtained from pig crosses of Large White, Landrace, and Duroc.

The PI observed in the TIB final product (18.58%; value not included in Table 1), was slightly lower than RIB and was like those described in other dry-cured hams [45].

An adequate control of the ripening phase of reduced salt dry-cured hams is essential to assess the prolongation of this processing stage, to avoid texture or aroma problems [46], because free amino acids—resulting from the intense proteolysis the product undergoes during manufacturing—will contribute greatly to developing the sensory characteristics of the final product [47].

NaCl and ash concentrations were also higher in RWC dry-cured ham ($p \leq 0.001$) for all the processing stages. Consistent with salt reduction, the NaCl content in RIB and RWC was less than the values reported by some authors for dry-cured ham from commercial crosses of Croatian white pigs (between 5.76% and 7.01%) [48] and other native breeds (5.75%) [49] for the final product (processing stage V).

The average NaCl concentration was 4.11% in the traditionally manufactured Iberian dry-cured hams, thus a reduction of 30% compared to RIB. In RWC dry-cured hams, a reduction of 27.5% was reached, with an average value considered of 5.20% in traditional white dry-cured ham [50]. According to the Annex of Regulation (EC) No 1924/2006 [19], the claim 'Reduced in salt' could be included in the labeling of these products, because the indicated 25% reduction has been exceeded. Pinna et al. [51] also achieved a considerable reduction in salt content in typical Italian dry-cured hams by modifying salt added and the salting time.

Despite reducing the salt content of dry-cured hams, it does not compromise the stability and safety of the final product, as they meet the required microbiological conditions established. In this way, the counts of *Listeria monocytogenes* (in 25 g), *Salmonella* (in 25 g), *E. coli* (cfu/g), *Staphylococcus* (cfu/g), *Clostridium* (cfu/g), Mesophilic aerobes (cfu/g), and Enterobacteria (cfu/g) complied with the limits established by Regulation (EC) No 2073/2005 [52], relative to the microbiological criteria applicable to food products.

Table 2 includes the evolution of the mineral composition of reduced boneless dry-cured ham obtained from commercial crosses of Iberian and white pigs throughout processing.

The processing stage ($p \leq 0.001$) and breed ($p \leq 0.001$) significantly modified the concentration of Na, K, Mg, and P. The amount of Zn was only significantly affected ($p \leq 0.001$) by the processing stage, showing higher values in the final stages. Na values increased from the beginning of postsalting (processing stage II) and were always higher in RWC than in RIB, as was observed for NaCl (Table 1). The concentration of the rest of the minerals did not change significantly ($p > 0.05$). The concentration of K, Mg, P, Fe, and Zn was higher than observed in a previous study [53], whereas Na and Mn were lower. Ca values were similar; however, no references could be found for B and Cu.

Table 1. Effect of processing stage and breed on the physicochemical parameters and salt content of boneless dry-cured ham. Results are expressed in g/100 g of product (means values ± SEM).

		Processing Stage					p-Value		
		I	II	III	IV	V	Processing Stage	Breed	Interaction
Moisture	RIB	53.12 ± 1.31 ^{a}	52.82 ± 1.77 ^{a}	47.12 ± 2.11 ^{a}	37.35 ± 1.83 ^{b}	31.59 ± 1.26 ^{b}	0.000	0.000	0.000
	RWC	57.82 ± 6.93 ^{a}	56.65 ± 1.58 ^{a}	53.49 ± 1.71 ^{a}	52.08 ± 1.29 ^{a}	51.46 ± 0.64 ^{a}			
Fat	RIB	25.00 ± 1.43 ^{bc}	21.10 ± 2.32 ^{abc}	22.77 ± 2.37 ^{abc}	27.42 ± 2.00 ^{cd}	33.87 ± 1.94 ^{d}	0.028	0.000	0.007
	RWC	17.34 ± 4.54 ^{abc}	16.18 ± 1.00 ^{ab}	17.61 ± 1.43 ^{ab}	16.72 ± 1.01 ^{ab}	15.99 ± 0.46 ^{a}			
Protein	RIB	15.00 ± 0.35 ^{b}	16.48 ± 0.90 ^{ab}	19.53 ± 0.30 ^{ac}	22.32 ± 0.73 ^{c}	22.13 ± 1.19 ^{c}	0.000	0.000	0.001
	RWC	16.10 ± 1.53 ^{ab}	17.92 ± 0.10 ^{ab}	20.43 ± 0.50 ^{ac}	28.31 ± 0.55 ^{d}	29.68 ± 0.52 ^{d}			
Total Nitrogen	RIB	2.40 ± 0.06 ^{b}	2.63 ± 0.14 ^{ab}	3.13 ± 0.05 ^{ac}	3.57 ± 0.12 ^{c}	3.54 ± 0.19 ^{c}	0.000	0.000	0.001
	RWC	2.57 ± 0.25 ^{ab}	2.87 ± 0.02 ^{ab}	3.27 ± 0.08 ^{ac}	4.53 ± 0.09 ^{d}	4.75 ± 0.08 ^{d}			
Nonprotein Nitrogen	RIB	0.25 ± 0.06 ^{a}	0.18 ± 0.07 ^{a}	0.30 ± 0.07 ^{a}	0.48 ± 0.31 ^{ab}	0.74 ± 0.16 ^{bc}	0.000	0.000	0.001
	RWC	0.34 ± 0.09 ^{ab}	0.26 ± 0.11 ^{a}	0.33 ± 0.13 ^{a}	1.25 ± 0.42 ^{d}	1.04 ± 0.18 ^{cd}			
Proteolysis Index	RIB	10.54 ± 0.86 ^{a}	6.73 ± 1.42 ^{a}	9.50 ± 1.10 ^{a}	13.88 ± 3.62 ^{ab}	20.90 ± 1.24 ^{bc}	0.000	0.012	0.071
	RWC	13.45 ± 2.24 ^{abc}	9.01 ± 1.87 ^{a}	10.07 ± 1.97 ^{a}	27.85 ± 5.82 ^{c}	22.02 ± 1.59 ^{bc}			
NaCl	RIB	0.51 ± 0.27 ^{d}	1.96 ± 0.69 ^{a}	1.99 ± 0.17 ^{a}	2.79 ± 0.14 ^{abc}	2.86 ± 0.21 ^{abc}	0.000	0.016	0.176
	RWC	0.16 ± 0.02 ^{d}	2.33 ± 0.08 ^{ab}	2.43 ± 0.13 ^{ab}	3.64 ± 0.18 ^{bc}	3.77 ± 0.20 ^{c}			
Ash	RIB	2.21 ± 0.51 ^{c}	5.58 ± 1.65 ^{abc}	5.59 ± 0.68 $^{o\ abc}$	5.44 ± 0.48 ^{ab}	5.68 ± 0.85 ^{ab}	0.000	0.000	0.012
	RWC	2.39 ± 0.44 ^{bc}	8.81 ± 0.88 ^{ad}	6.84 ± 0.61 ^{ad}	10.92 ± 0.85 ^{d}	10.41 ± 0.40 ^{d}			

Two-way ANOVA. ^{a,b,c,d} Values within a row with different superscripts differ significantly at $p \leq 0.05$ (Fisher LSD Test). SEM: standard error of the mean; RIB: reduced Iberian dry-cured ham; RWC: reduced dry-cured ham from white commercial pig crosses; I: Raw muscle; II: Start of postsalting; III: End of postsalting; IV: Drying stage; V: Final product.

Table 2. Effect of the processing stage and the breed on the mineral composition of boneless dry-cured ham.

		Processing Stage					p-Value			RDA
		I	II	III	IV	V	Processing Stage	Breed	Interaction	
Na [1]	RIB	0.23 ± 0.08 a	0.83 ± 0.32 b	0.81 ± 0.11 b	1.01 ± 0.11 bc	1.13 ± 0.14 c	0.000	0.000	0.072	0.006
	RWC	0.15 ± 0.00 a	1.24 ± 0.14 c	1.16 ± 0.11 c	1.75 ± 0.17 de	1.54 ± 0.08 d				
K [1]	RIB	0.23 ± 0.04 a	0.28 ± 0.03 a	0.30 ± 0.02 a	0.33 ± 0.03 a	0.45 ± 0.03 ab	0.000	0.000	0.000	2000
	RWC	0.28 ± 0.05 a	0.34 ± 0.01 a	0.39 ± 0.02 a	0.96 ± 0.04 b	0.64 ± 0.02 b				
Ca [1]	RIB	0.02 ± 0.01 a	0.01 ± 0.00 a	0.02 ± 0.00 a	0.01 ± 0.00 a	0.01 ± 0.00 a	0.536	0.673	0.675	800
	RWC	0.01 ± 0.00 a	0.01 ± 0.00 a	0.02 ± 0.00 a	0.01 ± 0.00 a	0.02 ± 0.01 a				
Mg [1]	RIB	0.02 ± 0.00 a	0.32 ± 0.00 a	0.02 ± 0.00 a	0.02 ± 0.00 a	0.03 ± 0.00 ab	0.000	0.001	0.061	375
	RWC	0.02 ± 0.00 a	0.02 ± 0.00 a	0.03 ± 0.00 a	0.04 ± 0.00 b	0.04 ± 0.00 b				
P [1]	RIB	0.15 ± 0.05 a	0.16 ± 0.01 a	0.18 ± 0.01 a	0.20 ± 0.01 a	0.23 ± 0.02 a	0.000	0.000	0.000	700
	RWC	0.16 ± 0.03 a	0.19 ± 0.01 a	0.23 ± 0.01 a	0.34 ± 0.01 b	0.31 ± 0.01 b				
Fe [2]	RIB	9.66 ± 0.56 a	6.75 ± 0.80 a	5.69 ± 1.05 a	14.13 ± 5.48 a	11.66 ± 1.03 a	0.133	0.737	0.978	14
	RWC	8.06 ± 1.68 a	7.75 ± 0.60 a	8.33 ± 1.60 a	14.26 ± 2.78 a	13.02 ± 3.83 a				
Cu [2]	RIB	1.39 ± 0.57 a	1.05 ± 0.26 a	0.70 ± 0.14 a	3.86 ± 1.96 a	1.5 ± 0.27 a	0.577	0.537	0.509	1
	RWC	0.32 ± 0.12 a	1.62 ± 0.69 a	1.41 ± 0.14 a	1.24 ± 0.59 a	1.79 ± 0.23 a				
Mn [2]	RIB	0.62 ± 0.38 a	0.15 ± 0.02 a	0.27 ± 0.04 a	0.29 ± 0.05 a	0.10 ± 0.03 a	0.478	0.541	0.673	2
	RWC	0.31 ± 0.17 a	0.2 ± 0.08 a	0.20 ± 0.04 a	0.12 ± 0.05 a	0.26 ± 0.011 a				
Zn [2]	RIB	21.64 ± 1.80 ab	15.91 ± 7.80 a	16.56 ± 2.42 a	21.53 ± 2.70 ab	24.59 ± 1.74 bc	0.000	0.169	0.251	10
	RWC	16.47 ± 3.22 a	19.76 ± 2.53 a	18.83 ± 2.44 a	26.69 ± 1.58 bc	29.76 ± 2.90 c				
B [2]	RIB	0.78 ± 0.53 a	0.36 ± 0.06 a	0.18 ± 0.06 a	0.34 ± 0.06 a	0.47 ± 0.08 a	0.882	0.538	0.598	Not declared
	RWC	0.14 ± 0.06 a	0.21 ± 0.06 a	0.36 ± 0.01 a	0.38 ± 0.19 a	0.51 ± 0.15 a				

Two-way ANOVA. a,b,c,d,e Values within a row with different superscripts differ significantly at $p \leq 0.05$ (Fisher LSD Test). [1] Results are expressed in g/100 g of product (means values ± standard error of mean). [2] Results are expressed in mg/100 g of product (means values ± standard error of mean). RIB: reduced Iberian dry-cured ham; RWC: reduced dry-cured ham from white commercial pig crosses; I: Raw muscle; II: Start of post-salting; III: End of post-salting; IV: D'ying stage; V: Final product; RDA: Recommended Daily Allowances of minerals.

3.2. Free Amino Acids

Results for the effect of Iberian dry-cured ham type and the effect of breed on free amino acid (FAA) content in the final product (processing stage V) are shown in Table 3.

Table 3. Effect of Iberian dry-cured ham type (processing) and effect of breed on free amino acid content (FAA). The results are expressed in g/kg of dry matter as mean values ± SEM.

FAA	Dry-Cured Ham Type			p-Value	
	TIB	RIB	RWC	Processing	Breed
Asp	2.08 ± 0.06	2.05 ± 0.54	1.94 ± 0.74	0.962	0.921
Glu	3.98 ± 0.11	4.26 ± 1.04	4.87 ± 0.92	0.809	0.706
Ser	1.51 ± 0.05	1.34 ± 0.21	1.83 ± 0.47	0.530	0.443
His	0.91 ± 0.02	1.00 ± 0.25	1.17 ± 0.25	0.760	0.677
Gly	1.23 ± 0.01	1.42 ± 0.40	1.79 ± 0.37	0.685	0.566
Thr	1.45 ± 0.03	1.32 ± 0.28	1.81 ± 0.30	0.685	0.352
Arg	1.75 ± 0.16	1.06 ± 0.02	1.32 ± 0.22	0.051	0.368
Ala	4.02 ± 0.14	4.70 ± 1.06	5.67 ± 0.46	0.590	0.489
Tyr	0.70 ± 0.01	0.89 ± 0.16	1.44 ± 0.47	0.377	0.384
Cys	nd	nd	nd	-	-
Val	2.10 ± 0.05	2.22 ± 0.53	2.51 ± 0.53	0.847	0.732
Met	0.53 ± 0.21	0.64 ± 0.23	0.79 ± 0.01	0.764	0.580
Phe	1.42 ± 0.15	1.56 ± 0.38	1.82 ± 0.35	0.765	0.669
Ile	1.48 ± 0.09	1.64 ± 0.44	1.90 ± 0.42	0.760	0.706
Leu	2.43 ± 0.19	2.65 ± 0.71	3.21 ± 0.79	0.786	0.654
Lys	3.73 ± 0.10	4.13 ± 1.15	5.00 ± 1.17	0.766	0.649
Pro	1.87 ± 0.01	1.96 ± 0.40	2.18 ± 0.25	0.837	0.688
Total FAA	31.19 ± 0.38	32.84 ± 7.76	39.26 ± 7.71	0.852	0.617

TIB: traditional Iberian dry-cured ham; RIB: reduced Iberian dry-cured ham; RWC: reduced dry-cured ham from white commercial pig crosses; SEM: standard error of the mean; p-value Processing: One-way ANOVA between TIB and RIB; p-value Breed: One-way ANOVA between RIB and RWC (p-value significant at $p \leq 0.05$); nd: nondetected.

None of the FAA studied was affected by the processing of different Iberian dry-cured ham (traditional and reduced salt boneless manufactured) ($p > 0.05$). The same was observed regarding the total FFA ($p > 0.05$). Therefore, peptidase activity was not significantly affected ($p > 0.05$) by salt reduction (30%) although total FAA content was slightly higher in RIB. These findings disagreed with the study by Cittadini et al. [54], in which an increase in proteolytic phenomenon was observed as the NaCl content decreased.

Abellán et al. [55] described that the concentration of amino acids reflects the proteolysis achieved during the ripening stage of dry-cured meat products. Considering the data obtained in PI, NPN (Table 1), and the total FFA (Table 3), the proteolysis of dry-cured Iberian ham followed an expected evolution, despite the reduction in salt content. According to Lorenzo et al. [56], the proteolytic reactions are promoted in meat products with a partial replacement of sodium.

The differences in amino acid concentration of boneless dry-cured ham of different breeds were not significant ($p > 0.05$). Krvavica et al. [57] also found no effect of breed on the FFA content in two types of dry-cured Croatian ham obtained from different genotypes of commercial white pig crosses.

The differences in the PI between the two breeds studied (Table 1) could be explained by a higher protease activity (calpain and cathepsins) of RWC dry-cured hams. However, no differences in FAA concentration were observed, probably because the breed did not affect peptidases activity.

3.3. Instrumental Color and Texture Profile

Table 4 shows the effect Iberian dry-cured ham type and the effect of breed on the instrumental color.

Table 4. Effect of Iberian dry-cured ham type (processing) and effect of breed on instrumental color. Results are expressed as mean values ± SEM.

Color Parameter	Dry-Cured Hams			p-Value	
	TIB	RIB	RWC	Processing	Breed
Lightness (L*)	47.22 ± 4.23	53.03 ± 1.79	57.88 ± 0.85	0.165	0.164
Redness (a*)	24.70 ± 2.96	23.36 ± 1.62	20.72 ± 1.06	0.692	0.392
Yellowness (b*)	27.34 ± 5.26	28.46 ± 1.24	31.09 ± 3.19	0.758	0.363
Chroma (C*)	37.26 ± 4.61	37.09 ± 1.30	37.47 ± 2.70	0.961	0.891
Hue angle (h°)	47.01 ± 6.44	50.75 ± 2.52	55.99 ± 3.04	0.519	0.298

TIB: traditional Iberian dry-cured ham; RIB: reduced Iberian dry-cured ham; RWC: reduced dry-cured ham from white commercial pig crosses; SEM: standard error of the mean.

The instrumental color parameters were not affected by different processes for Iberian dry-cured ham ($p > 0.05$ in all cases), agreeing with the data obtained by Lorenzo et al. [58], who studied the effect of partial replacement of NaCl with other salts on dry-cured *lacón*. In contrast, Tejada et al. [32] observed an effect of different salt formulation on the color parameters of another derived meat pig product (Spanish *chorizo*) describing a higher luminosity value (L*) in the product cured with a traditional formulation (with NaCl as the main ingredient), as well as higher values of b*, C*, and h*. No breed effect on color parameters was observed ($p > 0.05$ in all cases). The range of L*, a*, and b* values obtained in the two types of Iberian dry-cured ham studied (TIB and RIB) and in the reduced salt dry-cured ham, obtained from white commercial pig crosses, were higher than dry-cured ham obtained from the Celta pig by Bermúdez et al. [38].

Table 5 shows the effect Iberian dry-cured ham type and breed on the instrumental texture.

Table 5. Effect of Iberian dry-cured ham type (processing) and effect of breed on instrumental texture. Results are expressed as mean values ± SEM.

Texture Parameter	Dry-Cured Hams			p-Value	
	TIB	RIB	RWC	Processing	Breed
C1 Hardness (N)	6.89 ± 0.95	8.61 ± 0.31	5.84 ± 0.54	0.041	0.000
C1 Hardness deformation	2.95 ± 0.07	2.97 ± 0.00	2.93 ± 0.05	0.684	0.179
C1 Adhesiveness (mJ)	0.72 ± 0.09	1.03 ± 0.39	0.57 ± 0.09	0.249	0.121
C2 Cohesiveness	6.10 ± 0.74	7.93 ± 0.38	4.99 ± 0.03	0.021	0.000
C2 Recoverable deformation (mm)	0.53 ± 0.05	0.60 ± 0.03	0.56 ± 0.02	0.091	0.152
C2 Springiness	0.95 ± 0.19	1.14 ± 0.10	1.10 ± 0.01	0.122	0.558
C2 Gumminess (N)	1.56 ± 0.03	2.12 ± 0.08	1.81 ± 0.04	0.000	0.000
C2 Chewiness (mJ)	3.11 ± 0.36	5.16 ± 0.39	3.59 ± 0.60	0.000	0.023
C2 Hardness (N)	5.42 ± 0.90	10.97 ± 0.87	6.03 + 0.23	0.001	0.000

TIB: traditional Iberian dry-cured ham; RIB: reduced Iberian dry-cured ham; RWC: reduced dry-cured ham from white commercial pig crosses; SEM: standard error of the mean; N: Newton; mJ: millijoules; mm: millimeters; *p*-value Processing: One-way ANOVA between TIB and RIB; *p*-value Breed: One-way ANOVA between RIB and RWC (*p*-value significant at $p \leq 0.05$).

The processing of Iberian dry-cured ham and the breed had a significant effect on C1 hardness, C2 cohesiveness, C2 gumminess, C2 chewiness, and C2 hardness (Table 5). All cited texture profile parameters were higher in RIB compared to TIB. Despite the differences observed in the TPA, consumers did not report an effect of processing between the two Iberian dry-cured hams studied (Table 6). Although the TPA confirmed the differences found in the sensory analysis regarding breed, where consumers scored RIB texture better than RWC's (Table 6).

Table 6. Effect of Iberian dry-cured ham type (processing) and effect of breed on consumer acceptability by a consumer panel. Results are expressed as mean values ± SEM *.

	Dry-Cured Ham Type			p-Value	
	TIB	RIB	RWC	Processing	Breed
Appearance	3.66 ± 0.13	4.17 ± 0.15	2.62 ± 0.16	0.061	0.006
Color	3.83 ± 0.12	4.13 ± 0.13	2.68 ± 0.15	0.159	0.021
Odor	3.55 ± 0.15	3.87 ± 0.13	2.89 ± 0.13	0.200	0.008
Texture	3.81 ± 0.11	3.98 ± 0.14	2.83 ± 0.13	0.232	0.013
Salty taste	3.57 ± 0.13	3.87 ± 0.13	2.87 ± 0.13	0.252	0.001
Global taste	3.96 ± 0.12	4.06 ± 0.10	2.81 ± 0.14	0.224	0.002
Global acceptance	4.00 ± 0.12	4.09 ± 0.12	2.57 ± 0.123	0.220	0.005

* Attributes were scored assigning a numerical value through a verbal hedonic scale between 1 (I dislike very much) and 5 (I like very much); SEM: standard error of mean; TIB: traditional Iberian dry-cured ham; RIB: reduced Iberian dry-cured ham; RWC: reduced dry-cured ham from white commercial pig crosses; p-value Processing: One-way ANOVA between TIB and RIB; p-value Breed: One-way ANOVA between RIB and RWC (p-value significant at $p \leq 0.05$).

The data here are partially consistent with the study of Tejada et al. [32], in which the authors found an effect of salt reduction on hardness, cohesiveness, gumminess, and chewiness in another derived meat pig product. However, TPA hardness values where higher in the NaCl reduced product of the cited study, contrary to the data obtained in this study, as RIB showed higher values. The authors associated this phenomenon with the inhibition of cathepsins by NaCl, which reduces the proteolysis activity affecting the texture of the product. Therefore, we can conclude that proteolysis of RIB was not affected significantly, considering TPA hardness values (Table 5) and according to data obtained for the FFA (Table 3). Regarding breed, RIB's higher hardness values could be related to the lower moisture content obtained than the RWC dry-cured ham (Table 1).

Cittadini et al. [54] also studied the effect of NaCl replacement by other chloride salts on TPA parameters (hardness, springiness, cohesiveness, gumminess, and chewiness) of foal Cecina, a similar dry-cured product, but in contrast to our result, they only found significant differences in the springiness.

3.4. Consumer Sensory Acceptability and Preference

Table 6 shows the acceptability scores for TIB, RWC, and RIB dry-cured hams given by the consumer panel.

Regarding the type of processing, the panel of consumers scored all the attributes in RIB dry-cured ham higher than the TIB dry-cured ham, although none were significantly different ($p > 0.05$). Therefore, the consumer acceptability of sensory traits is similar in both types of dry-cured ham; thus, the reduction of the salt content and the deboning do not affect the organoleptic characteristics of the Iberian dry-cured ham. The results agree with other studies of cured meat in which the palatability and texture were not compromised with the reduction of salt in respect to the traditional method [59]. However, contrasting results have been reported in cooked ham products, where texture, flavor, and overall consumer acceptability were significantly affected by salt reduction [60].

In Italian dry-cured ham obtained from white commercial pig crosses, a greater acceptability was observed in salt-reduced dry-cured ham in respect to the same product processed after traditional manufacturing [44].

Both types of Iberian ham (TIB and RIB) obtained global acceptance scores above 4 (I like) on the scale of 1–5, so it can be asserted that the consumer accepts Iberian dry-cured ham more.

Regarding the effect of the breed on the consumer acceptability of dry-cured ham, all sensory traits were scored significantly high by the untrained panel in dry-cured RIB ham compared to dry-cured RWC ham ($p \leq 0.05$).

The intramuscular fat content of the product has been described among the main composition parameters that influence the organoleptic quality in dry-cured products [61].

As has been described, this parameter was significantly higher in RIB dry-cured ham compared to RWC dry-cured ham, thus data agreed with other studies on Iberian pig dry-cured products [62] and other native breeds [63], where it was observed that products obtained from autochthonous breeds were better valued by consumers.

In the preference study, 6.38% of consumers preferred the RWC dry-cured ham, 63.83% the RIB dry-cured ham, and 29.79% the TIB. Therefore, from a consumer viewpoint, the reduction of salt in dry-cured ham improved the perception.

Regarding the preference between the two Iberian products, 70% of the consumers chose the reduced salt product, although no significant differences were detected in the evaluation of the acceptance of the salty taste (Table 6).

4. Conclusions

The deboning of the dry-cured ham before processing and the reduction of the salting time produced dry-cured hams with lower salt content. A greater reduction in salt was achieved in Iberian dry-cured ham than in that from white commercial pig crosses due to the different physicochemical and biochemical characteristics of its meat. The decreased salt concentration achieved allows the inclusion of the nutritional claim "reduced sodium/salt content" compared to similar products.

The reduction in salt and deboning did not have a negative effect on the proteolysis of dry-cured ham (both Iberian and white commercial pig crosses), as no differences in FFA content were observed. Furthermore, the PI increased only slightly (which was higher in dry-cured hams from white commercial pig crosses).

Reduced salt dry-cured hams have adequate consumer acceptance, adequate instrumental color, and texture characteristics. Although the processes modified the texture of the reduced Iberian dry-cured hams, their sensory characteristics were better valued than those with bone and following the traditional manufacturing processes.

Author Contributions: Conceptualization, L.T., B.M.-R., and J.T.; methodology, L.T., B.M.-R., and B.P.; software, L.T. and B.M.-R.; validation, L.T., B.M.-R., and J.T.; formal analysis, L.T., B.M.-R., J.T., and E.S.; investigation, L.T., B.M.-R., B.P., and J.T.; resources, L.T., B.M.-R., and B.P.; data curation, L.T., B.M.-R., and E.S.; writing—original draft preparation, L.T., B.M.-R., and E.S.; writing—review and editing, L.T., B.M.-R., E.S., J.T., and B.P.; visualization, L.T., B.M.-R., E.S., J.T., and B.P.; supervision L.T., B.M.-R., E.S., J.T., and B.P.; project administration, L.T. and B.M.-R.; funding acquisition, L.T., B.M.-R., and B.P. All authors have read and agreed to the published version of the manuscript.

Funding: This research was funded by the project *Desarrollo de un nuevo jamón ibérico deshuesado bajo en sodio y rico en pétidos bioactivos* (RTC-2017-6319, RETOS-COLABORACIÓN 2017). Ministerio de Ciencia, Innovación y Universidades (Spain).

Institutional Review Board Statement: Not applicable.

Informed Consent Statement: Not applicable.

Conflicts of Interest: The authors declare no conflict of interest. The funders had no role in the design of the study; in the collection, analyses, or interpretation of data; in the writing of the manuscript, or in the decision to publish the results.

References

1. Martín-Gómez, A.; Arroyo-Manzanares, N.; Rodríguez-Estévez, V.; Arce, L. Use of a non-destructive sampling method for characterization of Iberian cured ham breed and feeding regime using GC-IMS. *Meat Sci.* **2019**, *152*, 146–154. [CrossRef] [PubMed]
2. Strazzullo, P.; D'Elia, L.; Kandala, N.-B.; Cappuccio, F.P. Salt intake, stroke, and cardiovascular disease: Meta-analysis of prospective studies. *BMJ* **2009**, *339*, b4567. [CrossRef] [PubMed]
3. Doyle, M.E.; Glass, K.A. Sodium reduction and its effect on food safety, food quality, and human health. *Compr. Rev. Food Sci. Food Saf.* **2010**, *9*, 44–56. [CrossRef] [PubMed]
4. Inguglia, E.S.; Zhang, Z.; Tiwari, B.K.; Kerry, J.P.; Burgess, C.M. Salt reduction strategies in processed meat products–A review. *Trends Food Sci. Technol.* **2017**, *59*, 70–78. [CrossRef]
5. Desmond, E. Reducing salt: A challenge for the meat industry. *Meat Sci.* **2006**, *74*, 188–196. [CrossRef] [PubMed]

6. Toldrá, F.; Etherington, D.J. Examination of cathepsins B, D, H and L activities in dry-cured hams. *Meat Sci.* **1988**, *23*, 1–7. [CrossRef]
7. Zhou, C.; Wang, C.; Tang, C.; Dai, C.; Bai, Y.; Yu, X.; Li, C.; Xu, X.; Zhou, G.; Cao, J. Label-free proteomics reveals the mechanism of bitterness and adhesiveness in Jinhua ham. *Food Chem.* **2019**, *297*, 125012. [CrossRef] [PubMed]
8. Zhou, C.; Wang, C.; Cai, J.; Bai, Y.; Yu, X.; Li, C.; Xu, X.; Zhou, G.; Cao, J. Evaluating the effect of protein modifications and water distribution on bitterness and adhesiveness of Jinhua ham. *Food Chem.* **2019**, *293*, 103–111. [CrossRef] [PubMed]
9. Liao, R.; Xia, Q.; Zhou, C.; Geng, F.; Wang, Y.; Sun, Y.; He, J.; Pan, D.; Cao, J. LC-MS/MS-based metabolomics and sensory evaluation characterize metabolites and texture of normal and spoiled dry-cured hams. *Food Chem.* **2022**, *371*, 131156. [CrossRef]
10. Frye, C.B.; Hand, L.W.; Calkins, C.R.; Mandigo, R.W. Reduction or Replacement of sodium chloride in a tumbled ham product. *J. Food Sci.* **1986**, *51*, 836–837. [CrossRef]
11. Armenteros, M.; Aristoy, M.C.; Toldrá, F. Evolution of nitrate and nitrite during the processing of dry-cured ham with partial replacement of NaCl by other chloride salts. *Meat Sci.* **2012**, *91*, 378–381. [CrossRef] [PubMed]
12. Armenteros, M.; Aristoy, M.C.; Barat, J.M.; Toldrá, F. Biochemical and sensory changes in dry-cured ham salted with partial replacements of NaCl by other chloride salts. *Meat Sci.* **2012**, 361–367. [CrossRef] [PubMed]
13. Hand, L.W.; Terreall, R.N.; Smith, G.C. Effects of complete or partial replacement of osodium chloride on processing and sensory properties of hams. *J. Food Sci.* **1982**, *47*, 1776–1778. [CrossRef]
14. Barat, J.M.; Pérez-Esteve, E.; Aristoy, M.C.; Toldrá, F. Partial replacement of sodium in meat and fish products by using magnesium salts. A review. *Plant Soil* **2013**, *368*, 179–188. [CrossRef]
15. Seong, P.N.; Seo, H.W.; Cho, S.H.; Kim, Y.S.; Kang, S.M.; Kim, J.H.; Hang, G.H.; Park, B.Y.; Moon, S.S.; Hoa, V.B. Potential use of glasswort poder as a salt replacer for the production of healthier dry-cured ham products. *Czech J. Food Sci.* **2017**, *35*, 149–159. [CrossRef]
16. Santos, B.; Campagnol, P.; Morgano, M.; Pollonio, M. Monosodium glutamate, disodium inosinate, disodium guanylate, lysine and taurine improve the sensor quality of fermented cooked sausages with 50% and 75% replacement of NaCl with KCl. *Meat Sci.* **2014**, *96*, 509–513. [CrossRef] [PubMed]
17. Barretto, T.L.; Rodrigues, M.A.; Telis-Romero, J.; da Silva, A.C. Improving sensory acceptance and physicochemical properties by ultrasound application to restructured cooked ham with salt (NaCl) reduction. *Meat Sci.* **2018**, *145*, 55–62. [CrossRef] [PubMed]
18. Sadeghi-Mehr, A.; Lautenschlaeger, R.; Drusch, S. Sensory, physicochemical and microbiological properties of dry-cured formed ham: Comparison of four different binding systems. *Eur. Food Res. Technol.* **2016**, *242*, 1379–1391. [CrossRef]
19. Regulation (EC) No. 1924/2006 of the European Parliament and of the Council of 20 December 2006 on Nutrition and Health Claims Made On Foods, (OJ L 404, 30.12.2006, p. 9). Available online: https://eur-lex.europa.eu/legal-content/EN/TXT/?uri=CELEX%3A02006R1924-20141213 (accessed on 1 December 2021).
20. Ventanas, J. *Jamón Ibérico y Serrano. Fundamentos de la Elaboración de la Calidad*; Mundi-Prensa: Madrid, Spain, 2012.
21. Phan, V.A.; Yven, C.; Lawrence, G.; Chabanet, C.; Reparet, J.M.; Salles, C. In vivo sodium reléase related to salty perception during eating model cheeses of different textures. *Int. Dairy J.* **2008**, *18*, 956–963. [CrossRef]
22. Ruusunen, M.; Puolanne, E. Reducing sodium intake from meat products. *Meat Sci.* **2005**, *70*, 531–541. [CrossRef] [PubMed]
23. Lorido, L.; Estévez, M.; Ventanas, J.; Ventanas, S. Comparative study between Serrano and Iberian dry-cured hams in relation to the application of high hydrostatic pressure and temporal sensory perceptions. *LWT Food Sci. Technol.* **2015**, *64*, 1234–1242. [CrossRef]
24. Aliño, M.; Grau, R.; Toldrá, F.; Blesa, E.; Pagán, M.J.; Barat, J.M. Physicochemical properties and microbiology of dry-cured loins obtained by partial sodium replacement with potassium, calcium and magnesium. *Meat Sci.* **2010**, *85*, 580–588. [CrossRef] [PubMed]
25. [ISO] 1442: 1997. *Meat and Meat Products. Determination of Moisture Content (Reference Method)*; International Organization for Standardization: Geneva, Switzerland, 1997.
26. Folch, J.; Lees, M.; Stanley, G. A simple method for the isolation of total lipides from animal tissues. *J. Biol. Chem.* **1957**, *226*, 495–509. [CrossRef]
27. Association of Official Analytical Chemists. [AOAC] Official Method 920.153. Ash in Meat. In *Official Methods of Analysis, Meat and Meat Products*, 16th ed.; Cunniff, P., Ed.; Association of Official Analytical Chemists: Gaithersburg, MD, USA, 2005; Volume 2.
28. [ISO] 1841-1: 1996. *Meat and Meat Products. Determination of chloride content–Part 1: Volhard Method (Reference Method)*; International Organization for Standardization: Geneva, Switzerland, 1996.
29. Association of Official Analytical Chemists [AOAC]. *Official Methods of Analysis*, 19th ed.; Association of Official Analytical Chemists: Gaithersburgh, MD, USA, 2012.
30. Harkouss, R.; Mirade, P.S.; Gatellier, P. Development a rapid, specific and efficient procedure for the determination of proteolytic activity in dry-cured ham: Definition of a new proteolysis index. *Meat Sci.* **2012**, *92*, 84–88. [CrossRef] [PubMed]
31. Aaslyng, M.D.; Vestergaard, C.; Koch, A.G. The effect of salt reduction on sensory quality and microbial growth in hotdog sausages, bacon, ham and salami. *Meat Sci.* **2014**, *96*, 47–55. [CrossRef] [PubMed]
32. Tejada, L.; Buendía-Moreno, L.; Álvarez, E.; Palma, A.; Salazar, E.; Muñoz, B.; Abellán, A. Development of an Iberian Chorizo Salted With a Combination of Mineral Salts (Seawater Substitute) and Better Nutritional Profile. *Front. Nutr.* **2021**, *8*, 642726. [CrossRef] [PubMed]

33. Abellán, A.; Cayuela, J.M.; Pino, A.; Martínez-Cachá, A.; Salazar, E.; Tejada, L. Free amino acid content of goat's milk cheese made with animal rennet and plant coagulant. *J. Sci. Food Agric.* **2012**, *92*, 1657–1664. [CrossRef] [PubMed]
34. Bourne, M.C. Texture profile analysis. *Food Technol.* **1978**, *32*, 62–66.
35. UNE-ISO 6658:2019. *Sensory Analysis. Methodology*; General Guidance; Asociación Española de Normalización: Madrid, Spain, 2019.
36. UNE-ISO 4121:2006. *Sensory Analysis–Guidelines for the Use of Quantitative Response Scales (ISO 4121:2003)*; Asociación Española de Normalización: Madrid, Spain, 2006.
37. Martín, L.; Córdoba, J.J.; Antequera, T.; Timón, M.L.; Ventanas, J. Effects of salt and temperature on proteolysis during ripening of Iberian ham. *Meat Sci.* **1998**, *49*, 145–153. [CrossRef]
38. Bermúdez, R.; Franco, D.; Carballo, J.; Lorenzo, J.M. Physicochemical changes during manufacture and final sensory characteristics of dry-cured Celta ham. Effect of muscle type. *Food Contr.* **2014**, *43*, 263–269. [CrossRef]
39. Sirtori, F.; Dimauro, C.; Bozzi, R.; Aquilani, C.; Franci, O.; Calamai, L.; Pezzati, A.; Pugliese, C. Evolution of volatile compounds and physical, chemical and sensory characteristics of Toscano PDO ham from fresh to dry-cured product. *Eur. Food Res. Technol.* **2020**, *246*, 409–424. [CrossRef]
40. Guàrdia, M.D.; Guerrero, L.; Gelabert, J.; Gou, P.; Arnau, J. Consumer attitude towards sodium reduction in meat products and acceptability of fermented sausages with reduced sodium content. *Meat Sci.* **2006**, *73*, 484–490. [CrossRef] [PubMed]
41. Pugliese, C.; Sirtori, F. Quality of meat and meat products produced from southern European pig breeds. *Meat Sci.* **2012**, *90*, 511–518. [CrossRef] [PubMed]
42. Rosell, C.; Toldrá, F. Comparison of Muscle Proteolytic and Lipolytic Enzyme Levels in Raw Hams from Iberian and White Pigs. *J. Sci. Food Agric.* **1998**, *76*, 117–122. [CrossRef]
43. Cordoba, J.J.; Antequera, T.; Garcia, C.; Ventanas, J.; Lopez Bote, C.; Asensio, M.A. Evolution of free amino acids and amines during ripening of Iberian cured ham. *J. Agric. Food Chem.* **1994**, *42*, 2296–2301. [CrossRef]
44. Schivazappa, C.; Virgili, R. Impact of salt levels on the sensory profile and consumer acceptance of Italian dry-cured ham. *J. Sci. Food Agric.* **2020**, *100*, 3370–3377. [CrossRef] [PubMed]
45. Pérez-Palacios, T.; Ruiz, J.; Martín, D.; Barat, J.M.; Antequera, T. Pre-cure Freezing Effect on Physicochemical, Texture and Sensory Characteristics of Iberian Ham. *Food Sci. Technol. Int.* **2011**, *17*, 127–133. [CrossRef] [PubMed]
46. Benedini, R.; Parolari, G.; Toscani, T.; Virgili, R. Sensory and texture properties of Italian typical dry-cured hams as related to maturation time and salt content. *Meat Sci.* **2012**, *90*, 431–437. [CrossRef] [PubMed]
47. Toldrá, F.; Flores, M. The role of muscle proteases and lipases in flavor development during the processing of dry-cured ham. *Crit. Rev. Food Sci. Nutr.* **1998**, *38*, 331–352. [CrossRef] [PubMed]
48. Petričević, S.; Radovčić, N.M.; Lukić, K.; Listeš, E.; Medić, H. Differentiation of dry-cured hams from different processing methods by means of volatile compounds, physico-chemical and sensory analysis. *Meat Sci.* **2018**, *137*, 217–227. [CrossRef]
49. Salazar, E.; Abellán, A.; Cayuela, J.M.; Poto, A.; Girón, F.; Zafrilla, P.; Tejada, L. Effect of processing time on the quality of dry-cured ham obtained from a native pig breed (Chato Murciano). *Anim. Prod. Sci.* **2014**, *55*, 113–121. [CrossRef]
50. ANICE, 2017. Compromiso de Reformulación para la Reducción de Sal y Grasa en los Derivados Cárnicos. Circular 13/17: Propuesta de Reducción de Sal y Grasa en los Derivados Cárnicos el 17/02/2017. Available online: https://www.anice.es/industrias/circulares-ano-2017/circular-1317---propuesta-de-reduccion-de-sal-y-grasa-en-los-derivados-carnicos_20518_228_28252_0_1_in.html (accessed on 1 December 2021).
51. Pinna, A.; Saccani, G.; Schivazappa, C.; Simoncini, N.; Virgili, R. Revision of the cold processing phases to obtain a targeted salt reduction in typical Italian dry-cured ham. *Meat Sci.* **2020**, *161*, 107994. [CrossRef] [PubMed]
52. Regulation (EC) No 2073/2005 of the European Parliament and of the Council of 15 November 2005 on Microbiological Criteria for Foodstuffs, (OJ L 338, 22.12.2005, p. 1). Available online: https://eur-lex.europa.eu/eli/reg/2005/2073/oj (accessed on 1 December 2021).
53. Jiménez-Colmenero, F.; Ventanas, J.; Toldrá, F. Nutritional composition of dry-cured ham and its role in a healthy diet. *Meat Sci.* **2010**, *84*, 585–593. [CrossRef] [PubMed]
54. Cittadini, A.; Domínguez, R.; Gómez, B.; Pateiro, M.; Pérez-Santaescolástica, C.; López-Fernández, O.; Sarriés, M.V.; Lorenzo, J.M. Effect of NaCl replacement by other chloride salts on physicochemical parameters, proteolysis and lipolysis of dry-cured foal "cecina". *J. Food Sci. Technol.* **2020**, *57*, 1628–1635. [CrossRef] [PubMed]
55. Abellán, A.; Salazar, E.; Vázquez, J.; Cayuela, J.M.; Tejada, L. Changes in proteolysis during the dry-cured processing of refrigerated and frozen loin. *LWT Food Sci. Technol.* **2018**, *96*, 507–512. [CrossRef]
56. Lorenzo, J.M.; Cittadini, A.; Bermúdez, R.; Munekata, P.E.; Domínguez, R. Influence of partial replacement of NaCl with KCl, CaCl2 and MgCl2 on proteolysis, lipolysis and sensory properties during the manufacture of dry-cured lacón. *Food Control* **2015**, *55*, 90–96. [CrossRef]
57. Krvavica, M.; Lasić, D.; Kljusurić, J.G.; Đugum, J.; Janović, Š.; Milovac, S.; Bošnir, J. Chemical Characteristics of Croatian Traditional Istarski pršut (PDO) Produced from Two Different Pig Genotypes. *Molecules* **2021**, *26*, 4140. [CrossRef]
58. Lorenzo, J.M.; Bermúdez, R.; Domínguez, R.; Guiotto, A.; Franco, D.; Purriños, L. Physicochemical and microbial changes during the manufacturing process of dry-cured lacón salted with potassium, calcium and magnesium chloride as a partial replacement for sodium chloride. *Food Control.* **2015**, *50*, 763–769. [CrossRef]

59. Gómez, I.; Janardhanan, R.; Ibañez, F.C.; Beriain, M.J. The Effects of Processing and Preservation Technologies on Meat Quality: Sensory and Nutritional Aspects. *Foods* **2020**, *9*, 1416. [CrossRef] [PubMed]
60. Delgado-Pando, G.; Fischer, E.; Allen, P.; Kerry, J.P.; O'Sullivan, M.G.; Hamill, R.M. Salt content and minimum acceptable levels in whole-muscle cured meat products. *Meat Sci.* **2018**, *139*, 179–186. [CrossRef] [PubMed]
61. Affentranger, P.; Gerwig, C.; Seewer, G.J.F.; Schwiirer, D.; Kiinzi, N. Growth and carcass characteristics as well as meat and fat quality of three types of pigs under different feeding regimens. *Lives. Prod. Sci.* **1996**, *45*, 187–196. [CrossRef]
62. Ventanas, S.; Ruiz, J.; García, C.; Ventanas, J. Preference and juiciness of Iberian dry-cured loin as affected by intramuscular fat content, crossbreeding and rearing system. *Meat Sci.* **2007**, *77*, 324–330. [CrossRef] [PubMed]
63. Salazar, E.; Cayuela, J.M.; Abellán, A.; Poto, A.; Peinado, B.; Tejada, L. A comparison of the quality of dry-cured loins obtained from the native pig breed (Chato Murciano) and from a modern crossbreed pig. *Anim. Prod. Sci.* **2013**, *53*, 352–359. [CrossRef]

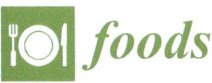

Article

Effects of Drying Process on the Volatile and Non-Volatile Flavor Compounds of *Lentinula edodes*

Lijia Zhang [1], Xiaobo Dong [1,2], Xi Feng [3], Salam A. Ibrahim [4], Wen Huang [1] and Ying Liu [1,*]

1. College of Food Science and Technology, Huazhong Agricultural University, Wuhan 430070, China; 13297021290@163.com (L.Z.); xbdong@nwafu.edu.cn (X.D.); huangwen@mail.hzau.edu.cn (W.H.)
2. College of Food Science and Engineering, Northwest A&F University, Xianyang 712100, China
3. Department of Nutrition, Food Science and Packaging, San Jose State University, San Jose, CA 95192, USA; xi.feng@sjsu.edu
4. Department of Family and Consumer Sciences, North Carolina A&T State University, 171 Carver Hall, Greensboro, NC 27411, USA; ibrah001@ncat.edu
* Correspondence: yingliu@mail.hzau.edu.cn; Tel.: +86-13407161906

Abstract: In this study, fresh *Lentinula edodes* was dehydrated using freeze-drying (FD), hot-air drying (HAD), and natural drying (ND), and the volatile and non-volatile flavor compounds were analyzed. The drying process changed the contents of eight-carbon compounds and resulted in a weaker "mushroom flavor" for dried *L. edodes*. HAD mushrooms had higher levels of cyclic sulfur compounds (56.55 µg/g) and showed a stronger typical shiitake mushroom aroma than those of fresh (7.24 µg/g), ND (0.04 µg/g), and FD mushrooms (3.90 µg/g). The levels of 5′-nucleotide increased, whereas the levels of organic acids and free amino acids decreased after the drying process. The dried *L. edodes* treated with FD had the lowest levels of total free amino acids (29.13 mg/g). However, it had the highest levels of umami taste amino acids (3.97 mg/g), bitter taste amino acids (6.28 mg/g) and equivalent umami concentration (EUC) value (29.88 g monosodium glutamate (MSG) per 100 g). The results indicated that FD was an effective drying method to produce umami flavor in dried mushrooms. Meanwhile, HAD can be used to produce a typical shiitake mushroom aroma. Our results provide a theoretical basis to manufacture *L. edodes* products with a desirable flavor for daily cuisine or in a processed form.

Keywords: *Lentinula edodes*; drying methods; volatile compounds; non-volatile compounds; sulfur compounds; free amino acids; 5′-nucleotide

1. Introduction

Lentinula edodes (Berk.) Sing or Shiitake mushroom, accounting for about 17% of global mushroom production, is the second largest cultivated edible mushroom in the world [1,2]. The global production of cultivated mushrooms has increased more than 73% in the last 10 years (FAOSTAT, 2019). *L. edodes* is one of the most popular edible and medicinal mushrooms in East Asia for its rich nutrients, favorable medicinal properties as well as desirable flavor [3,4]. Shiitake mushroom has been widely used as a flavor enhancer in meat and fermented products due to its unique flavor [5,6].

The desirable flavor of shiitake mushrooms is composed of volatile and non-volatile components [3]. It has been identified with various volatile compounds from *L. edodes*. The major volatile components are eight-carbon (C8) compounds and sulfur compounds [1]. Both C8 and sulfur compounds are produced by enzymatic reactions, in which lipoxygenase and hydroperoxide lyase catalyze linoleic acid to produce C8 compounds, such as 1-octen-3-one and 1-octen-3-ol, whereas γ-glutamyl transpeptidase and cysteine sulfoxide lyase catalyze lenthinic acid to produce sulfur compounds, including 1,2,4-trithiolane and lenthionine [7,8]. Among these volatile compounds, 1-octen-3-ol, widely present in mushrooms, is responsible for a typical mushroom-like odor, whereas lenthionine, a cyclic 5-sulfur compound, also contributes to the aroma of *L. edodes* [9,10]. Fresh shiitake mushroom gives off a slight odor by the abundance of 1-octen-3-ol. However, the unique aroma of shiitake mushroom develops due to the increase of sulfur compounds after drying [1]. The taste of mushrooms is mainly triggered by several small water-soluble substances, including organic acids, 5'-nucleotides and free amino acids [11]. Thus, it is vital to investigate the effects of processing methods on volatile and non-volatile compounds of shiitake mushrooms.

Drying is a convenient and effective technique to prolong the shelf life of fresh shiitake mushrooms by decreasing the moisture content [12,13]. However, the quality of mushrooms (flavor, nutrients, texture and color) is affected by the drying method [12]. Hot-air drying (HAD), freeze-drying (FD) and natural drying (ND) are the three most typical drying methods for shiitake mushrooms. Lu et al. [14] studied the changes of volatile components in *L. edodes* during the vacuum freeze-drying process. Qin et al. [15] evaluated the changes in aroma profile of *L. edodes* during different stages of HAD. Politowicz et al. [12] investigated the effects of different drying methods (CD (convective drying), FD (freeze-drying), VMD (vacuum-microwave drying) and CPD-VMFD (vacuum–microwave finish-drying)) on volatile composition and sensory profile (inner color and sponginess) of *L. edodes*. However, the influence of the drying methods of hot-air drying (HAD), freeze drying (FD) and natural drying (ND) on both the volatile and non-volatile flavor compounds in *L. edodes* has never been studied.

The objectives of this work were to analyze the volatile and non-volatile flavor components' profile of *Lentinula edodes* by three drying methods (HAD, FD and ND). The results could provide theoretical evidence for new product developments with *Lentinula edodes*.

2. Materials and Methods

2.1. Material

Fresh shiitake mushrooms were obtained from a local market (Wuhan, China). The samples with uniform size (including the cap and stipe) and maturity were selected. The moisture contents of shiitake mushrooms were $87.50 \pm 1.30\%$ (g/g, w.b.). Internal standard solution (cyclohexanone (99.50% purity)) was purchased from FLUKA (Seelze, Germany). The n-alkane standards (C_7–C_{30}) were purchased from Sigma Chemical Company (St. Louis, MO, USA).

2.2. Drying Methods

2.2.1. Freeze-Drying (FD)

Fresh shiitake mushrooms (1000 g) were dried by a freeze drier (Betr 2–8 LD plus, Christ, Germany). The vacuum degree was 20–40 Pa. Cold trap temperature was $-50\ °C$. The drying chamber was $-35\ °C$. Drying was carried out for 72 h until the moisture content was less than 10% (g/g, w.b.) [11].

2.2.2. Hot Air Drying (HAD)

Fresh shiitake mushrooms (1000 g) were directly dried in a forced air circulation oven (GZX-9240MBE, Yuhua Equipment Ltd., Gongyi, China). The temperature was set at $50\ °C$ and the air velocity was at 0.45 m/s. Samples were dried until the final moisture content was below 10% (g/g, w.b.).

2.2.3. Natural Drying (ND)

Fresh shiitake mushrooms (1000 g) were placed on trays in a single layer. Samples were then placed outdoors in a well-ventilated location with abundant sunlight. The average temperature was $25 \pm 5\ °C$ and the relative humidity was $70 \pm 10\%$. The drying lasted for about 3 days until the final moisture content was below 10% (g/g, w.b.).

2.3. Electronic Nose Analysis

An FOX 4000 electronic nose system from Alpha M.O.S. (Toulouse, France) was used for electronic nose analysis [16]. The instrument comprised of 18 metal oxide sensors and combined with a headspace auto-sampler HS100. Dried shiitake mushroom samples were ground to a fine powder and screened by a 60-meshes sifter. Then, fresh mushroom and different dried powders were homogenized in saturated sodium chloride solution (1:20), respectively. Sample of 2 mL were added into a 10 mL vial and capped with a Teflon rubber cap, equilibrated at 40 °C for 120 s under agitation (500 rpm). Dry air was used at a flow of 150 mL/min as carrier gas. Equilibrated headspace (2500 µL) was injected into the electronic nose at the rate of 2500 µL/s by a 2500 µL gas-tight syringe (50 °C). The acquisition time and delay time between consecutive injections were set as 120 s and 300 s, respectively.

2.4. HS-SPME-GC-MS Analysis

The volatile compounds were analyzed following Jing-Nan et al.'s methods with a minor modification [17]. An SPME (solid-phase micro-extraction) manual device equipped with a 50 µm/30 µm divinylbenzene/carboxen/polydimethylsiloxane (DVB/CAR/PDMS) fiber (Supelco, Bellfonte, PA, USA) was used to extract volatile compounds from samples. Mushroom homogenate (1.8 g mushroom powder in 20 mL NaCl saturated solution) was added into 40 mL-vial containing a magnetic stirring bar. After being spiked with 25 µL of cyclohexanone (0.95 mg/mL of ethyl alcohol) as internal standard, the vials were immediately seal with a PTFE septa (Supelco, Bellfonte, PA, USA). Samples were balanced at 50 °C for 15 min, then the fiber was inserted into the vial to extract volatile compounds for 1 h. Finally, the fiber was inserted into the injection port of GC and desorbed for 5 min under the splitless mode.

An Agilent 7890A GC coupled with an Agilent 5975 MS was used to analyze volatile compounds. A HP-5MS fused silica capillary column (30 m × 0.25 mm I.D., 0.25 mm film thickness, Agilent technologies, Santa Clara, CA, USA) was installed in GC. GC conditions were set as follows: the carrier gas of helium with a flow rate of 1 mL/min; the injector temperature was 250 °C; the oven temperature programming was set at 40 °C for 3 min initially, then 3 °C/min to 150 °C, held for 1 min, finally 5 °C/min to 220 °C, maintained for 2 min. The ionization source temperature was set at 230 °C. The MS was obtained by electron impact mode at 70 eV in a range from 30 amu to 395 amu.

Volatile compounds were identified by Kovats retention index (RI) and the database (Wiley7.0 and NIST05) [15]. The Kovats retention index (RI) of unknown compounds was calculated using n-alkanes (C7-C30) injected under the same conditions. The quantity of volatiles was calculated with the internal standard (cyclohexanone) [18].

2.5. Assay of Organic Acids

Organic acids were extracted and analyzed as the cited method [19]. A sample (500 mg) was used to extract organic acids with 25 mL of KH_2PO_4 (pH = 2.65) in 75 °C water bath for 25 min. The solution was centrifuged 20 min at 10,000 rpm, then filtered and analyzed by HPLC system. The HPLC system is equipped with an InertSustain AQ-C18 column (4.6 × 250 mm, 5 µm) (Shimadzu, Shanghai, China). Dipotassium phosphate (0.01 mol/L, pH = 2.65) was used as mobile phase with a flow rate at 0.4 mL/min. The injection volume was 20 µL and wavelength of the UV detector was 214 nm. Organic acids in the samples were identified by the retention time of the standard organic acids (Sinopharm Chemical Reagent Co. Ltd., Shanghai, China) and quantified with their standard curves.

2.6. Assay of Free Amino Acids

According to the report [11], 1 g of mushroom powder and extract was obtained with 50 mL of hydrochloric acid (0.10 mol/L) at 25 °C for 45 min. Then, centrifuged for 30 min at 12,000 rpm. The free amino acids were analyzed by an L-8900 high-speed amino acid analyzer (Hitachi High-Tech. Corp., Tokio, Japan).

2.7. Assay of 5′-Nucleotides

5′-nucleotides was extracted and analyzed following the cited method [11]. Sample power (500 mg) was used to extract 5′-nucleotides with distilled water (25 mL) at $100 \pm 5\ °C$ for 1 min. After centrifugation (10,000 rpm, 15 min), the supernatant was evaporated. Then, the residue was re-dissolved in deionized water (10 mL). Sample of 20 μL was injected to the same HPLC system as described in Section 2.5. 5′-nucleotide in the samples were identified by the retention time of the standard 5′-nucleotide (Sigma, USA) and quantified with their standard curves.

2.8. Statistical Analysis

Principal component analysis (PCA) was performed by XLSTAT 2010 (Microsoft Corporation, Washington, DC, USA). One way analysis of variance (ANOVA) was used to analyze the differences among samples at a significant level of 0.05 by SPSS 25 (IBM, Armonk, NY, USA).

3. Results and Discussion

3.1. Electronic Nose Analysis of L. edodes Samples

The electronic nose obtains comprehensive flavor information within a short time by mimicking the human olfactory system [20]. It was used for classifying and monitoring the drying process of *L. edodes* [14,21]. Principal component analysis (PCA) is a multivariate chemometric method that can be used to identify the correlation patterns of constituent variables involved in the distinction between samples [16]. PCA also can provide a better visualization and highlight the differences in volatile profiles. As shown in Figure 1, the accumulative variance contribution rate of the first two PCs was 93% (PC1 accounted for 81.67% and PC2 accounted for 16.29%), which indicated the feasibility of PCA and the two main components contained most of the information about volatile compounds [22]. Despite sensor instability among replications, volatile profiles from different samples were located into four separated areas. FD samples located in the positive axis of PC1, while both ND and HAD samples were in the negative axis of PC1, which indicated that the volatile compounds of ND and HAD samples were significantly different from those of FD samples. These results also showed that the drying processes altered shiitake mushroom aroma profiles.

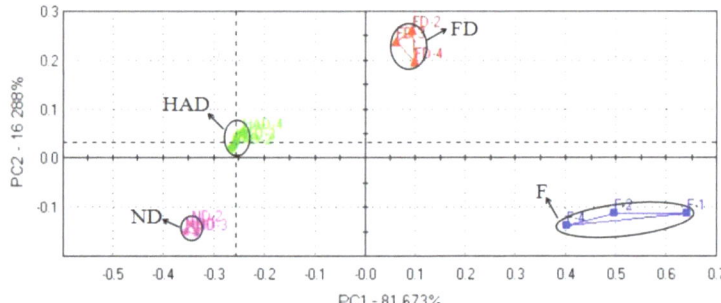

Figure 1. PCA of E-nose data for fresh and dried *L. edodes*; F: fresh sample; FD: freeze drying sample; HAD: hot-air drying sample; ND: natural drying sample.

3.2. HS-SPME-GC-MS Analysis of Volatile Compounds of L. edodes

In order to further investigate the effects of different drying methods on the flavor of *L. edodes*, the specific volatile components of different mushroom samples were measured by HS-SPME-GC-MS. Semi-quantitative analysis with an internal standard was used to compare differences among samples. The volatile compounds of fresh and dried mushroom samples were shown in Table 1. A total of 55 volatile compounds from *L. edodes* were tentatively identified and quantified, including 11 alcohols, 9 aldehydes, 6 ketones, 11 sulfur compounds and 17 hydrocarbons. A total of 41, 36 and 24 compounds were detected in FD, HAD and ND samples, with contents of 171.29 μg/g, 206.88 μg/g and 256.67 μg/g, respectively. It is notable that only 22 compounds were detected in fresh mushroom (1451 μg/g). It was consistent with the reports that more volatile compounds were formed in dried *L. edodes* [1]. After drying treatment, the total volatile components increased, but the total volatile compounds content decreased.

Table 1. Contents of volatile compounds in fresh and different dried *L. edodes*.

	Compounds	RI [a]	Contents (μg/g)				ID [e]
			F [b]	FD	HAD	ND	
Alcohols (11)	1-Hexanol	871	nd [d]	0.40	0.56	1.17	A
	1-Octen-3-ol [c]	983	857.02	103.78	5.72	105.30	B
	2-Cyclohexen-1-ol	985	nd	nd	7.22	nd	A
	3-Octanol [c]	998	6.09	1.93	nd	1.40	B
	2-Octen-1-ol [c]	1071	132.99	6.35	2.59	13.86	B
	1-Octanol [c]	1077	19.89	1.99	0.68	2.06	B
	Linalool	1100	nd	2.13	nd	nd	A
	Phenylethyl Alcohol	1117	nd	0.08	0.95	nd	A
	4-Methyl-benzeneethanol	1173	nd	nd	0.66	nd	A
	α-Terpineol	1188	nd	0.43	nd	nd	B
	Cedrol	1596	nd	0.11	nd	nd	B
	Total alcohols		1015.99	117.20	18.39	123.79	
Aldehydes (9)	Hexanal	803	nd	0.34	4.62	0.02	A
	(E)-Hept-2-enal	958	nd	nd	nd	0.18	A
	Benzaldehyde	965	0.69	0.62	1.30	0.15	A
	Octanal [c]	1004	nd	nd	0.18	nd	A
	Benzeneacetaldehyde	1046	0.48	3.44	0.93	0.32	A
	(E)-2-Octenal [c]	1058	11.78	nd	1.76	1.72	A
	2-Phenylpropenal	1157	nd	0.67	5.64	0.07	A
	Decanal	1206	0.69	0.42	0.27	0.09	A
	(z)-3,7-Dimethylocta-2,6-dienal	1241	nd	1.18	nd	nd	A
	Total aldehydes		13.64	6.67	14.70	2.55	
Ketones (6)	1-Octen-3-one [c]	981	237.99	5.52	21.17	118.24	B
	3-Octanone [c]	991	6.09	11.61	6.79	nd	B
	3-Octen-2-one [c]	1042	nd	nd	nd	0.11	A
	Acetophenone	1066	nd	nd	0.14	0.02	A
	(+)-Camphor	1139	0.18	0.08	0.05	0.02	B
	2-Undecanone	1297	nd	0.06	0.34	0.01	A
	Total ketones		244.26	17.27	28.49	118.40	
Sulfur compounds (11)	Carbon disulfide	<700	148.36	12.51	66.31	11.01	A
	Dimethyl disulfide	700	nd	nd	2.58	nd	B
	Dimethyl trisulfide	973	nd	0.80	0.26	nd	B
	1,2,4-Trithiolane	1083	7.00	2.79	32.21	nd	B
	2,4,5-Trithiahexane	1121	nd	nd	4.87	nd	A
	Dimethyl tetrasulfide	1209	nd	nd	2.27	nd	A
	1,2,4,5-Tetrathiane	1362	nd	0.11	7.23	nd	B
	1,2,4,6-Tetrathiepane	1504	nd	0.01	3.22	nd	B
	Lenthionine	1615	0.24	1.00	17.11	0.04	B
	Hexathiepane	1615	nd	nd	0.25	nd	B
	Cyclic octaatomic sulfur	2000	nd	nd	0.29	nd	A
	Total sulfur compounds		155.60	17.22	136.60	11.05	

Table 1. Cont.

Compounds		RI [a]	Contents (μg/g)				ID [e]
			F [b]	FD	HAD	ND	
Hydrocarbons (17)	1,3-Xylene	865	nd	0.05	0.04	0.03	A
	P-Isopropyltoluene	1021	1.06	0.32	nd	0.03	A
	D-Limonene	1025	17.43	10.54	7.74	0.78	A
	Naphthalene	1176	0.30	0.33	0.54	0.02	A
	Dodecane	1199	0.16	0.38	nd	nd	A
	5-Ethyl-2-methyl-octane	1280	0.95	nd	nd	nd	A
	3-Carene	1283	nd	0.07	nd	nd	B
	Decane	1288	nd	0.13	nd	nd	A
	b-Elemen	1390	nd	0.08	nd	nd	A
	Tetradecane	1400	0.56	0.14	0.09	0.00	A
	Germacrene D	1477	nd	0.08	nd	nd	A
	(-)-a-Selinenea-	1491	nd	0.20	nd	nd	A
	Pentadecane	1501	0.91	0.39	nd	nd	A
	Hexadecane	1600	nd	0.11	0.05	0.02	A
	Heptadecane	1697	nd	0.05	nd	nd	A
	Eicosane	2000	0.14	0.06	nd	nd	A
	Total hydrocarbons		21.51	12.93	8.46	0.88	

RI [a], retention index. F [b], fresh shiitake mushroom; FD, freeze drying sample; HAD, hot-air drying sample; ND, natural drying sample. eight-carbon [c] compounds. nd [d], not detected. Identification [e]: A, a comparison of mass spectrum and RI with authentic standards; B, comparison of mass spectrum and RI with published data and Wiley 7.0 and NIST05 MS library.

It has been reported that alcohols, aldehydes and ketones played important roles in flavor profiles of foods [9,10,23,24]. As shown in Table 1, the contents of alcohols, aldehydes and ketones in fresh, FD, HAD and ND were 1273.89 μg/g, 141.14 μg/g, 61.58 μg/g, and 244.74 μg/g, respectively. However, the contents of alcohols and ketones significantly decreased after the drying process. Similar results were reported in other mushrooms [9,10]. As shown in Figure 2, alcohols were the highest in fresh samples, but decreases were shown, especially in HAD mushroom samples. The content of aldehydes in HAD mushroom samples increased slightly in comparison with fresh samples. This may be due to aldehydes mainly derived from the oxidation and degradation of unsaturated fatty acids [25]. In addition, increasing the temperature of *L. edodes* samples may also promote Maillard reaction, including Strecker degradation, which increased aldehyde content [26]. The content of ketones in FD samples was the lowest. It was reported that ketones are mainly obtained from the Maillard reaction and the oxidation and degradation of unsaturated fatty acids [27], and ketones can also be produced by degradation of esters [28]. However, in this study, the most probable route may be through enzymatic reactions. The preservation or formation of ketones in *L. edodes* was not conducive when the FD temperature was not appropriate [14].

The flavor differences between fresh and dried *L. edodes* were obvious. The "mushroom flavor" of fresh *L. edodes* is described as a sweet, earthy and cheesy aroma, while the shiitake flavor of dried *L. edodes* is similar to that of onion and garlic [29]. Eight-carbon compounds are ubiquitous among mushrooms, which are a key contributor to mushroom flavor [9,30]. As shown in Table 1, the contents of eight-carbon compounds in fresh, FD, HAD, and ND mushrooms were 1271.85 μg/g, 131.18 μg/g, 38.89 μg/g and 242.69 μg/g, respectively. The contents of 1-octen-3-ol in in fresh, FD, HAD, and ND mushrooms were 857.02 μg/g, 103.78 μg/g, 5.72 μg/g and 105.30 μg/g, respectively. The contents of 1-octen-3-one and 3-octanone in in fresh, FD, HAD, and ND mushrooms were 244.08 μg/g, 17.13 μg/g, 27.96 μg/g and 118.24 μg/g, respectively. Generally, 1-octen-3-ol, 1-octen-3-one and 3-octanone were the major C8 compounds in mushrooms. 1-octen-3-ol, also called mushroom alcohol, feature with a typical odor of mushrooms [29]. 1-octen-3-one and 3-octanone could produce a similar odor like 1-octen-3-ol [31]. As shown in Table 1, 1-octen-3-ol and 1-octen-3-one were detected in all of the four mushrooms, and fresh mushrooms had the highest level of 1-octen-3-ol and 1-octen-3-one. 3-octanone was detected in fresh, FD, and HAD mushrooms, and FD mushrooms had the highest amount. However, other research reported that 1-octen-3-ol and 3-octanone were the dominant compounds in the dried *L. edodes* (vacuum, microwave, microwave vacuum, convective drying, vacuum-microwave drying and freeze-drying) [1,12]. The differences were possibly due to the different volatile compound extraction methods. In sum, drying processes changed the contents of C8 compounds, which resulted in weaker "mushroom flavor" for dried *L. edodes* compared with fresh *L. edodes*. This interesting finding could be helpful to further understand the biosynthesis of C8 compounds in mushrooms.

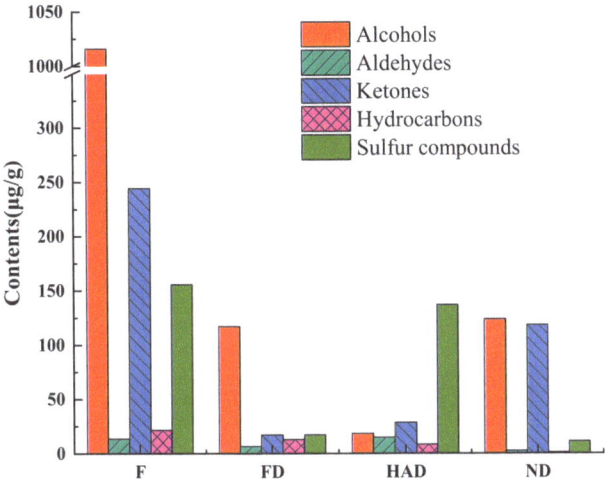

Figure 2. Contents of different types of volatile compounds in fresh and different dried *L. edodes*; F: fresh sample; FD: freeze drying sample; HAD: hot-air drying sample; ND: natural drying sample.

Volatile sulfur compounds are important aroma-active compounds in vegetables and processed meats, and they can offer unique aroma in *L. edodes* differing from many other commonly consumed mushrooms [22,32]. As shown in Table 1, the contents of sulfur compounds in mushrooms decreased after the drying process. However, more types of sulfur compounds were detected from dried mushrooms compared with fresh mushrooms. which was similar to that reported by Lu et al. [14]. Carbon disulfide from mushrooms had little influence in relation to the overall aroma [33]. The straight chain sulfur compounds and cyclic sulfur compounds were reported to greatly contribute to the unique aroma of *L. edodes* [34]. As shown in Table 1, the straight chain sulfur compounds, dimethyl disulfide and dimethyl trisulfide, were not detected in fresh and ND mushrooms, while dimethyl disulfide was detected in HAD mushrooms, and dimethyl trisulfide was detected in both FD and HAD mushrooms. The results showed that 1,2,4-trithiolane, 1,2,4,5-tetrathiane and lenthionine were the main cyclic sulfur compounds detected in the four kinds of mushroom samples. HAD mushrooms had the highest level of cyclic sulfur compounds (56.55 µg/g) among the four mushroom samples, and the content of cyclic sulfur compounds in fresh shiitake mushroom, FD and ND were 7.24 µg/g, 3.90 µg/g and 0.04 µg/g, respectively. Tian et al. [1] reported that HAD increased the content of cyclic sulfur compounds compared with fresh shiitake mushrooms. The formation of these cyclic sulfur compounds included two steps: the enzymic reactions of lenthinic acid catalyzed by cysteine sulfoxide lyase and γ-glutamyl transpeptidase; and the nonenzymatic polymerization of methylene disulfide [8]. In addition, lenthionine can decompose to dimethyl disulfide and dimethyl trisulfide [35]. Therefore, the differences of sulfur compounds in FD, HAD, and ND mushrooms might be attributed to enzyme activities and drying temperature during drying processes.

In sum, different drying processes significantly affected the volatile profiles of *L. edodes*, especially the C8 and sulfur compounds. HAD mushrooms had weaker "mushroom flavor" and strong shiitake flavor. In fact, the volatile content of L. edodes was different in each stage (fresh, early, middle and late stage) of HAD [21]. The above complicated changes of volatile compounds in mushrooms may be attributed to typical drying conditions, such as higher temperature for HAD, long-time exposure in the sunlight for ND and vacuum evaporation for FD, which could affect volatile compounds formation and precursor degradation.

3.3. Effects of Drying Methods on Organic Acids of L. edodes

Organic acids (tartaric acid, malic acid, ascorbic acid, citric acid, fumaric acid and succinic acid) were detected (Table 2). As shown in Table 2, succinic acid (472.61–645.25 mg/g) was the most abundant organic acid in the samples, accounting for more than 70% of the organic acid content, followed by citric acid (107.65–142.31 mg/g) and malic acid (21.00–36.22 mg/g). Chen et al. [36] reported that the content of main organic acids was highest, in descending order, with succinic acid, citric acid and malic acid in L. edodes. These results were consistent with our results. The total content of organic acids in fresh and different dried L. edodes ranged from 621.32 mg/g to 875.82 mg/g and were in the descending order of fresh (875.82 mg/g), ND (695.30 mg/g), HAD (667.82 mg/g), FD (621.32 mg/g). The result was higher than that of the organic acids in other species (*Agrocybe cylindracea, Pleurotus cystidiosus, Agaricus blazei, Pleurotus eryngii, Coprinus comatus*), which ranged from 59.42 mg/g in to 237.81 mg/g [19]. However, compared with total organic acids of fresh L. edodes, the drying process decreased the relative contents, and FD samples were the lowest.

Table 2. Organic acid contents of fresh and different dried L. edodes.

Organic Acids (mg/g)	F [a]	FD	HAD	ND
Tartaric acid	41.91 ± 1.97 [A]	Nd [b]	12.18 ± 0.19 [B]	Nd [b]
Malic acid	36.22 ± 0.70 [A]	27.82 ± 0.77 [B]	23.57 ± 2.35 [BC]	21.00 ± 0.38 [C]
Ascorbic acid	6.27 ± 0.28 [A]	5.00 ± 0.27 [C]	5.66 ± 0.11 [B]	4.88 ± 0.18 [C]
Citric acid	134.49 ± 0.45 [C]	107.65 ± 2.17 [D]	138.13 ± 1.90 [B]	142.31 ± 1.09 [A]
Fumaric acid	11.68 ± 0.03 [A]	8.23 ± 0.03 [B]	6.57 ± 0.02 [D]	7.61 ± 0.02 [C]
Succinic acid	645.25 ± 3.03 [A]	472.61 ± 3.34 [D]	481.71 ± 1.72 [C]	519.51 ± 2.11 [B]
Total	875.82 ± 2.04 [A]	621.32 ± 3.42 [D]	667.82 ± 0.48 [C]	695.30 ± 0.96 [B]

Mean ± SD (n = 3). Means with different superscript (A, B, C, D) in the same row are significantly different ($p < 0.05$). F [a], fresh shiitake mushroom; FD, freeze drying sample; HAD, hot-air drying sample; ND, natural drying sample. nd [b], not detected.

3.4. Effects of Drying Methods on Free amino Acids of L. edodes

Lentinus edodes contains a variety of amino acids. They can provide strong umami and pleasant sweet flavors [37]. As shown in Table 3, the contents of total free amino acids in fresh and dried L. edodes ranged from 29.13 to 32.82 mg/g dry weight. The total free amino acids content of the fresh samples was 32.817 mg/g dry weight, which was consistent with the reported value (31.70 mg/g) [38]. The content of total free amino acids in FD samples was the lowest. This may be due to the high temperature promoting protein hydrolysis.

Free amino acids were classified into umami, sweet, bitter and tasteless based on their taste properties [39]. As shown in Table 3, threonine was the highest sweet amino acid, accounting for 77% to 87%, while glutamic acid was the highest umami taste amino acid. The results are similar to others [36]. The contents of aspartic acid were significantly increased in FD samples compared with fresh, HAD and ND. As revealed in Figure 3, fresh *Lentinus edodes* contained the sweetest amino acid taste, while the FD sample was the most umami-like and bitter tasting amino acid.

Table 3. The content of free amino acids in fresh and different dried *L. edodes*.

	Free Amino Acids (mg/g)	F [a]	FD	HAD	ND
Umami Taste Amino Acids	Asp [b]	0.56 ± 0.01 [B]	1.57 ± 0.001 [A]	0.10 ± 0.01 [C]	0.10 ± 0.001 [C]
	Glu	3.33 ± 0.02 [A]	2.40 ± 0.001 [C]	3.26 ± 0.01 [A]	2.76 ± 0.003 [B]
	total	3.89 ± 0.02 [AB]	3.97 ± 0.001 [A]	3.36 ± 0.02 [AB]	2.86 ± 0.003 [B]
Sweet Taste Amino Acids	Ala	0.74 ± 0.003 [D]	1.27 ± 0.003 [B]	1.80 ± 0.01 [A]	0.95 ± 0.003 [C]
	Gly	0.77 ± 0.003 [A]	0.85 ± 0.001 [A]	0.80 ± 0.01 [A]	0.57 ± 0.003 [B]
	Ser	0.76 ± 0.01 [A]	0.72 ± 0.003 [A]	0.46 ± 0.003 [B]	0.39 ± 0.003 [C]
	Thr	14.89 ± 0.01 [A]	10.57 ± 0.05 [B]	10.59 ± 0.07 [AB]	13.10 ± 0.08 [A]
	total	17.16 ± 0.02 [A]	13.41 ± 0.06 [B]	13.65 ± 0.06 [AB]	15.00 ± 0.07 [A]
Bitter Taste Amino Acids	Arg	2.77 ± 0.002 [A]	2.07 ± 0.003 [C]	1.51 ± 0.01 [C]	2.45 ± 0.01 [B]
	His	0.68 ± 0.001 [A]	0.55 ± 0.001 [B]	0.37 ± 0.01 [C]	0.36 ± 0.001 [C]
	Ile	0.11 ± 0.001 [B]	0.43 ± 0.001 [A]	0.42 ± 0.001 [A]	0.15 ± 0.001 [B]
	Leu	0.20 ± 0.001 [B]	0.71 ± 0.001 [A]	0.66 ± 0.01 [AB]	0.14 ± 0.003 [B]
	Met	0.10 ± 0.001 [A]	0.08 ± 0.01 [A]	0.07 ± 0.003 [A]	0.08 ± 0.01 [A]
	Phe	0.67 ± 0.09 [A]	0.79 ± 0.01 [A]	0.92 ± 0.03 [A]	0.56 ± 0.01 [B]
	Val	1.33 ± 0.01 [B]	1.64 ± 0.003 [A]	1.36 ± 0.01 [AB]	1.10 ± 0.003 [C]
	total	5.85 ± 0.10 [AB]	6.28 ± 0.02 [A]	5.30 ± 0.07 [AB]	4.83 ± 0.02 [B]
Tasteless Amino Acids	Lys	1.16 ± 0.003 [B]	1.43 ± 0.003 [A]	1.17 ± 0.001 [B]	0.86 ± 0.003 [C]
	Tyr	0.28 ± 0.01 [A]	0.34 ± 0.003 [A]	0.42 ± 0.03 [A]	0.18 ± 0.02 [A]
	total	1.44 ± 0.02 [B]	1.77 ± 0.001 [A]	1.59 ± 0.03 [B]	1.04 ± 0.02 [B]
Others	GABA	0.20 ± 0.001 [B]	0.13 ± 0.003 [B]	0.41 ± 0.003 [A]	0.51 ± 0.001 [A]
	Orn	4.29 ± 0.01 [C]	3.57 ± 0.01 [D]	5.32 ± 0.01 [B]	6.25 ± 0.01 [A]
Total Amino Acids		32.81 ± 0.09 [A]	29.13 ± 0.06 [C]	29.61 ± 0.08 [BC]	30.48 ± 0.03 [B]

Mean ± SD (n = 3). Means with different superscript (A, B, C, D) within a row are significantly different (p < 0.05). F [a], fresh shiitake mushroom; FD, freeze drying sample; HAD, hot-air drying sample; ND, natural drying sample. Asp [b], L-Aspartic acid; Glu, L-Glutamic acid; Ala, L-Alanine; Gly, Glycine; Ser, L-Serine; Thr, L-Threonine; Arg, L-Arginine; His, L-Histidine; Ile L-Isoleucine; Leu, L-Leucine; Met, L-Methionine; Phe, L-Phenylalanine; Val, L-Valine; Lys, L-Lysine; Tyr, L-Tyrosine; GABA, γ-Aminobutyric Acid; Orn, L-Ornithine.

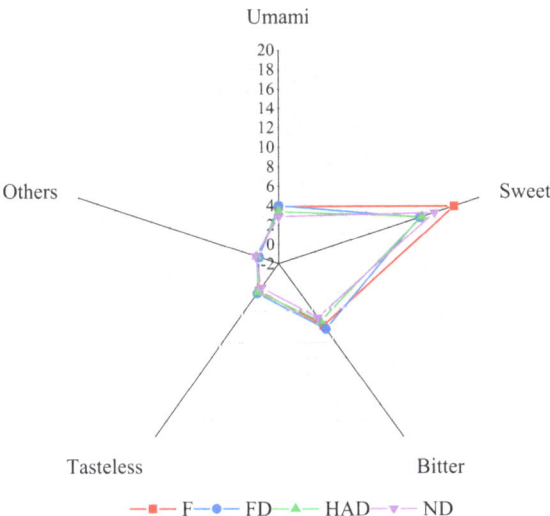

Figure 3. Radar graph of the sensory results of fresh and different dried *L. edodes*; F: fresh sample; FD: freeze drying sample; HAD: hot-air drying sample; ND: natural drying sample; Uma-mi = ASP + GLU; Sweet = Ala + Gly + Ser + Thr; Bitter = Arg + His + Ile + Leu + Met + Phe + Val; Tasteless = Lys + T-yr; Other = GABA + Orn.

3.5. Effects of Drying Methods on 5′-Nucleotides of L. edodes

5′-nucleotides in mushrooms contribute to umami taste [1]. 5′-nucleotides (5′-CMP, 5′-UMP, 5′-GMP, 5′-AMP) were detected in this study (Table 4). As shown in Table 4, the total content of 5′-nucleotides in fresh and different dried *L. edodes* ranged from 7.94 to 14.41 mg/g, which indicated the 5′-nucleotide increased after drying. In addition, 5′-CMP (3.14–8.36 mg/g) and 5′-AMP (2.60–4.92 mg/g) were found as the main 5′-nucleotide in *L. edodes* samples.

Table 4. 5′-nucleotides in fresh and different dried *L. edodes*.

5′-Nucleotides [a]	F [b]	FD	HAD	ND
5′-CMP	3.14 ± 0.03 [B]	2.96 ± 0.03 [B]	7.78 ± 0.03 [A]	8.38 ± 0.06 [A]
5′-UMP	0.27 ± 0.02 [C]	0.39 ± 0.004 [B]	0.92 ± 0.03 [B]	1.92 ± 0.09 [A]
5′-GMP	0.33 ± 0.004 [A]	0.22 ± 0.003 [A]	0.39 ± 0.03 [A]	0.57 ± 0.03 [A]
5′-AMP	4.25 ± 0.01 [A]	4.92 ± 0.02 [A]	2.60 ± 0.01 [B]	3.69 ± 0.26 [B]
Flavor 5′-nucleotides [c]	0.33 ± 0.004 [A]	0.22 ± 0.003 [A]	0.39 ± 0.03 [A]	0.57 ± 0.03 [A]
MSG-like 5′-nucleotide [d]	4.58 ± 0.002 [A]	5.14 ± 0.02 [A]	2.99 ± 0.02 [B]	4.26 ± 0.29 [A]
Total	7.94 ± 0.05 [B]	8.48 ± 0.00 [B]	11.61 ± 0.08 [A]	14.41 ± 0.14 [A]

Mean ± SD (n = 3). Means with different superscript (A, B, C) within a row are significantly different ($p < 0.05$). 5′-CMP [a], 5-cytosine monophosphate; 5′-UMP, 5-uridine monophosphate; 5′-GMP, 5-guanosine monophosphate; 5′-AMP, 5-adenosine monophosphate. F [b], fresh shiitake mushroom; FD, freeze drying sample; HAD, hot-air drying sample; ND, natural drying sample. Flavor 5′-nucleotides [c]: 5′-GMP + 5′-IMP + 5′-XMP, while only 5′-GMP was detected in this study. MSG-like 5′-nucleotide [d]: 5′-AMP + 5′-GMP + 5′-IMP + 5′-XMP, while 5′-IMP and 5′-XMP was not detected in this study.

3.6. Equivalent Umami Analysis

The equivalent umami concentration (EUC) represents the MSG concentration, based on the synergistic effect of MSG-like components (Asp and Glu) and 5′-nucleotide (5′-AMP, 5′-GMP and 5′-IMP), which may enhance the umami taste of mushrooms [3]. As shown in Figure 4, the EUC value of fresh and different dried *L. edodes* ranged from 5.84 to 29.88 g MSG/100 g, which were similar to the reported results [19]. It is reported that the EUC values defined at four levels: <10% (<10 g MSG/100 g dry matter), 10–100% (10–100 g MSG/100 g), 100–1000% (100–1000 g MSG/100 g) and >1000% (>1000 g MSG/100 g) [40]. The EUC values of the HAD and ND samples at the first level (<10 g MSG/100 g), fresh and FD samples at the second level (10–100 g MSG/100 g) (Figure 4). Among the four samples, the FD dried *L. edodes* had the highest EUC value (29.88 g MSG/100 g) and were in the descending order of FD > fresh (15.12 g MSG/100 g) > ND (7.46 g MSG/100 g) > HAD (5.84 g MSG/100 g), which proved FD as an effective drying method to produce umami tasting dried *L. edodes*.

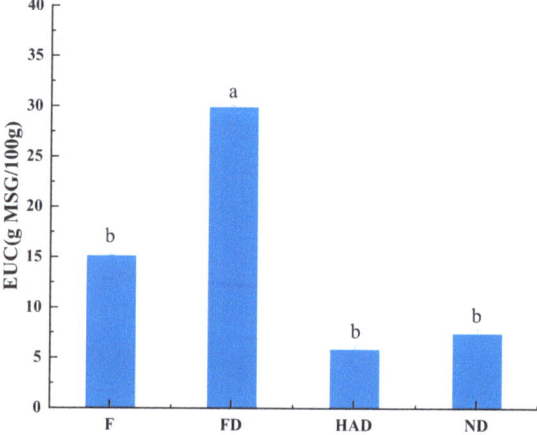

Figure 4. Equivalent umami concentration (EUC) values of fresh and different dried *L. edodes*; F: fresh sample; FD: freeze drying sample; HAD: hot-air drying sample; ND: natural drying sample. Means with different letters (a, b) are significantly different ($p < 0.05$).

4. Conclusions

In the present study, volatile and non-volatile compound profiles of L. edodes were modified by three typical drying methods (FD, HAD and ND). After drying, the content of C8 volatile compounds decreased, but sulfur compounds (straight chain and cyclic sulfurs) were increased, especially in the HAD mushrooms, which resulted in strong shiitake flavor. The drying process increased the relative contents of total 5′-nucleotide of L. edodes as well as the freeze-drying L. edodes had the highest levels of umami taste amino acids, bitter taste amino acids and EUC value. Hot-air drying would be a better method to produce typical shiitake mushroom aroma, while FD was an effective drying method to produce umami tasting dried L. edodes.

The growth of the global dried mushroom market is driven by the demands of organic and healthy food with a clean label. In order to provide nutrient and high-quality final products to consumers, fundamental research should be conducted to better understand the mechanisms of macro and micro-nutrient changes and flavor formation during processing. This research provided up-to-date information about the formation of volatile and non-volatile compounds during different drying processing, which could provide useful information to the mushroom industry to select the optimum method to process dried mushrooms without any preservatives and additives. Future research will focus on understanding the contribution of volatile and non-volatile compounds to sensory perception.

Author Contributions: Conceptualization, Y.L. and W.H.; methodology, L.Z. and X.D.; software, L.Z.; validation, L.Z. and W.H.; formal analysis, L.Z.; investigation, L.Z. and X.D.; resources, W.H.; data curation, L.Z.; writing—original draft preparation, L.Z. and X.D.; writing—review and editing, X.F. and S.A.I.; visualization, L.Z.; supervision, L.Z.; project administration, W.H.; funding acquisition, Y.L. All authors have read and agreed to the published version of the manuscript.

Funding: This research was funded by the Natural Science Foundation of China (No. 31601434), the Agricultural Science and Technology Innovation Center of Hubei Province (2016-620-000-001-044), Hubei Agriculture Research System (HBHZDZB-2021-023).

Institutional Review Board Statement: Not applicable.

Informed Consent Statement: Not applicable.

Data Availability Statement: Not applicable.

Conflicts of Interest: The authors declare no conflict of interest.

References

1. Tian, Y.; Zhao, Y.; Huang, J.; Zeng, H.; Zheng, B. Effects of different drying methods on the product quality and volatile compounds of whole shiitake mushrooms. *Food Chem* **2016**, *197*, 714–722. [CrossRef]
2. Mleczek, M.; Budka, A.; Siwulski, M.; Mleczek, P.; Gasecka, M.; Jasinska, A.; Kalac, P.; Sobieralski, K.; Niedzielski, P.; Proch, J.; et al. Investigation of differentiation of metal contents of Agaricus bisporus, Lentinula edodes and Pleurotus ostreatus sold commercially in Poland between 2009 and 2017. *J. Food Compos. Anal.* **2020**, *90*, 103488. [CrossRef]
3. Gao, S.S.; Huang, Z.C.; Feng, X.; Bian, Y.B.; Huang, W.; Liu, Y. Bioconversion of rice straw agro-residues by Lentinula edodes and evaluation of non-volatile taste compounds in mushrooms. *Sci. Rep.* **2020**, *10*, 1814. [CrossRef]
4. Reis, G.C.L.; Custodio, F.B.; Botelho, B.G.; Guidi, L.R.; Gloria, M.B.A. Investigation of biologically active amines in some selected edible mushrooms. *J. Food Compos. Anal.* **2020**, *86*, 103375. [CrossRef]
5. Pil-Nam, S.; Park, K.-M.; Kang, G.-H.; Cho, S.-H.; Park, B.-Y.; Van-Ba, H. The impact of addition of shiitake on quality characteristics of frankfurter during refrigerated storage. *LWT-Food Sci. Technol.* **2015**, *62*, 62–68. [CrossRef]
6. Zhang, Y.Y.; Hartung, N.M.; Fraatz, M.A.; Zorn, H. Quantification of key odor-active compounds of a novel nonalcoholic beverage produced by fermentation of wort by shiitake (*Lentinula edodes*) and aroma genesis studies. *Food Res. Int.* **2015**, *70*, 23–30. [CrossRef]
7. Holighaus, G.; Weissbecker, B.; von Fragstein, M.; Schutz, S. Ubiquitous eight-carbon volatiles of fungi are infochemicals for a specialist fungivore. *Chemoecology* **2014**, *24*, 57–66. [CrossRef]
8. Liu, Y.; Lei, X.Y.; Chen, L.F.; Bian, Y.B.; Yang, H.; Ibrahim, S.A.; Huang, W. A novel cysteine desulfurase influencing organosulfur compounds in *Lentinula edodes*. *Sci. Rep.* **2015**, *5*, 10047. [CrossRef]

9. Pei, F.; Yang, W.; Ma, N.; Fang, Y.; Zhao, L.; An, X.; Xin, Z.; Hu, Q. Effect of the two drying approaches on the volatile profiles of button mushroom (*Agaricus bisporus*) by headspace GC-MS and electronic nose. *LWT-Food Sci. Technol.* **2016**, *72*, 343–350. [CrossRef]
10. Yang, W.; Yu, J.; Pei, F.; Mariga, A.M.; Ma, N.; Fang, Y.; Hu, Q. Effect of hot air drying on volatile compounds of Flammulina velutipes detected by HS-SPME-GC-MS and electronic nose. *Food Chem.* **2016**, *196*, 860–866. [CrossRef] [PubMed]
11. Hu, S.; Feng, X.; Huang, W.; Ibrahim, S.A.; Liu, Y. Effects of drying methods on non-volatile taste components of Stropharia rugoso-annulata mushrooms. *LWT-Food Sci. Technol.* **2020**, *127*, 109428. [CrossRef]
12. Politowicz, J.; Lech, K.; Lipan, L.; Figiel, A.; Carbonell-Barrachina, A.A. Volatile composition and sensory profile of shiitake mushrooms as affected by drying method. *J. Sci. Food Agric.* **2018**, *98*, 1511–1521. [CrossRef]
13. Cheng, S.S.; Li, R.; Yang, H.M.; Wang, S.Q.; Lin, R.; Tan, M.Q. Characterisation of moisture migration of shiitake mushroom (*Lentinula edodes*) during storage and its relationship to quality deterioration. *Int. J. Food Sci. Technol.* **2020**, *55*, 2132–2140. [CrossRef]
14. Lu, X.; Hou, H.; Fang, D.; Hu, Q.; Chen, J.; Zhao, L. Identification and characterization of volatile compounds in Lentinula edodes during vacuum freeze-drying. *J. Food Biochem.* **2021**, e13814. [CrossRef] [PubMed]
15. Qin, L.; Gao, J.-X.; Xue, J.; Chen, D.; Lin, S.-Y.; Dong, X.-P.; Zhu, B.-W. Changes in Aroma Profile of Shiitake Mushroom (*Lentinus edodes*) during Different Stages of Hot Air Drying. *Foods* **2020**, *9*, 444. [CrossRef]
16. Yao, Y.; Pan, S.; Fan, G.; Dong, L.; Ren, J.; Zhu, Y. Evaluation of volatile profile of Sichuan dongcai, a traditional salted vegetable, by SPME-GC-MS and E-nose. *LWT-Food Sci. Technol.* **2015**, *64*, 528–535. [CrossRef]
17. Ren, J.N.; Tai, Y.N.; Dong, M.; Shao, J.H.; Yang, S.Z.; Pan, S.Y.; Fan, G. Characterisation of free and bound volatile compounds from six different varieties of citrus fruits. *Food Chem.* **2015**, *185*, 25–32. [CrossRef]
18. Paraskevopoulou, A.; Chrysanthou, A.; Koutidou, M. Characterisation of volatile compounds of lupin protein isolate-enriched wheat flour bread. *Food Res. Int.* **2012**, *48*, 568–577. [CrossRef]
19. Li, X.; Feng, T.; Zhou, F.; Zhou, S.; Liu, Y.; Li, W.; Ye, R.; Yang, Y. Effects of drying methods on the tasty compounds of Pleurotus eryngii. *Food Chem.* **2015**, *166*, 358–364. [CrossRef]
20. Hotel, O.; Poli, J.P.; Mer-Calfati, C.; Scorsone, E.; Saada, S. A review of algorithms for SAW sensors e-nose based volatile compound identification. *Sens. Actuators B-Chem.* **2018**, *255*, 2472–2482. [CrossRef]
21. Zhang, H.; Peng, J.; Zhang, Y.R.; Liu, Q.; Pan, L.Q.; Tu, K. Discrimination of volatiles of shiitakes (*Lentinula edodes*) produced during drying process by electronic nose. *Int. J. Food Eng.* **2020**, *16*, 20190233. [CrossRef]
22. Liu, M.; Wang, J.; Li, D.; Wang, M. Electronic Tongue Coupled with Physicochemical Analysis for the Recognition of Orange Beverages. *J. Food Qual.* **2012**, *35*, 429–441. [CrossRef]
23. Choi, S.M.; Lee, D.-J.; Kim, J.-Y.; Lim, S.-T. Volatile composition and sensory characteristics of onion powders prepared by convective drying. *Food Chem.* **2017**, *231*, 386–392. [CrossRef] [PubMed]
24. Rajkumar, G.; Shanmugam, S.; Galvao, M.d.S.; Dutra Sandes, R.D.; Santos Leite Neta, M.T.; Narain, N.; Mujumdar, A.S. Comparative evaluation of physical properties and volatiles profile of cabbages subjected to hot air and freeze drying. *LWT-Food Sci. Technol.* **2017**, *80*, 501–509. [CrossRef]
25. Tan, H.R.; Lau, H.; Liu, S.Q.; Tan, L.P.; Sakumoto, S.; Lassabliere, B.; Leong, K.-C.; Sun, J.; Yu, B. Characterisation of key odourants in Japanese green tea using gas chromatography-olfactometry and gas chromatography-mass spectrometry. *LWT-Food Sci. Technol.* **2019**, *108*, 221–232. [CrossRef]
26. Shi, Y.; Li, X.; Huang, A. A metabolomics-based approach investigates volatile flavor formation and characteristic compounds of the Dahe black pig dry-cured ham. *Meat Sci.* **2019**, *158*, 107904. [CrossRef] [PubMed]
27. Giri, A.; Osako, K.; Ohshima, T. Identification and characterisation of headspace volatiles of fish miso, a Japanese fish meat based fermented paste, with special emphasis on effect of fish species and meat washing. *Food Chem.* **2010**, *120*, 621–631. [CrossRef]
28. Cao, J.; Zou, X.-G.; Deng, L.; Fan, Y.-W.; Li, H.; Li, J.; Deng, Z.-Y. Analysis of nonpolar lipophilic aldehydes/ketones in oxidized edible oils using HPLC-QqQ-MS for the evaluation of their parent fatty acids. *Food Res. Int.* **2014**, *64*, 901–907. [CrossRef] [PubMed]
29. Cheng, Y.; Sun, J.; Ye, X.; Lv, B.; Chu, Y.; Chen, J. Advances on flavor substances of edible mushrooms. *Sci. Technol. Food Ind.* **2012**, *33*, 412–414.
30. Jung, M.Y.; Lee, D.E.; Baek, S.H.; Lim, S.M.; Chung, I.-M.; Han, J.-G.; Kim, S.-H. An unattended HS-SPME-GC-MS/MS combined with a novel sample preparation strategy for the reliable quantitation of C8 volatiles in mushrooms: A sample preparation strategy to fully control the volatile emission. *Food Chem.* **2021**, *347*, 128998. [CrossRef]
31. Combet, E.; Henderson, J.; Eastwood, D.C.; Burton, K.S. Eight-carbon volatiles in mushrooms and fungi: Properties, analysis, and biosynthesis. *Mycoscience* **2006**, *47*, 317–326. [CrossRef]
32. Corral, S.; Leitner, E.; Siegmund, B.; Flores, M. Determination of sulfur and nitrogen compounds during the processing of dry fermented sausages and their relation to amino acid generation. *Food Chem.* **2016**, *190*, 657–664. [CrossRef] [PubMed]
33. Ito, Y.; Toyoda, M.; Suzuki, H.; Iwaida, M. Gas-liquid-chromatographic determination of lenthionine in shiitake mushroom (lentinus-edodes) with special reference to relation between carbon-disulfide and lenthionine. *J. Food Sci.* **1978**, *43*, 1287–1289. [CrossRef]
34. Hiraide, M.; Miyazaki, Y.; Shibata, Y. The smell and odorous components of dried shiitake mushroom, Lentinula edodes I: Relationship between sensory evaluations and amounts of odorous components. *J. Wood Sci.* **2004**, *50*, 358–364. [CrossRef]

35. Chen, C.C.; Wu, C.M. Studies on the enzymic reduction of 1-octen-3-one in mushroom (agaricus-bisporus). *J. Agric. Food Chem.* **1984**, *32*, 1342–1344. [CrossRef]
36. Chen, W.; Li, W.; Yang, Y.; Yu, H.; Zhou, S.; Feng, J.; Li, X.; Liu, Y. Analysis and Evaluation of Tasty Components in the Pileus and Stipe of Lentinula edodes at Different Growth Stages. *J. Agric. Food Chem.* **2015**, *63*, 795–801. [CrossRef] [PubMed]
37. Pei, F.; Yang, W.-J.; Shi, Y.; Sun, Y.; Mariga, A.M.; Zhao, L.-Y.; Fang, Y.; Ma, N.; An, X.-X.; Hu, Q.-H. Comparison of Freeze-Drying with Three Different Combinations of Drying Methods and Their Influence on Colour, Texture, Microstructure and Nutrient Retention of Button Mushroom (*Agaricus bisporus*) Slices. *Food Bioprocess Technol.* **2014**, *7*, 702–710. [CrossRef]
38. Xu, L.; Fang, X.; Wu, W.; Chen, H.; Mu, H.; Gao, H. Effects of high-temperature pre-drying on the quality of air-dried shiitake mushrooms (*Lentinula edodes*). *Food Chem.* **2019**, *285*, 406–413. [CrossRef]
39. Yin, C.; Fan, X.; Fan, Z.; Shi, D.; Yao, F.; Gao, H. Comparison of non-volatile and volatile flavor compounds in six Pleurotus mushrooms. *J. Sci. Food Agric.* **2019**, *99*, 1691–1699. [CrossRef] [PubMed]
40. Yang, J.H.; Lin, H.C.; Mau, J.L. Non-volatile taste components of several commercial mushrooms. *Food Chem.* **2001**, *72*, 465–471. [CrossRef]

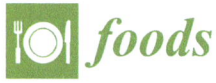

Article

Effect of Osmotic Pretreatment Combined with Vacuum Impregnation or High Pressure on the Water Diffusion Coefficients of Convection Drying: Case Study on Apples

Monika Janowicz, Agnieszka Ciurzyńska * and Andrzej Lenart

Department of Food Engineering and Process Management, Institute of Food Sciences, Warsaw University of Life Sciences, SGGW, 159c Nowoursynowska St., 02-776 Warsaw, Poland; monika_janowicz@sggw.edu.pl (M.J.); andrzej_lenart@sggw.edu.pl (A.L.)
* Correspondence: agnieszka_ciurzynska@sggw.edu.pl; Tel.: +48-22-59-375-77

Abstract: The paper presents water diffusion coefficients as providing a significant contribution to the creation of a comprehensive database and knowledge of weight variation during the drying process of raw plant materials that is used for modelling the technological process and designing innovative products. Dehydration is one of the most widely used methods for improving the stability and durability of fruit and vegetables because it reduces water activity and microbial activity, and minimises the physical and chemical changes during storage. The considerable impact of pressure on heat exchange and weight during the convection drying process of osmotically pretreated apples is demonstrated. The course of the drying curves and the drying rate is determined by the use of pressures of 0.02 and 500 MPa. Varied pressure applied during osmotic impregnation significantly influences the value of the diffusion coefficient: the average determined for the entire course of the drying curve and the average determined in the intervals of the reduced water content. The lowest values of the average water diffusion coefficient are obtained for apples preboiled under overpressure conditions and, at the same time, the determined diffusion coefficients in the water content are characterised on the drying curve by a clearly decreasing course until the reduced water content reaches approximately 0.2.

Keywords: diffusion coefficient; drying convection; pressure pretreatment; osmotic dehydration; apples

Citation: Janowicz, M.; Ciurzyńska, A.; Lenart, A. Effect of Osmotic Pretreatment Combined with Vacuum Impregnation or High Pressure on the Water Diffusion Coefficients of Convection Drying: Case Study on Apples. *Foods* **2021**, *10*, 2605. https://doi.org/10.3390/foods10112605

Academic Editors: Antonio José Pérez-López and Luis Noguera-Artiaga

Received: 15 September 2021
Accepted: 24 October 2021
Published: 28 October 2021

Publisher's Note: MDPI stays neutral with regard to jurisdictional claims in published maps and institutional affiliations.

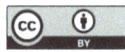

Copyright: © 2021 by the authors. Licensee MDPI, Basel, Switzerland. This article is an open access article distributed under the terms and conditions of the Creative Commons Attribution (CC BY) license (https://creativecommons.org/licenses/by/4.0/).

1. Introduction

To determine the quality of foods of plant origin, especially processed as a result of water removal, the following characteristics are most often used: structure, including density, porosity and consistency, optical—colour, general appearance, sensory—taste, smell, rehydration ability and nutritional value. They depend on many process factors, but, most of all, they depend on the properties of the raw material [1,2]. The attractiveness of dried food products based on the raw materials of plant origin depends on their quality. The raw materials of an appropriate quality allow products to be obtained that meet the expectations of a prospective consumer. Changes occurring in the plant material during drying may be modified by controlling the process parameters. Significant changes in the properties of the raw material are prevented by appropriate preliminary treatment. Various types of pretreatment are applied prior to drying in order to later reduce the undesirable effects of temperature gradients in the tissue structure during convection drying. Fruit and vegetables preserved by the osmotic–convection method retain the colour, smell and taste almost unchanged, despite being treated for a long time at an increased temperature. The unchanged colour of the material results from the inhibition of the activity of polyphenyl oxidase, which causes the enzymatic browning process. The preservation of the smell, and in many cases its intensification compared to the material obtained only by convection, is associated with the formation of a layer of osmotic substance on the surface of the plant material. This hinders the movement of moisture and, thus, also the possibility of a loss of aromatic compounds. The osmotic treatment removes some salt and organic acids from the raw material. As a result, there is a change in the ratio of sugar to acids, affecting the organoleptic assessment of the finished product [3–8]. In addition to the many advantages mentioned above, the material treated with this method is characterised by a porous structure, smooth surface, and almost unchanged shape and size, which affects the visual impression of the potential consumer and facilitates its rehydration in water [9–11].

Conventional drying techniques and the possibility of combining traditional drying with unconventional methods of food preservation, create new opportunities for the food industry. The aim of these techniques is, nowadays, to meet the increasing demands of the consumer, as well as to provide safe, comfortable products characterised by the repeatability and functionality of properties, as well as high nutritional value. The search for new methods of fixation causes new process parameters to be tested, resulting in combined methods being used in order to give favourable results. Therefore, food is preserved on an industrial scale by both temperature changing and non-thermal methods. High hydrostatic pressure (HHP) techniques belong to the group of unconventional methods of ensuring adequate food quality. The use of the HHP treatment allows not only to extend the shelf life of food by eliminating pathogenic microorganisms but also to change its properties, thus giving the possibility of creating new food products. The high hydrostatic pressure technology is a processing method characterised by its short time, high efficiency, low energy consumption and simple operation process, which has been recognised as an environmentally friendly method by the American Food and Drug Administration [12]. The use of high hydrostatic pressure treatment significantly improves the conditions of heat and weight exchange in diffusion processes. This happens regardless of the diversity of plant tissue at which the action is directed and regardless of the combination of the parameters used [13–15]. The previous work has mainly focused on the kinetics and modelling of the HHP technique [16], its drying efficiency and water permeation rate, and the microstructure changes after the HHP pretreatment. The combination of osmotic dehydration, treatment under varied pressure and drying makes it interesting to understand the conditions of weight exchange occurring during the removal of water from the plant tissue.

Water diffusion coefficients constitute an indispensable contribution to the creation of a comprehensive database of weight variation during the drying process of plant raw materials. Knowledge in this area is necessary for modelling technological processes and designing innovative products. A number of technological processes in the food industry are based on the movement of specific components at the boundary of a solid–liquid or inside a sample. Dehydration, due to both osmotic pressure and evaporation as a result of drying, is one of the most commonly used methods of improving the stability and durability of fruit and vegetables because it reduces the water activity, reduces microbial activity and minimises physical and chemical changes during storage [17,18]. The authors' own research [19] and many other research projects [13,20–26] on the impact of osmotic dehydration on the convection drying process of apples have confirmed that the heat and weight exchange mechanism in this process resembles diffusion. The results of the research on drying pre-dehydrated apples under varied process parameters (a type of osmotic substance, pressure) under convection have proven a decreasing rate of water removal along with reaching the equilibrium water content in the sample. The efficiency rate of water removal depends on the factors directly affecting the diffusion conditions. The extent of changes is influenced by the parameters of the dewatering process as well as the changes in the composition and internal structure occurring in the dehydrated matter.

The vast majority of existing scientific publications have focused on the effect of osmotic dehydration performed at atmospheric pressure, a vacuum or high pressure, on the subsequent drying process. However, the presented research is the only one that has studied the osmotic dehydration process under a wide range of pressures—both low and high values in different variants. In this manner, the article can serve as a source of valuable knowledge so important before process optimization.

The aim of the research is to explain the influence of the pressure used during pretreatment on the course of the convection drying process, and the change in the water diffusion coefficient resulting from the use of varied pressure during the osmotic treatment. The work included the use of reduced and elevated pressure relative to atmospheric pressure. At the same time an attempt was made to determine the water diffusion coefficient during the convective drying of apples.

2. Materials and Methods

2.1. Characteristics of Raw Materials

The test samples comprised "Idared" variety apples stored in a cold store at a temperature of +5–+8 °C at an air humidity of 80–90%. The variety was chosen for the research purpose because during the long availability period in the market, they keep concise and strong structure. They also constitute a model plant tissue with a porous structure, thanks to which they store various substances well.

Apples were washed, peeled and cut into cubes (10 mm) (Figure 1). The chopped material was immersed in a 0.5% citric acid solution to protect against enzymatic browning reactions, then dried on a filter paper. The apple cubes prepared in this way underwent the technological treatment using osmotic dehydration in a sucrose solution (61.5°Bx) at a pressure ranging from 0.02 to 500 MPa, followed by convection drying.

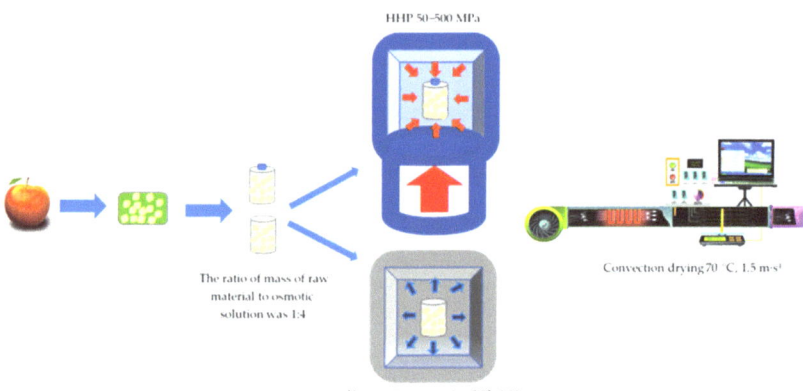

Figure 1. The diagram of the conducted experiments.

Vacuum impregnation under varied pressure was carried out in a sucrose solution characterised by the water activity of 0.9. The ratio of raw material weight to osmotic solution was 1:4. The process time under varied pressure conditions was 180 min. The whole of the range of pressure in vacuum impregnation was 0.02–0.08, the apples were dehydrated throughout the process (180 min) under the pressure and at the temperature pre-set at the level of 25 ± 1 °C. The vacuum impregnation process was carried out in the laboratory chamber of the SPT-200 vacuum dryer (ZUT Colector, Kraków, Poland).

Pretreatment of the apples with high hydrostatic pressures was carried out using a high-pressure chamber owned by the Institute of High Pressure Physics (IWC) in Warsaw, also known as "Unipress". Pretreatment of samples with the HHP was carried out in two stages: the first stage, obtaining the initial pressure of 80–150 MPa, and the second stage, obtaining the desired pressure (50, 100, 200, 500 MPa), holding for 5 min, and the remaining part of the osmotic dehydration was carried out under the atmospheric pressure of 0.1 MPa. The temperature of the samples during pressure, depending on the applied pressure, ranged from 23–27 °C and was higher corresponding to higher pressure.

The convection drying of apples was carried out in a laboratory dryer with forced air flow. The raw material was laid on metal nets in a single layer and dried at a temperature of about 70 °C with a drying air velocity of 1.5 m·s^{-1}. Drying was carried out until a constant weight was obtained under the given drying conditions for 20 min of the process. The weight loss was recorded continuously using the Axis electronic scale by Radwag AR-2000 with an accuracy of 0.1 g and "Measurement" software in the DOS (disk operating system) system. Water content in the tested sample at each stage of treatment was determined on the basis of the sample weight and the dry substance weight obtained by the drying method according to the AOAC [27] in vacuum dryer (Memmert VO400, Schwabach, Germany) (10 mPa, 70 °C, for 24 h).

The calculations were performed in triplicate for all technological operations.

2.2. Changes in the Structure of Apples

Changes in the structure of apples resulting from the applied technological procedures were determined on the basis of the analysis of photos taken at the Analytical Centre of the Warsaw University of Life Sciences, using the FEI Quanta 200 ESEM scanning electron microscope with the EDS micro-analyser and digital image recording. Observations were made without pretreatment of the samples at a pressure of 100–133 Pa, with an accelerating voltage of 25 or 30 kV. Equipping the microscope with a Peltier device for the purpose of controlling the temperature of samples allows for the examination of wet samples.

Calculation of water loss (WL) and the increase in dry matter (SG) [28]

$$WL = \frac{(m_o - m_{i.d.m}) - (m_1 - m_{d.m.})}{m_o} * 100\% \quad (1)$$

$$SG = \frac{(m_{d.m.} - m_{i.d.m})}{m_o} * 100\% \quad (2)$$

where:

m_o—weight of apples before the dehydration process (g),
m_{o1}—weight of apples after the dehydration process (g),
$m_{i.d.m}$—the initial dry matter content in apples (g),
$m_{d.m.}$—dry matter content in apples after the osmotic dehydration process (g).

2.3. Mathematical and Statistical Analysis of Research Results

The mathematical elaboration of the results was performed using Excel and Table-Curve2D software that allows an equation to be found describing data by searching for solutions from among a wide range of models. The statistical analysis of results was conducted using the analysis of variance based on the ANOVA (the one-way analysis of variance) summary table (StatSoft-Statistica 13.1. Inc., Tulusa, OK, USA). Tests were applied to verify the assumption of homogeneity of single- and multi-factor variance (adopted level of significance, $p = 0.05$). If many dependent and accompanying variables occurred in the statistical analysis, tests were presented for each dependent variable and accompanying variable. The least significant difference (LSD) test was carried out to compare the study results and correlations between them.

3. Results

3.1. Convection Drying of Osmotically Dehydrated Apples under Varied Pressure Conditions

Figure 2 shows the course of drying curves for apples osmotically impregnated using varied pressure. Changes in the initial water content resulted from the osmotic impregnation of apples in the sucrose solution. The osmotic dehydration affected the course of the process by changing its mechanism and the value of the diffusion coefficient of water in the sample. It was found that the use of osmotic dehydration under varied pressures influenced the achievement of a different level of dehydration and, thus, a different value of the initial water content after osmotic dehydration of the samples.

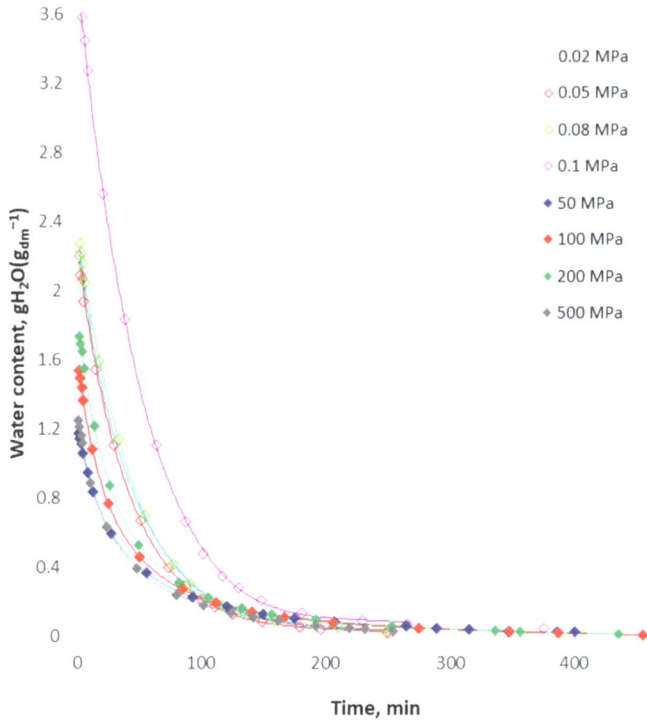

Figure 2. The course of the drying curves of apples initially osmotically dehydrated under varied pressure.

In addition, the pressure under which the pretreatment process takes place affects the final equilibrium water content of apples and the time of the drying process, which can be better seen in Table 1. As a result of the convection drying of apples vacuum impregnated under varied pressure (0.02–500 MPa), droughts with significantly different final equilibrium water content were obtained after significantly different drying times. The final equilibrium water content ranged from 0.015 to 0.050 g $H_2O \cdot$(g d.m.)$^{-1}$, which corresponds with the moisture range of 1.5–4.8%. At the same time, the drying time for apples ranged from 250 to 455 min depending on whether vacuum, atmospheric pressure or HHP was used for the osmotic dehydration, which was confirmed by setting three homogeneous groups (Table 1).

Table 1. Process and sample parameters in the obtained dried apples from osmotically dehydrated apples. Mean values marked with the same letter index (a–c) and (A–D) do not differ statistically significantly at the level of $p = 0.05$.

Pressure (MPa)	Final Equilibrium Water Content $gH_2O \cdot$(g d.m.)$^{-1}$	Time Drying (min)
0.02	0.040 ± 0.005 [C]	250 ± 5 [a]
0.05	0.039 ± 0.003 [BC]	250 ± 9 [a]
0.08	0.041 ± 0.006 [C]	250 ± 2 [a]
0.1	0.050 ± 0.001 [D]	375 ± 2 [c]
50	0.032 ± 0.003 [B]	400 ± 2 [b]
100	0.015 ± 0.004 [A]	455 ± 5 [b]
200	0.020 ± 0.007 [A]	435 ± 5 [b]
500	0.035 ± 0.004 [BC]	255 ± 3 [a]

It was found that the use of the pressure above atmospheric pressure (50–200 MPa) during the vacuum impregnation significantly extended the time of convection drying to obtain the equilibrium water content in the dried apples at a temperature of 70 °C with an air flow of 1.5 m·s^{-1}. At the same time, the droughts after overpressure pretreatment were characterised by a significantly lower final equilibrium water content in the entire range of applied overpressure conditions (50–500 MPa) (Table 1).

An inverse trend in the drying time was observed in the case of the samples vacuum impregnated under lower than atmospheric pressure as compared to the treatment under atmospheric pressure. The application of osmotic pretreatment under lower than atmospheric pressure significantly reduced the time of convection drying to obtain the equilibrium water content (Table 1).

The statistical analysis of the obtained results confirmed a significant reduction in the equilibrium water content for dried apples vacuum impregnated under lower than atmospheric pressure and a significant reduction in drying time compared to apples osmotically dehydrated under atmospheric pressure. The analysis of the results obtained for the vacuum impregnation only in the range of reduced pressure (0.02–0.08 MPa) did not prove the impact of the applied osmotic dehydration on the parameters under consideration (final equilibrium water content and drying time).

The statistical effect of the applied HHP on the final equilibrium water content in the dried apples and drying time was also demonstrated, both in relation to the apples subjected to osmotic treatment under atmospheric pressure and in the range of 50–200 MPa. A significant effect on the extension of the process time was proven for the overpressure range of 50–200 MPa. In the case of the application of the osmotic treatment under the pressure of 500 MPa, the drying time of the apples was significantly shortened as compared to the other conditions at issue, such as overpressure and atmospheric pressure.

Figure 3 shows the course of the drying efficiency rate curves of osmotically dehydrated apples under varied pressure. It was found that the drying of apples osmotically dehydrated under atmospheric pressure was characterised by the lowest drying rates at a certain water content as compared to the dehydrated sample both under and over the atmospheric pressure and higher than the atmospheric one. The analysis of the curves also allowed a change to be observed in the shape of the drying efficiency rate curves depending on whether the osmotic dehydration process was carried out under overpressure. The change in the course is clearly visible in the period of decreasing the drying efficiency rate below the water content in the sample at the level below 0.03 g $H_2O·(g\ d.m.)^{-1}$, which may be seen in the enlargements attached to the drawing (Figure 3). When defining the course of the curves according to the type of dried material, it may be assumed that the structure of apples obtained as a result of vacuum impregnation under lower than atmospheric pressure corresponds to the type of tissue with capillary–porous properties of a complex structure. The shape of the drying curves of osmotically dehydrated apples under higher than atmospheric pressure (50–200 MPa) characterises the sample with a clay-like structure during the drying process. As a result of such structural changes in the sample, not only the weight and heat exchange that determine the course of the process are changed but also the characteristics of ready-made droughts (structure, mechanical properties). Changes of this nature may be explained by the diffusivity of apple tissue. As a result of the two-way weight exchange phenomenon that occurs as a result of changes in the osmotic pressure in the diffusion system, an apple tissue, a hypertonic substance, cell sap is only superficially replaced with a sucrose solution, the presence of which in the material is clearly visible in the photos of the structure of the dried material compared to fresh material and not osmotically dehydrated (Figure 4). At the same time, the weight exchange causes a significant reduction in the initial water content in the material, regardless of the pressure applied, as compared to the sample dewatered under atmospheric pressure ($\approx$3.6 g $H_2O·(g\ d.m.)^{-1}$) (Figure 2).

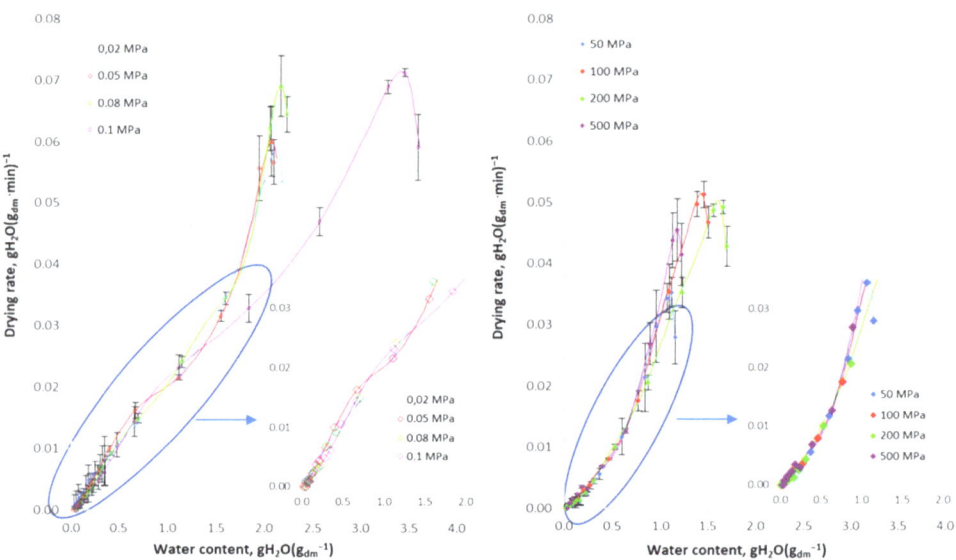

Figure 3. The course of the drying efficiency rate curves of apples initially osmotically dehydrated under varied pressure.

It was shown that as a result of diffusive mass movement, water loss (WL) was greater than the increase in dry matter weight (SG) (Table 2).

Table 2. Effectiveness of $WL \cdot (SG)^{-1}$ osmotic dehydration of apples and increase in dry matter weight in fruit tissue under varied pressure. Mean values marked with the same letter index (a–d) do not differ statistically significantly at the level of $p = 0.05$.

Pressure (MPa)	$WL \cdot (SG)^{-1}$ $gH_2O \cdot (g\ d.m.)^{-1}$	SG $g\ d.m. \cdot (g\ i.d.m.)^{-1}$
0.02	1.56 ± 0.17 [c]	13.24 ± 0.40 [c]
0.05	2.06 ± 0.39 [a]	11.18 ± 0.18 [b]
0.08	2.35 ± 0.38 [b]	10.16 ± 0.15 [a]
0.1	2.80 ± 0.43 [b]	9.91 ± 0.10 [a]
50	1.37 ± 0.18 [c]	11.88 ± 1.39 [bc]
100	2.08 ± 0.06 [a]	13.41 ± 0.67 [c]
200	2.19 ± 0.78 [ab]	13.12 ± 1.40 [c]
500	2.09 ± 0.26 [a]	15.27 ± 0.77 [d]

WL—water loss; SG—increase in dry matter weight.

It was also found that in the case of drying apples osmotically dehydrated under lower than atmospheric pressure, a reduction in the initial water content was recorded, which resulted in a significant reduction in the drying time to obtain the equilibrium water content. The tendency was also confirmed in the case of using osmotic dehydration under pressure higher than atmospheric at the level of 500 MPa, while for higher than atmospheric pressure in the range of 50–200 MPa the relationship was reversed (Table 1).

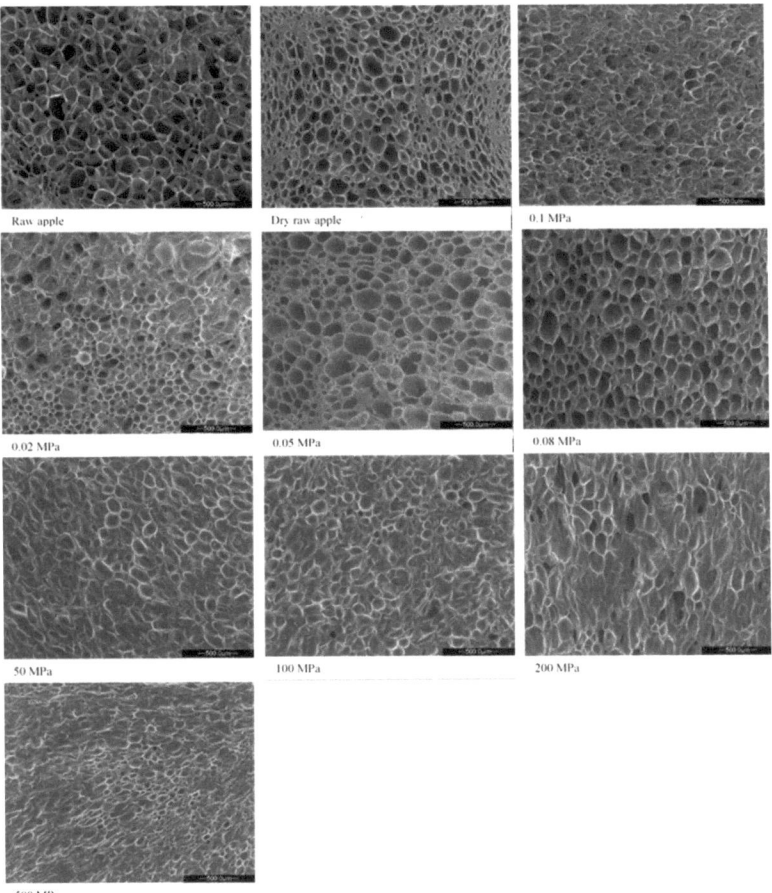

Figure 4. Structure of convectional dried apples non-dehydrated and osmotically dehydrated under lower than atmospheric pressure and higher than atmospheric pressure.

3.2. An Attempt to Determine the Water Diffusion Coefficient during the Drying of Osmotically Dehydrated Apples under Varied Pressure

The diversity of considerations on the drying process resulted in the necessity to choose a parameter that would describe the drying process in an unambiguous manner and independent of the method of weight variation at a given moment. Therefore, the mechanisms, regardless of the technical mode, are described by the effective diffusion coefficient. The knowledge of this parameter allows for an appropriate interpretation of the drying process, as well as for a legal description of it in terms of mathematics. In order to determine the diffusivity not only during drying but also in other weight variation processes (rehydration, extraction, osmotic dehydration, etc.), the Fick equation is used, the analytical solution of which, taking into account the geometry of the sample and under certain assumptions, allows simplification of the interpretation of the weight variation process. The correct determination of water diffusivity during drying requires the assumption that the water content on the surface of the material is in equilibrium with the air humidity. It should also be assumed that the drying conditions and diffusivity remain unchanged, regardless of the variability of the water content and temperature in the dried sample.

Based on the assumptions of the second Fick's law, assuming the initial and boundary conditions of the first type and taking into account the shape of the initial material (infinite plate) in the equation, and making the appropriate simplification to the form of Equation (3), the water diffusion coefficient was calculated as described below. The proposed mathematical description of the second drying period allowed the determination of the water diffusion coefficient (D_{ff}) using the regression method for each measurement series by determining the constant k. The coefficient D_{ff} was determined from the dependence (3) in the entire tested drying range, i.e., within the range of changes in the relative water content (MR) from 1 to 0.0025. The range of variability of the relative water content (MR) was divided into ranges from 1 to 0.1, every 0.05, and from 0.05 to 0.005, every 0.005. Depending on the experiment carried out, in some cases two adjacent compartments were joined, which facilitated the determination of the water diffusion coefficient for the average value of the relative water content in a given compartment.

Drying curves obtained as a result of experiments (Figure 2) are exponential and are described by the following equation formula

$$MR = \frac{u_\tau - u_r}{u_0 - u_r} = \Psi * e^{-K\tau} \quad (3)$$

where:

$\Psi = \frac{8}{\pi^2}$—the aspect ratio of the infinite plate of double-sided dried samples,
u_0 = initial water content, $gH_2O \cdot (g\ d.m.)^{-1}$,
u_τ = temporary water content, $gH_2O \cdot (g\ d.m.)^{-1}$,
τ = time, min,
K = drying constant.

In order to perform a comparative analysis of convection drying curves, a correction factor A was introduced into the general equation describing the drying kinetics. This allowed differences in water content to be taken into account in osmotically dehydrated apples, which were also the initial water content in the convection drying process by modifying the equation to

$$MR = (\Psi - A) * e^{-K\tau} \quad (4)$$

where:

A = correction factor,
MR = relative water content.

After taking into account, in the above equation, the shape of the research input and the correction coefficient defined above as well as boundary conditions commonly used in the description of heat exchange and weight of the second drying period in convection conditions, a new dependence is obtained

$$MR = \left(\frac{8}{\pi^2} - A\right) * exp\left(\frac{\pi^2 * D_{ff}}{2 * l^2} * \tau\right) \quad (5)$$

where:

D_{ff} = diffusion coefficient of water ($m^2 \cdot s$),
l = length (m).

The proposed mathematical description of the second drying period allows for the determination of the conventional diffusion coefficient of water. Using the regression method for each series of measurements, the constant K was determined according to the scheme

$$MR = \left(\frac{8}{\pi^2} - A\right) * exp(-K * \tau) \quad (6)$$

where:

$$K = \frac{\pi^2 * D_{ff}}{2 * l^2}$$

The mean values for the whole apple drying process determined in this way and calculated on the basis of the above dependences, indirectly allowed assessment of the influence of osmotic dehydration parameters on the convective drying kinetics.

Fruit subjected to varied pressure is characterised by a different value of the diffusion coefficients D_{ff} as compared to the sample dewatered at atmospheric pressure, which may indicate a greater permeability of cell walls caused by pressure stress. As a result, it may facilitate mass exchange during pretreatment, which results in the penetration of the hypertonic solution into the apple tissue (Figure 4) and provides higher values of the weight and heat variation coefficient during convection drying (Figure 5).

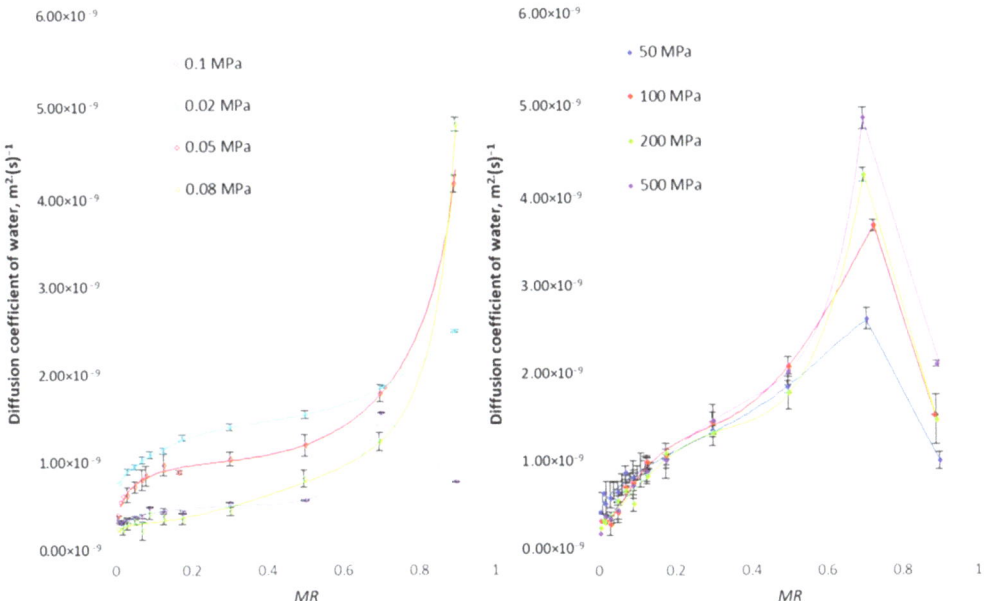

Figure 5. Change in the water diffusion coefficient during drying of apples pre-osmotically dehydrated under varied pressure.

It was found that the use of a hypertonic solution as a medium allowed the reduction in the initial water content in the plant tissue (osmotic dehydration) before drying, and, at the same time, increased the rate of weight movement during the drying process, which resulted in a higher value of the water diffusion coefficient calculated in individual ranges of the relative water content MR. It was observed that for the osmotically dehydrated sample under high hydrostatic pressure, the course of changes in water diffusion during drying is similar to the course of changes in the tissue of dehydrated fruit under atmospheric pressure. The tendency characteristic for the discussed courses of [29] is a significant increase in the water diffusion rate in the range of the relative water content from 0.9 to 0.7. In the case of osmotically dehydrated apples under negative pressure (0.02–0.08 MPa) in the entire range of changes in the relative water content, the diffusivity of apples' tissue significantly decreases. The values of the water diffusion coefficient for MR values at the level of about 0.9 are significantly higher than those for apples with initially reduced content water under the conditions of using high-pressure osmotic tissue treatment (50–500 MPa). It was found that the tissue mobility to weight variation increased as a result of pressure-induced stress, regardless of its value and the presence of a hypertonic substance in the tissue, as evidenced not only by photos of the internal structure of drained and dried apples (Figure 4) but also the value of the dewatering efficiency coefficients defined as the ratio water loss (*WL*) and the increase in dry substance weight (*SG*) presented in Table 2.

4. Discussion

In order to ensure the appropriate quality and microbiological stability, dried vegetables should have a water content of 10–15%, and fruit, 20–25%. It may be assumed that thanks to the application of pretreatment under different pressures, it is possible to obtain droughts with a high degree of water (1.5–4.8%) removal and, therefore, more stability during storage (Table 1). The selected method and type of technological processes have an impact on the amount of water contained in the dried material and the course of pretreatment and drying. This is confirmed by the authors' own and other researchers' investigations on drying: osmotic dehydration in varied conditions and drying using various methods [2,7,8,19,30–36]. The research results clearly indicate that the optimisation of technological processes in order to obtain the appropriate product quality should be the result of the analysis of several factors including, among others, processing conditions, preparation methods and physical properties of the processed raw material, and their integration in order to increase the acceptance of the dried product. The methodology and results of this type of research may be used for developing new food products and optimising existing ready-to-eat dried products [2,8,19,23,24,31,37,38].

The degree of water removal during osmotic dehydration is determined by two-way diffusion weight movement, process parameters (osmotically dehydrated under lower than atmospheric pressure and higher than atmospheric pressure) and the internal structure of plant materials. The diffusion rate of water from any material with tissue structure depends on factors such as the temperature and osmotic concentration of the solution, the size and geometry of the sample, the ratio of the weight of the sample to the weight of the solution, and the degree of damage resulting from the osmotic dehydration pretreatment [6]. Scientific research confirms the influence of variable weight movement parameters (osmotically dehydrated under lower than atmospheric pressure and higher than atmospheric pressure) on the course of fruit and vegetable dehydration [4,5]. Osmotic treatment without varied pressure support has little effect on the modification of the structure of plant raw materials and their sensory characteristics, but the use of varied pressure in combination with the reduced water content prolongs the shelf life of products and improves their quality. As a result, the product prepared in this way may become a raw material in a different type of technological process at a later stage of processing [5,7–10]. The action of the vacuum causes the internal gas to expand and flow out of the product, which carries the water with it. During relaxation, gas is reduced and the external substance enters the pore structure. Vacuum dehydration allows control of the solution introduction into the pores of the fruit [31]. The mixture may contain active compounds, antimicrobial agents, substances used to control food stability, freshness, nutritional or flavour value, minerals and vitamins. These products can enlarge the functional food market.

Mathematical models describing the absorption of the osmotic substance as exemplified by calcium and iron ions were developed, allowing for the process to be carried out in a controlled manner [39–41]. The effect of high hydrostatic pressure on food ingredients causes a strong strengthening and intensification of the processes taking place during the treatment processes [19,24,37,38,42]. The influence of high pressure on hydrogen, ionic and hydrophobic (non-covalent) bonds is ambiguous. They may be destroyed or formed under the action of the HHP, depending on the volumetric changes in the system [19,37,43–45]. Therefore, proteins, nucleic acids and starches, the quaternary structures of which are formed using these bonds, are denatured, coagulated or gelatinised. It may be concluded that the most frequently mentioned effects of the use of non-thermal food preservation and high pressures is, above all, the destruction of microorganisms ensuring the appropriate quality of food. However, it should be remembered that the HHP also denatures proteins or is responsible for their structural modification. Enzymes may be both inactivated and activated by the HHP treatment, depending both on the pressure applied and on the type of enzyme. As a result of pressure, the properties of polymers also change [13,19,25,26,29,36,38,45,46].

Weight variation studies on the osmotic dehydration of mango under varied pressure (Sulistyawati et al.) [25] found that the factor determining the degree of water removal from plant tissue depended not only on the value of the applied pressure but also on fruit ripeness. They observed that after negative pressure had been applied, gas was removed from the pores of the tissue, and excess pressure increased its permeability, which explained the changes in the efficiency factor of osmotic dehydration. In the case of mangoes, Tedjo et al. [20] also found a greater increase in dry matter weight in relation to the loss of water from fruit tissue in terms of weight variation during osmotic dehydration under elevated pressure. However, for the process carried out under negative pressure, it was confirmed by Torres et al. [21]. In studies conducted with the use of bananas [22], tomatoes [24], peaches and apricots [38], it was found that in the case of tissues of this type, as a result of diffusive mass movement, water loss (WL) was greater than the increase in dry matter weight (SG), which was also confirmed in the study of apple tissue in the presented considerations.

The research clearly shows the effect of water removal, with the use of diffusion in the process of osmotic dehydration in hypertonic solutions supported by varied pressure (osmotic dehydrated under lower than atmospheric pressure and higher than atmospheric pressure), on the course of convective drying. The effect of this influence is a change in the drying course, especially in the drying time necessary to obtain an equilibrium water content in the dried apples and in the course of the drying efficiency rate curves. In particular, in the case of drying efficiency rate, characteristic curves are observed [29], which indicate significant changes in the weight variation process during diffusion in the drying process, resulting from varied processing conditions. Yucel et al. [13] also found that conventional drying of fruits and vegetables affected the physical and biochemical properties of the dried material, which in turn led to a significant tissue shrinkage and a change in structure, colour and taste. Therefore, the high pressure may be used for pretreatment prior to drying and, by its action, ensuring the permeability of the cell membrane and, thus, enhancing the weight variation, largely preserving the properties of the plant tissue. At the same time, the application of high pressure at the level of 100 MPa resulted in a significant reduction in the drying time of apples and carrots, while in the case of green peas, this effect was achieved by increasing the pretreatment temperature from 20 to 35 °C in addition to the HHP. In the studies of Yucel et al. [13], it was shown, however, that the higher the pressure used during the pretreatment, the shorter the drying time of the tested tissues of fruit and vegetables, which was not clearly confirmed in the studies carried out on "Idared" variety apples in this study. The results obtained by Zhang et al. [26] for strawberries suggest that the HHP pretreatment disrupted the integrity of the fruit tissue, which increased the efficiency of vacuum drying and freeze-drying. The HHP significantly increased the diffusivity of strawberry tissue, reducing the drying time by 9–24%. It seems that the lack of confirmation of the drying time reduction in the case of the research carried out on the tissue of apples of "Idared" variety apples, dehydrated in the pressure range of 50–200 MPa, may result from the osmotic pretreatment applied. The pressure both lowered and increased relative to atmospheric conditions during osmotic dehydration, in addition to changing the kinetics of weight movement and the structure of the product, but it depended on the elasticity and flexibility of the raw material matrix [46]. This is the effect of pressure during the osmotic dehydration of fruit tissue with a sucrose solution in place of cell juice, which is more difficult to drain from the material matrix due to drying. In addition, during osmotic dehydration under varied pressure, gas is removed from the fruit tissues, which make up 25% of apples, affecting the pressure inside the pores of the fruit. According to the hydromechanical effect, the osmotic solution penetrating in place of the gas removed increases the surface of the interfacial contact [47], but at the same time has worse thermal properties than the proper cell juice for apple tissue, the properties of which are similar to those of water and are much better than the properties of a hypertonic solution (sucrose 61.5%). The presented arguments may explain the phenomena and the results obtained in this research. The presented images of the structure (Figure 4) and the results of the efficiency of osmotic dehydration (Table 2) testify to the higher concentration of the solution inside the tissue structures.

According to the research carried out on strawberry tissue to determine the effect of fruit processed under the pressure range of 0–250 MPa before drying, Zhang et al. [26] found that pressure stress affected the distribution of moisture in fruit tissue. They observed greater uniformity in tissue hydration in its individual places and found that with increasing pressure during treatment before drying, the availability of water increased, which was the direct cause of reduced vacuum drying and freeze-drying time.

The mechanism of water migration may vary depending on the nature of the raw material being dried and the relationship between the matrix and the amount of moisture that may be removed. There are many descriptions explaining the specificity and dynamics of water movement during drying. One of the mechanisms is the removal of water as a result of capillary interactions, resulting from the difference in concentration, another is surface diffusion using the porous surface theory, describing the diffusion of vapour in pores partially filled with air on the basis of the difference in resilience [1,17,18,48–50]. We can also talk about the mechanism of water diffusion under the influence of temperature difference.

Tissue relaxation caused by the action of pressure is an effect of cell walls' destruction and the partial release of substances from inside the cells that form the structure and maintain the turgor of the plant tissue. The effect is similar to that of blanching [28,51]. At the same time, it is the result of pressure stress, and not a sudden rise in temperature, such as in blanching. Pretreatment with the use of hypertonic solutions carried out at atmospheric pressure and the effects during drying, as well as the properties of drought, resulting from its use with pressure changes (atmospheric—negative pressure, overpressure), pulsed electric field, ultrasound, gamma radiation, high hydrostatic pressures, ohmic heating is confirmed by numerous studies [16,23,25,34,35,37–43,52–55]. The properties of dried plant tissue depend not only on the pretreatment but above all on its type, state of ripeness, water content and activity as well as the content of active ingredients at a given moment, which is shown, inter alia, by studies conducted for strawberries [32], apples and bananas [56], apples [19], pomegranate arils [33], goji berry [23], mango [25], persimmon fruit [34,35] and apricot [57].

5. Conclusions

The weight variation during osmotic dehydration under varied pressure depends on the process parameters used. The use of lower than and higher than atmospheric pressure during osmotic dehydration results in a reduction in the initial water content. At the same time, the application of varied pressure, regardless of its value, changes the rate of the penetration of the hypertonic solution (osmotic substance) into the tissue of the tested apples, which has an influence on the properties of the final dried product and the drying process. The action of pressure causes the destruction of cell walls and the release of the cell sap. It was found that water diffusivity during drying increased as a result of pressure-induced stress, regardless of its value and the presence of a hypertonic substance in the tissue. By changing the internal structure of osmo-dehydrated and dried apples, the drainage efficiency, defined as the ratio of water loss to solid gain, increases. The structure of apples obtained during osmotic dehydration under negative pressure causes the drying characteristics of materials with a complex capillary–porous structure to be obtained. On the other hand, the course of the drying curves of osmotically dehydrated apples under high pressure is characteristic for materials with a structure similar to clay.

Author Contributions: Conceptualization, M.J.; methodology, M.J.; software, M.J. and A.C.; validation, M.J. and A.C.; formal analysis, M.J.; investigation, M.J.; resources, M.J. and A.C.; data curation, M.J. and A.C.; writing—original draft preparation, M.J., A.C. and A.L.; writing—review and editing, M.J., A.C. and A.L.; visualization, M.J. and A.C.; supervision, M.J. and A.L. All authors have read and agreed to the published version of the manuscript.

Funding: This research received no external funding.

Institutional Review Board Statement: Not applicable.

Informed Consent Statement: Not applicable.

Data Availability Statement: Data of investigations are available from the authors.

Conflicts of Interest: The authors declare no conflict of interest.

References

1. Khalloufi, S.; Ratti, C. Quality deterioration of freeze-dried foods as explained by their glass transition temperature and internal structure. *J. Food Sci.* **2003**, *68*, 892–903. [CrossRef]
2. Deng, L.Z.; Mujumdar, A.S.; Zhang, Q.; Yang, X.H.; Wang, J.; Zheng, Z.A.; Gao, Z.J.; Xiao, H.W. Chemical and physical pretreatments of fruits and vegetables: Effects on drying characteristics and quality attributes—A comprehensive review. *Critial Rev. Food Sci. Nutr.* **2019**, *59*, 1408–1432. [CrossRef] [PubMed]
3. Yu, Y.; Jin, T.Z.; Xiao, G. Effects of pulsed electric fields pretreatment and drying method on drying characteristics and nutritive quality of blueberries. *J. Food Process. Preserv.* **2017**, *41*, e13303. [CrossRef]
4. Ahmed, I.; Qazi, I.M.; Jamal, S. Developments in osmotic dehydration technique for the preservation of fruits and vegetables. *Innov. Food Sci. Emerg. Technol.* **2016**, *34*, 29–43. [CrossRef]
5. Yadav, A.K.; Singh, S.V. Osmotic dehydration of fruits and vegetables: A review. *J. Food Sci. Technol.* **2014**, *51*, 1654–1673. [CrossRef] [PubMed]
6. Phisut, N. Factors affecting mass transfer during osmotic dehydration of fruits. *Int. Food Res. J.* **2012**, *19*, 7.
7. Akbarian, M.; Ghasemkhani, N.; Moayedi, F. Osmotic dehydration of fruits in food industrial: A review. *Int. J. Biosci.* **2014**, *4*, 42–57. [CrossRef]
8. Jansrimanee, S.; Lertworasirikul, S. Synergetic effects of ultrasound and sodium alginate coating on mass transfer and qualities of osmotic dehydrated pumpkin. *Ultrason. Sonochem.* **2020**, *69*, 105256. [CrossRef] [PubMed]
9. Tabtiang, S.; Prachayawarakon, S.; Soponronnarit, S. Effects of osmotic treatment and superheated steam puffing temperature on drying characteristics and texture properties of banana slices. *Dry. Technol.* **2012**, *30*, 20–28. [CrossRef]
10. Zou, K.; Teng, J.; Huang, L.; Dai, X.; Wei, B. Effect of osmotic pretreatment on quality of mango chips by explosion puffing drying. *LWT* **2013**, *51*, 253–259. [CrossRef]
11. Liu, Z.; Zhang, M.; Bhandari, B.; Wang, Y. 3D printing: Printing precision and application in food sector. *Trends Food Sci. Technol.* **2017**, *69*, 83–94. [CrossRef]
12. Joo, C.G.; Lee, K.H.; Park, C.; Joo, I.W.; Choe, T.B.; Lee, B.C. Correlation of increased antioxidation with the phenolic compound and amino acids contents of Camellia sinensis leaf extracts following ultra high pressure extraction. *J. Ind. Eng. Chem.* **2012**, *2*, 623–628. [CrossRef]
13. Yucel, U.; Alpas, H.; Bayindirli, A. Evaluation of high pressure pretreatment for enhancing the drying rates of carrot, apple, and green bean. *J. Food Eng.* **2010**, *98*, 266–272. [CrossRef]
14. Jangam, S.V. An overview of recent developments and some R&D challenges related to drying of foods. *Dry. Technol.* **2011**, *29*, 1343–1357. [CrossRef]
15. Swami Hulle, N.R.; Rao, P.S. Effect of high pressure pretreatments on structural and dehydration characteristics of aloe vera (Aloe barbadensis Miller) cubes. *Dry. Technol.* **2016**, *34*, 105–118. [CrossRef]
16. Dash, K.K.; Balasubramaniam, V.M.; Kamat, S. High pressure assisted osmotic dehydrated ginger slices. *J. Food Eng.* **2019**, *247*, 19–29. [CrossRef]
17. Chen, Z.; Zhao, J.C. Recommendation for reliable evaluation of diffusion coefficients from diffusion profiles with steep concentration gradients. *Materialia* **2018**, *2*, 63–67. [CrossRef]
18. Sun, Y.; Zhang, M.; Mujumdar, A. Berry Drying: Mechanism, Pretreatment, Drying Technology, Nutrient Preservation, and Mathematical Models. *Food Eng. Rev.* **2019**, *11*, 61–77. [CrossRef]
19. Janowicz, M.; Lenart, A. Selected physical properties of convection dried apples after HHP treatment. *LWT* **2015**, *63*, 828–836. [CrossRef]
20. Tedjo, W.; Taiwo, K.A.; Eshtiaghi, M.N.; Knorr, D. Comparison of pretreatment methods on water and solid diffusion kinetics of osmotically dehydrated mangos. *J. Food Eng.* **2002**, *53*, 133–142. [CrossRef]
21. Torres, J.; Talens, P.; Escriche, I.; Chiralt, A. Influence of process conditions on mechanical properties of osmotically dehydrated mango. *J. Food Eng.* **2006**, *74*, 240–246. [CrossRef]

22. Verma, D.; Kaushik, N.; Rao, P.S. Application of high hydrostatic pressure as a pretreatment for osmotic dehydration of banana slices (Musa cavendishii) Finish–dried by dehumidified air drying. *Food Bioprocess. Technol.* **2014**, *7*, 1281–1297. [CrossRef]
23. Dermesonlouoglou, E.; Chalkia, A.; Dimopoulos, G.; Taoukis, P. Combined effect of pulsed electric field and osmotic dehydration pre–treatments on mass transfer and quality of air dried goji berry. *Innov. Food Sci. Emerg. Technol.* **2018**, *49*, 106–115. [CrossRef]
24. Dermesonlouoglou, E.K.; Andreou, V.; Alexandrakis, Z.; Katsaros, G.J.; Giannakourou, M.C.; Taoukis, P.S. The hurdle effect of osmotic pretreatment and high–pressure cold pasteurisation on the shelf–life extension of fresh–cut tomatoes. *Int. J. Food Sci. Technol.* **2017**, *4*, 916–926. [CrossRef]
25. Sulistyawati, I.; Dekker, M.; Fogliano, V.; Verkerk, R. Osmotic dehydration of mango: Effect of vacuum impregnation, high pressure, pectin methylesterase and ripeness on quality. *LWT* **2018**, *98*, 179–186. [CrossRef]
26. Zhang, L.; Qiao, Y.; Wang, C.; Liao, L.; Shi, D.; An, K.; Hu, J.; Wang, J.; Shi, L. Influence of high hydrostatic pressure pretreatment on properties of vacuum–freeze dried strawberry slices. *Food Chem.* **2020**, *331*, 127203. [CrossRef]
27. AOAC. *Official Methods of Analysis*, 17th ed.; The Association of Official Agricultural Chemists: Arlington, VA, USA, 2002.
28. Panagiotou, N.; Karathanos, V.; Maroulis, Z. Effect of osmotic agent on osmotic dehydration of fruits. *Dry. Technol.* **1999**, *17*, 175–189. [CrossRef]
29. Emelyanov, A.B.; Kononov, N.R.; Yusupov, S.; Myagkov, A.A. On the development of research on resource and energy saving processes in chemical and related industries. *Proc. VSUET* **2017**, *79*, 148–153.
30. Al-Khuseibi, M.K.; Sablani, S.S.; Perera, C.O. Comparison of water blanching and high hydrostatic pressure effects on drying kinetics and quality of potato. *Dry. Technol.* **2005**, *23*, 2449–2461. [CrossRef]
31. Janowicz, M.; Lenart, A. Some physical properties of apples after low-pressure osmotic dehydration and convective drying. *Chem. Eng. Sci.* **2010**, *2*, 237–252.
32. Ciurzyńska, A.; Lenart, A. Rehydration and sorption properties of osmotically pretreated freeze–dried strawberries. *J. Food Eng.* **2010**, *97*, 267–274. [CrossRef]
33. Allahdad, Z.; Nasiri, M.; Varidi, M.; Varidi, M.J. Effect of sonication on osmotic dehydration and subsequent air–drying of pomegranate arils. *J. Food Eng.* **2019**, *244*, 202–211. [CrossRef]
34. Bozkir, H.; Ergün, A.R. Effect of sonication and osmotic dehydration applications on the hot air drying kinetics and quality of persimmon. *LWT* **2020**, *131*, 109704. [CrossRef]
35. Bozkir, H.; Rayman Ergun, A.; Serdar, E.; Metin, G.; Baysal, T. Influence of ultrasound and osmotic dehydration pretreatments on drying and quality properties of persimmon fruit. *Ultrason. Sonochem.* **2019**, *54*, 135–141. [CrossRef] [PubMed]
36. Cava, R.; García-Parra, J.; Ladero, L. Effect of high hydrostatic pressure processing and storage temperature on food safety, microbial counts, colour and oxidative changes of a traditional dry-cured sausage. *LWT* **2020**, *128*, 109462. [CrossRef]
37. Nuñez-Mancilla, Y.; Pérez-Won, M.; Uribe, E.; Vega-Gálvez, A.; Di Scala, K. Osmotic dehydration under high hydrostatic pressure: Effects on antioxidant activity, total phenolics compounds, vitamin C and colour of strawberry (Fragaria vesca). *LWT* **2013**, *52*, 151–156. [CrossRef]
38. Dermesonlouoglou, E.; Angelikaki, F.; Giannakourou, M.C.; Katsaros, G.J.; Taoukis, P.S. Minimally processed fresh–cut peach and apricot snacks of extended shelf-life by combined osmotic and high pressure processing. *Food Bioprocess. Technol.* **2018**, *12*, 371–386. [CrossRef]
39. Moraga, M.J.; Moraga, G.; Fito, P.J.; Martínez-Navarrete, N. Effect of vacuum impregnation with calcium lactate on the osmotic dehydration kinetics and quality of osmodehydrated grapefruit. *J. Food Eng.* **2009**, *90*, 372–379. [CrossRef]
40. Suliburska, J.; Krejpcio, Z. Evaluation of the content and bioaccessibility of iron, zinc, calcium and magnesium from groats, rice, leguminous grains and nuts. *J. Food Sci. Technol.* **2014**, *51*, 589–594. [CrossRef] [PubMed]
41. Kulczyński, B.; Suliburska, J.; Rybarczyk, M.; Gramza-Michałowska, A. The effect of osmotic dehydration conditions on the calcium content in plant matrice. *Food Chem.* **2021**, *343*, 128519. [CrossRef]
42. Yordanov, D.; Angelova, G. High pressure processing for foods preserving. *Biotechnol. Biotechnol. Equip.* **2010**, *24*, 1940–1945. [CrossRef]
43. Nuñez-Mancilla, Y.; Perez-Won, M.; Vega-Gálvez, A.; Arias, V.; Tabilo-Munizaga, G.; Briones-Labarca, V.; Lemus-Mondaca, R.; Di Scala, K. Modeling mass transfer during osmotic dehydration of strawberries under high hydrostatic pressure conditions. *Innov. Food Sci. Emerg. Technol.* **2011**, *12*, 338–343. [CrossRef]
44. Knorr, D. High pressure processing for preservation, modification and transformation of foods. *High Press. Res.* **2002**, *22*, 595–599. [CrossRef]
45. Ramya, V.; Jain, N.K. A review on osmotic dehydration of fruits and vegetables: An integrated approach. *Int. J. Food Process. Eng.* **2017**, *40*, e12440. [CrossRef]
46. Rastogi, N.K. Effect of high pressure on textural and microstructural properties of fruits and vegetables. In *Novel Food Processing Effects on Rheological and Functional Properties*; Ahmed, J., Ramaswamy, H.S., Kasapis, S., Boye, J.I., Eds.; CRC Press: Boca Raton, FL, USA, 2010; pp. 301–319.
47. Deng, Y.; Zhao, Y. Effects of pulsed-vacuum and ultrasound on the osmodehydration kinetics and microstructure of apples (Fuji). *J. Food Eng.* **2008**, *85*, 84–93. [CrossRef]
48. Jayaraman, K.; Gupta, D.D. Drying of fruits and vegetables. In *Handbook of Industrial Drying*, 3rd ed.; Arun, S.M., Ed.; CRC Press: Boca Raton, FL, USA, 2006; pp. 630–659.
49. Lewicki, P.P. Design of hot air drying for better foods. *Trends Food Sci. Technol.* **2006**, *17*, 153–163. [CrossRef]

50. Rahman, M.S. *Handbook of Food Preservation*, 2nd ed.; CRC Press: Boca Raton, FL, USA, 2007.
51. Xin, Y.; Zhang, M.; Xu, B.; Adhikari, B.; Sun, J. Research trends in selected blanching pretreatments and quick freezing technologies as applied in fruits and vegetables: A review. *Int. J. Refrig.* **2015**, *57*, 11–25. [CrossRef]
52. Mayor, L.; Moreira, R.; Sereno, A. Shrinkage, density, porosity and shape changes during dehydration of pumpkin (Cucurbita pepo L.) fruits. *J. Food Eng.* **2011**, *103*, 29–37. [CrossRef]
53. Moreno, J.; Simpson, R.; Estrada, D.; Lorenzen, S.; Moraga, D.; Almonacid, S. Effect of pulsed–vacuum and ohmic heating on the osmodehydration kinetics, physical properties and microstructure of apples (cv. Granny Smith). *Innov. Food Sci. Emerg. Technol.* **2011**, *4*, 562–568. [CrossRef]
54. Oliver, L.; Betoret, N.; Fito, P.; Meinders, M.B. How to deal with visco-elastic properties of cellular tissues during osmotic dehydration. *J. Food Eng.* **2012**, *110*, 278–288. [CrossRef]
55. Prithani, R.; Dash, K.K. Mass transfer modelling in ultrasound assisted osmotic dehydration of kiwi fruit. *Innov. Food Sci. Emerg. Technol.* **2020**, *64*, 102407. [CrossRef]
56. Moraga, G.; Talens, P.; Moraga, M.; Martínez-Navarrete, N. Implication of water activity and glass transition on the mechanical and optical properties of freeze–dried apple and banana slices. *J. Food Eng.* **2011**, *106*, 212–219. [CrossRef]
57. Sakooei-Vayghan, R.; Peighambardoust, S.H.; Hesari, J.; Peressini, D. Effects of osmotic dehydration (with and without sonication) and pectin–based coating pretreatments on functional properties and color of hot–air dried apricot cubes. *Food Chem.* **2020**, *311*, 125978. [CrossRef] [PubMed]

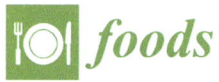

Article

Effects of Roasting Sweet Potato (*Ipomoea batatas* L. Lam.): Quality, Volatile Compound Composition, and Sensory Evaluation

Yu-Jung Tsai [1], Li-Yun Lin [2], Kai-Min Yang [3], Yi-Chan Chiang [1], Min-Hung Chen [4] and Po-Yuan Chiang [1,*]

[1] Department of Food Science and Biotechnology, National Chung Hsing University, 250 Kuokuang Road, Taichung 40227, Taiwan; a0983592262@gmail.com (Y.-J.T.); chiangyichan@gmail.com (Y.-C.C.)
[2] Department of Food Science and Technology, Hungkuang University, Taichung 433304, Taiwan; lylin@hk.edu.tw
[3] Department of Hospitality Management, Mingdao University, 369 Wen Hua Road, Changhua 52345, Taiwan; a9241128@gmail.com
[4] Agriculture & Food Agency Council of Agriculture Executive Yuan Marketing & Processing Division, Taipei City 10050, Taiwan; cmh@mail.afa.gov.tw
* Correspondence: pychiang@dragon.nchu.edu.tw; Tel.: +886-4-2285-1665

Citation: Tsai, Y.-J.; Lin, L.-Y.; Yang, K.-M.; Chiang, Y.-C.; Chen, M.-H.; Chiang, P.-Y. Effects of Roasting Sweet Potato (*Ipomoea batatas* L. Lam.): Quality, Volatile Compound Composition, and Sensory Evaluation. *Foods* **2021**, *10*, 2602. https://doi.org/10.3390/foods10112602

Academic Editors: Antonio José Pérez-López and Luis Noguera-Artiaga

Received: 2 October 2021
Accepted: 26 October 2021
Published: 27 October 2021

Publisher's Note: MDPI stays neutral with regard to jurisdictional claims in published maps and institutional affiliations.

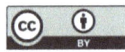

Copyright: © 2021 by the authors. Licensee MDPI, Basel, Switzerland. This article is an open access article distributed under the terms and conditions of the Creative Commons Attribution (CC BY) license (https://creativecommons.org/licenses/by/4.0/).

Abstract: Roasting can increase the Maillard reaction and caramelization of sweet potatoes to create an attractive appearance, color, aroma, and taste, and is rapidly increasing in the commercial market. This study mainly analyzed the influence of roasting sweet potatoes, with and without the peel, on sweet potato quality and flavor characteristics combined with sensory qualities. The results showed that the a* value (1.65–8.10), browning degree (58.30–108.91), total acidity (0.14–0.21 g/100 g, DW), and maltose content (0.00–46.16 g/100 g, DW) of roasted sweet potatoes increased with roasting time. A total of 46 volatile compounds were detected and 2-furanmethanol, furfural, and maltol were identified as the main sources of the aroma of roasted sweet potatoes. A sensory evaluation based on a comprehensive nine-point acceptance test and descriptive analysis showed that roasting for 1 to 2 h resulted in the highest acceptance score (6.20–6.65), including a golden-yellow color, sweet taste, and fibrous texture. The sweet potatoes became brown after roasting for 2.5 to 3 h and gained a burnt and sour taste, which reduced the acceptance score (4.65–5.75). These results can provide a reference for increased quality in the food industry production of roasted sweet potatoes.

Keywords: sweet potato; roasting color; total acidity; sugar content; GC/MS; sensory evaluation

1. Introduction

Sweet potato (*Ipomoea batatas* L. Lam) is one of the most popular root crops. There are many kinds of sweet potato, all containing carbohydrates, dietary fiber, protein, minerals, and vitamins. They also contain β-carotene, chlorogenic acid, flavonoids, anthocyanins, 3,5-dicaffeoylquinic acid, and polyphenolic compounds [1]. Blessington et al. [2] noted that roasting can increase the antioxidant content, reduce sugar, and form volatile compounds to enhance the flavor. Roasting has become one of the most popular cooking treatments [3]. The high temperature and low humidity used in roasting can easily lead to protein denaturation, starch gelatinization, caramelization, and thermal degradation products with a variety of volatiles [4]. Corrales et al. [5] mentioned that a pleasant aroma is produced by the volatile compounds released by the Maillard reaction after roasting, which bears a critical influence on the overall flavor and consumer acceptance of the food.

In recent years, roasted sweet potatoes have become a snack food, moving from traditional markets to convenience store and supermarket systems, including frozen roasted sweet potato products, in many countries. This change has increased the demand for sweet potatoes. It is important to optimize the thermal process and keep the quality stable [6]. However, different processing conditions during the roasting process may greatly affect the quality of the products. Changes in appearance, aroma, flavor, taste, and aftertaste may affect consumer acceptance, and different consumer groups will be attracted by different sensory characteristics [7]. Hou et al. [8] showed a positive correlation between the color, sugar composition, free amino acids, volatile compounds, and overall acceptability of roasted sweet potatoes, especially between 2-furanmethanol and overall acceptability. Leksrisompong et al. [9] analyzed consumer preference and descriptive analysis and found that, overall, preference for roasted sweet potatoes is mainly dominated by flavor preference, followed by taste preference. In addition, studies have explored the sensory properties of sweet potato varieties with different colors, finding that yellow varieties are correlated with fibrous texture and sweet taste [10,11]. This shows that the composition of volatile compounds will affect the flavor, and thus consumer preference, and the above studies are aimed at the characteristics of different varieties of sweet potatoes before and after roasting. No study has yet investigated different roasting times or the effect of processing methods (unpeeled and peeled) on the quality of roasted sweet potatoes, so it is necessary to discuss the color, sugar composition, and volatile compounds in combination with sensory qualities of roasted sweet potatoes that have been processed in different ways.

Based on the different tastes of consumers, there is a difference between eating unpeeled and peeled sweet potatoes. If the roasting temperature is too high or the process too long, scorching, acidification, and quality deterioration result [12]. Therefore, quality standardization has become an important issue. In addition, roasting whole sweet potatoes with the peel results in better color, aroma, and flavor than other processed sweet potato products made from peeled vegetables. This study analyzed the results of different sweet potato processing methods during the roasting process. It combined the color, total acidity, sugar analysis, and volatile compound changes with sensory evaluation, and used agglomerative hierarchical clustering (AHC) and principal component analysis (PCA) to explore the consumer preference impact of quality changes in peeled and unpeeled sweet potatoes prepared with different roasting times to improve quality control and consumer competitiveness.

2. Materials and Methods

2.1. Materials Preparation

Fresh sweet potato roots (TN57) were purchased from Guarantee responsibility Qiongpu Cooperative Farm (Yunlin, Taiwan) and a similar weight of sample was selected (180 ± 20 g), washed, placed in a roaster (Model K-5, Chung Pu Baking Machinery Co., Ltd., Taichung, Taiwan) at 220 °C for (0, 0.5, 1, 1.5, 2, 2.5, 3 h), and cooled to room temperature. In this process, sweet potatoes were divided into unpeeled and peeled, which refers to baking with and without peel, respectively.

2.2. Color Analysis

Color values were measured by a color meter (Model NE-4000, Nippon Denshku Industries Co., Ltd., Tokyo, Japan) and were expressed in L*, a*, and b* values, where L* indicates lightness, a* represents red (>0) or green (<0), and b* expresses yellow (>0) or blue (<0). Moreover, the browning index (B.I.) was calculated by the following equation (Equations (1) and (2)) [13]:

$$B.I. = \{100(x - 0.31)\}/0.17 \qquad (1)$$

$$x = (a^* + 1.75L^*)/(5.645L + a^* - 3.012b^*) \qquad (2)$$

2.3. Quality Index

2.3.1. Total Starch Content

This analysis method was modified from Liu et al. [14], which was determined using a method derived from the Megazyme kit (Megazyme K-TDFR, Wicklow, Ireland).

2.3.2. Sugar Composition

This analysis method was modified from Chan et al. [15]. A 1 g measure of each lyophilized powder sample was mixed with 60% ethanol. Content of sugar was analyzed by HPLC (Model L-600, Hitachi Co., Tokyo, Japan) equipped with a column (DC-613, 6 µm, 6 mm × 150 mm, Shodex Co., Tokyo, Japan). The method employed a refractive index detector (5450 RI Detector, Hitachi Co., Tokyo, Japan). The column temperature was held at 70 °C. The mobile phase was a mixture of HPLC grade acetonitrile (80%) with 1.5 mM NaOH (20%). A 10 µL measure was used for HPLC-RI and the flow rate was 1.5 mL/min [16].

2.3.3. Total Acidity

This analysis was evaluated by titration with 0.1 N NaOH and expressed citric acid according to the methods by Chemists and Horwitz [17].

2.4. GC/MS Analysis

The volatile composition of roasted sweet potatoes was modified from Hou et al. [8] and identified with an HP-6890 gas chromatograph combined with a 5973 Turbo Pump Mass Selective Detector (MSD), and a DB-wax capillary column (60 m × 0.25 mm × 0.25 µm), were purchased by Agilent Technologies Co. (Santa Clara, CA, USA). Each 1.5 g sample was heated to 60 °C in a vial and the headspace was sampled with a DVB/CAR/PDMS fiber (Supelco Inc., Bellefonte, PA, USA) for 60 min. The injection temperature was 240 °C, the oven temperature was held at 40 °C for 1 min, and was increased to 160 °C at a rate of 2 °C/min and further increased to 240 °C at a rate of 5 °C/min. Retention indices were calculated from the retention times of *n*-alkanes (C_8–C_{25}) that were run under the same chromatographic conditions. The identification of volatile compounds was compared with the mass spectral data obtained with those in the NIST library.

2.5. Sensory Evaluation

Sensory evaluation was measured by the method of previous studies [8,15,18]. In this study, 60 panelists (students and staff of NCHU) were inducted in the evaluation room in batches. Most of these panelists were between 19 and 25 years old, including 14 males (23%) and 46 females (67%). A total of 25 members (42%) were accustomed to eating roasted sweet potatoes with their peels, and 35 (58%) were not. Samples were evaluated on a 9-point hedonic scale ranging from 1 (extremely dislike) to 9 (extremely like) [19]. The results of overall acceptability were based on the comprehensive sensory attributes, including visual, aroma, flavor, texture, and aftertaste. In addition, the comprehensive sensory attributes definition of the description analysis test needed to be mentioned three times and each time for 30 min to ensure the correct understanding of the sensory attributes' description terminology. This evaluation took 30–60 min and these participants needed to clean their palates with crackers and water before tasting the next new sample (Table A1) [11,19,20].

2.6. Statistical Analysis

Each test was carried out in triplicate and the data are expressed as mean ± standard deviation. One-way analysis of variance (ANOVA) was conducted using Duncan's multiple range test and correlation analysis was performed using SPSS software (version 19 (2018), IBM Co., Armonk, NY, USA). The data were subjected to an AHC with squared Euclidean distances. Subsequently, the data were analyzed using PCA combined with VARIMAX rotation. For the AHC and PCA analyses, XLSTAT software (version in 2020, Addinsoft Institute Inc., New York, NY, USA) was used.

3. Results and Discussion

3.1. Appearance and Color Analysis

Sweet potatoes are mainly composed of starch, crude protein, crude fiber, and polysaccharides. They are easily heated during the roasting process to gelatinize the starch, caramelize, and undergo the Maillard reaction to create a good color and flavor [20]. The cut surface of fresh sweet potato has a milky white, firm appearance and structure. With the extension of roasting time, the internal temperature rises from 27 °C to 101 °C, causing the sweet potato to "grill", forming a softer texture and gradually more golden color. The color change to yellow is relatively stable after roasting for 1 to 1.5 h, but after roasting for 2 to 2.5 h, the outer peel of the sweet potato is likely to be scorched, and the flesh will shrink and change due to the evaporation of water. A peeled sweet potato will form a crusty surface due to the evaporation of water after roasting for 1 h. The cooking phenomena were more extreme after roasting for 3 h (Figure 1). Fresh sweet potatoes have higher brightness due to higher water and starch content. The L*, a*, b*, and B.I. values of unpeeled sweet potato were 70.35, 4.40, 28.99, and 56.38, and those of peeled sweet potato were 67.50, 5.51, 30.84, and 65.30. As the roasting time increased (0.5 to 3.0 h), the L* value of peeled sweet potato decreased from 49.90 to 40.98, and that of peeled sweet potato from 47.33 to 44.62; the a* value increased significantly after 1.5 h of roasting, and the b* value showed a significant increase after 1.5 h of roasting (Table 1). During roasting, peeled sweet potatoes' starch and polysaccharides will form a secondary crusty peel. The sweet potatoes undergoing the two treatments were dark brown due to the decrease in L* value and the increase in a* value, and the degree of browning rises rapidly [8]. After roasting for more than 2.5 h, the two sweet potatoes exhibited similar roasting effects, and both were brown with a hard-shell surface. There was no significant difference ($p > 0.05$) in B.I. and L* values, which is mainly due to roasting at high temperatures for a long time. Roasting causes caramelization and the Maillard reaction, producing dark polymers [8,21] and affecting the acceptability of the final products [22,23].

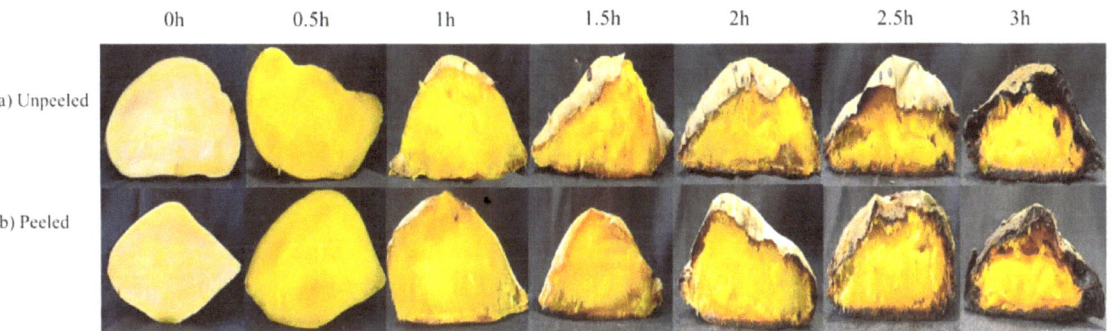

Figure 1. The appearance of roasted sweet potatoes. (**a**) Unpeeled; (**b**) Peeled.

Table 1. The influence of different roasting treatments on the color change of sweet potatoes.

Time (h)	L*		a*		b*		B.I.	
	Unpeeled	Peeled	Unpeeled	Peeled	Unpeeled	Peeled	Unpeeled	Peeled
0	70.35 ± 0.27 gA	67.50 ± 0.33 fA	4.40 ± 0.16 cA	5.51 ± 0.08 dA	28.99 ± 0.12 eA	30.84 ± 0.41 eA	56.38 ± 0.62 aA	65.30 ± 1.06 aA
0.5	49.90 ± 0.16 eB	47.33 ± 0.23 cA	1.65 ± 0.07 aA	3.33 ± 0.35 cB	27.94 ± 0.15 dB	26.90 ± 0.41 bA	80.39 ± 0.29 bA	85.08 ± 1.80 bB
1	50.83 ± 0.38 fB	49.85 ± 0.83 eA	1.47 ± 0.10 aB	0.54 ± 0.26 aA	29.83 ± 0.19 eA	29.91 ± 0.28 fA	85.55 ± 0.60 cA	86.77 ± 1.13 bA
1.5	45.16 ± 0.59 dA	48.73 ± 0.67 dB	3.27 ± 0.62 bB	2.22 + 0 30 bA	26.58 ± 0.39 cA	30.45 ± 0.33 gB	89.43 ± 1.63 dA	95.01 ± 1.96 cB
2	39.62 ± 0.37 aA	41.14 ± 0.22 aB	5.98 ± 0.29 dA	6.10 ± 0.51 eB	23.54 ± 0.20 aA	25.81 ± 0.18 aB	96.92 ± 0.37 eA	103.69 ± 2.03 dB
2.5	42.23 ± 0.61 cA	42.76 ± 0.44 bA	7.63 ± 0.11 eB	7.06 ± 0.32 fA	25.25 ± 0.65 bA	26.26 ± 0.32 bB	104.17 ± 2.73 fA	108.07 ± 0.64 dA
3	40.98 ± 3.03 bA	44.62 ± 1.08 aA	8.10 ± 0.15 fB	7.52 ± 0.23 gA	22.08 ± 0.87 cA	27.60 ± 0.46 dB	106.32 ± 4.74 fA	103.34 ± 1.25 eA

1. Each value is expressed as mean ± standard deviation ($n = 3$). 2. Values (a–g) with different letters within the same column ($p < 0.05$). 3. Values (A,B) with different letters within the same roasting time ($p < 0.05$).

3.2. Quality Index

Changes occurred in sugar composition during sweet potato roasting. The total starch content before roasting was around 64.62 g/100 g (Table 2). As the roasting time increased, starch gradually transformed into monosaccharides and disaccharides, so the total starch content decreased significantly (64.62 g–51.10 g/100 g). However, there was no significant difference in the total starch content of sweet potatoes after ripening. This may be due to the use of heat-stable amylase to convert starch into maltodextrin during the determination of total starch content, and then the use of high-purity amyloglucosidase to quantify glucose, which is degraded by dextrin [24]. While heat treatment changes the structure of starch, the structure of glucose does not change [25]. Chan et al. [15] pointed out that sweetness is one of the most important factors in determining the overall appeal of roasted sweet potatoes. In unroasted sweet potatoes, sucrose content is the highest (11.49 g/100 g, DW), followed by glucose (2.23 g/100 g, DW), and fructose (1.60 g/100 g, DW), as Lai et al. [26] reported, while the maltose content is affected by heat treatment and β-amylase, which decomposes starch into maltose and wheat maltodextrin, so the maltose content tends to increase rapidly after roasting [27]. Among the tested samples, the highest maltose content (51.82 g–55.28 g/100 g, DW) was found in sweet potatoes that were peeled and roasted for 1 to 2 h, which may be the cause of the difference in the volatile compound content found in sweet potatoes under the subsequent high temperature and long-term roasting treatment. However, the content of sucrose decreased (12.51 g–10.01 g/100 g, DW) after roasting for 1.5 h. Sucrose may participate in caramelization during heat treatment to produce caramel and polymerized dark substances, which will affect the sweet potato color, aroma, and flavor [8].

Roasted sweet potatoes tended to have a sour taste when over-roasted (Table 2). The group that was roasted for 2.5 to 3 h had the highest total acidity value (0.18–0.21 g/100 g, DW) and the total acidity of peeled potatoes was significantly higher than unpeeled samples (0.21 g/100 g and 0.19 g/100 g, DW, respectively), which may be related to water loss, sugar molecule cleavage, and interactions between polyphenol compounds and polysaccharides in the cell wall [12] Other studies have reported that the pH and total acidity of sweet potatoes will also change during the roasting process [28–30].

3.3. GC/MS Analysis

The aroma and flavor of roasted sweet potatoes mainly come from thermal pyrolyzes, such as the thermal release of terpene glycosidic bonds, carotenoid degradation, caramelization, the Maillard reaction, and Strecker degradation [4,31]. A total of 46 volatile compounds were detected in roasted sweet potatoes (Table 3), including sesquiterpenoids and their oxides (13), furan compounds (12), ketones (6), nitrogen-containing compounds (4), and other volatile compounds (11), including benzeneacetaldehyde, acetic acid, and γ-decalactone, which together form the unique flavor of roasted sweet potatoes. The aroma compounds detected in fresh sweet potatoes mainly come from nerolidol (floral odor), trans-β-ionone (violet-like, floral odor), and γ-decalactone (fruity odor) [32,33]. After roasting for 0.5 to 2 h, the aroma is mainly derived from trans-β-ionone, β-damascenone (sweet odor) [34,35], which is formed by the degradation of carotenoids, and benzeneacetaldehyde (floral, honey-like), which is formed by the degradation of phenylalanine in Strecker degradation [36]. Carbohydrates degrade into dark polymers and form 5-hydroxymethylfurfural (sweet odor), furfural (roasted nut odor), 2-furanmethanol (caramel-like, roasted odor), and maltol (caramel-like odor). These and other furans and their derivatives are important aroma compounds in roasted sweet potatoes and often appear with the Maillard reaction, which makes the aroma composition produced by the Maillard reaction more complex [37,38]. 2-furanmethanol, a source of sweetness and caramel odor, is positively correlated with overall preference [8]. However, after a long roasting time (2.5 to 3 h), the α-dicarbonyl compound and amino acids undergo Strecker degradation and participate in the Maillard reaction after polymerization, which affects the color and aroma by forming 2-pyrrolecarbaldehyde, 4-methyl-5-thiazoleethanol, and 1-(1H-pyrrol-2-yl)-ethanone, among other nitrogen-containing compounds providing roasting aromas [39]. The roasting process may degrade monosaccharides or oxidize aldehydes during the caramelization process; acetic acid generates a sour taste, which in turn changes the quality of roasted sweet potatoes and affects consumer preference [40]. Qin et al. [41] pointed out that aroma plays an important role in the overall flavor and sensory acceptance to consumers. To explain the aroma characteristics more completely, many studies now use PCA to analyze GC/MS data and identify important volatile compounds. By reducing the multi-dimensional data, it is easy to observe the differences between samples [42]. In this experiment, PCA was used to determine the important volatile compounds of peeled and unpeeled sweet potatoes roasted for different times to establish the relationship between the treatment method and the volatile compounds [43]. The first. principal component (F1 of two dimensions) and the second principal component (F2) combined can explain about 63.56% of the raw data (Figure 2). F1 accounts for 44.21%, explaining the distribution of the roasting time. The group roasted for 2 h is distributed in the negative direction of the X-axis, and the group roasted for 2.5 to 3 h is distributed in the positive direction of the X-axis, and displays increasing pyrolysis products such as β-damascenone and furan derivatives (Table 3, No. 5, 8, 14, 16, 17, 27, 31, 36, 38, 41, 42, 46) and N-containing compounds (Table 3, No. 29, 32, 34, 45). F2 accounted for 19.36%, explaining the difference between the two processing conditions. In Figure 2, the unpeeled sweet potatoes are distributed in the positive direction of the Y-axis, and they are rich in sesquiterpene compounds and carotenoid oxidation products. The peeled sweet potatoes are distributed in the negative direction of the Y-axis. In addition, during the roasting process, AHC was used to identify the aroma characteristics of three clusters. Cluster I contained unroasted and peeled potatoes roasted for 0.5 to 2 h; cluster II contained unpeeled potatoes roasted for 0.5 to 2.5 h and peeled potatoes roasted for 2.5 h; cluster III contained unpeeled and peeled potatoes roasted for 3 h, which are positively correlated with caramelization and the formation of Maillard reaction products. In addition, the distribution of volatile compounds shows that as the roasting time increased, the thermal degradation cracked and polymerized more organic compounds to generate more volatile compounds, thus increasing the diversity of volatile compounds [44,45].

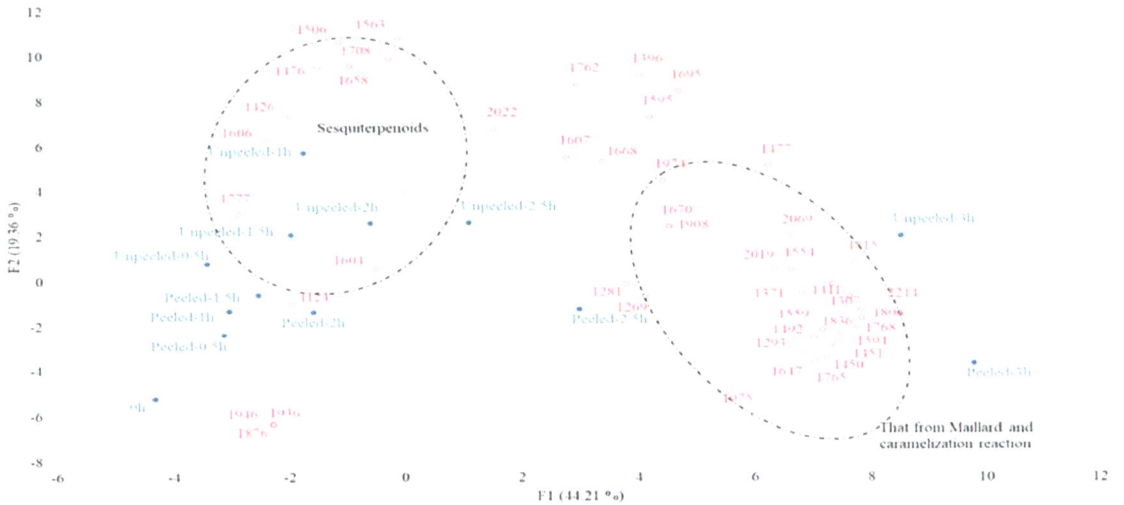

Figure 2. PCA plots of the volatile compound formation of sweet potato during roasting process; the hollow dots indicate the compounds responsible for the perceived aroma of sweet potatoes.

Table 2. Analysis of sugar composition and total titratable acidity of sweet potatoes by different roasting treatments.

Time (h)	Total Starch (g/100 g)		Fructose (g/100 g, DW)		Glucose (g/100 g, DW)		Sucrose (g/100 g, DW)		Maltose (g/100 g, DW)		Total Titratable Acidity (g/100 g, DW)	
Type	Unpeeled	Peeled	Unpeeled	Peeled	Unpeeled	Peeled	Unpeeled	Peeled	Unpeeled	Peeled	Unpeeled	Peeled
0	64.62 ± 0.46 [d]	64.62 ± 0.46 [d]	1.60 ± 0.29 [a]	1.82 ± 0.24 [ab]	2.23 ± 0.10 [a]	2.60 ± 0.18 [a]	11.49 ± 0.02 [c]	12.68 ± 1.10 [a]	ND	ND	0.14 ± 0.01 [b]	0.14 ± 0.01 [abc]
0.5	50.57 ± 0.13 [a]	51.84 ± 0.06 [a]	1.70 ± 0.06 [a]	1.56 ± 0.12 [a]	2.54 ± 0.02 [ab]	2.62 ± 0.05 [ab]	10.63 ± 0.21 [a]	11.12 ± 0.46 [a]	41.45 ± 0.45 [a]	45.92 ± 2.21 [a]	0.11 ± 0.01 [a]	0.09 ± 0.01 [a]
1	53.36 ± 0.06 [c]	53.94 ± 3.57 [c]	1.87 ± 0.06 [ab] *	1.97 ± 0.26 [ab] *	2.61 ± 0.00 [ab]	3.19 ± 0.43 [cd]	11.66 ± 0.34 [bc]	11.79 ± 0.69 [a]	39.04 ± 0.16 [a] *	52.70 ± 2.69 [ab] *	0.11 ± 0.01 [a]	0.11 ± 0.01 [ab]
1.5	52.28 ± 0.03 [b]	53.38 ± 0.42 [bc]	2.39 ± 0.01 [c] *	2.13 ± 0.26 [b] *	3.61 ± 0.23 [c]	3.37 ± 0.02 [c]	12.01 ± 0.14 [bc]	12.51 ± 0.91 [a]	39.79 ± 0.37 [a] *	55.28 ± 3.30 [b] *	0.13 ± 0.01 [b]	0.14 ± 0.01 [abc]
2	51.79 ± 0.06 [b]	52.47 ± 0.25 [abc]	1.94 ± 0.12 [b]	2.00 ± 0.47 [b]	2.79 ± 0.23 [ab]	3.38 ± 0.28 [c]	11.63 ± 0.16 [bc]	12.09 ± 1.40 [a]	39.71 ± 0.93 [a] *	51.82 ± 2.70 [ab] *	0.14 ± 0.01 [b]	0.16 ± 0.01 [abc]
2.5	51.20 ± 0.90 [b]	52.90 ± 0.93 [abc]	2.02 ± 0.09 [b]	1.98 ± 0.15 [ab]	2.75 ± 0.01 [ab]	3.01 ± 0.14 [bcd]	11.12 ± 0.24 [abc]	12.36 ± 2.09 [a]	40.00 ± 0.71 [a] *	49.82 ± 1.69 [ab] *	0.14 ± 0.01 [b] *	0.18 ± 0.01 [bc] *
3	51.10 ± 0.91 [b]	51.42 ± 0.73 [ab]	2.05 ± 0.05 [b] *	1.77 ± 0.13 [ab] *	2.89 ± 0.12 [b]	2.72 ± 0.19 [abc]	10.01 ± 0.01 [a] *	10.79 ± 0.04 [a] *	38.13 ± 0.20 [a]	46.16 ± 3.00 [a]	0.19 ± 0.01 [c] *	0.21 ± 0.01 [c] *

1. Each value is expressed as mean ± standard deviation ($n = 3$). 2. Values (a–d) with different letters within the same column. ($p < 0.05$). 3. ND: not detected. (*) Indicates the significant difference in the same roasting time. 4. DW: dry weight.

Table 3. Volatile compounds of sweet potatoes identified during roasting process.

No	Compound [a]	RI [b]	No	Compound [a]	RI [b]
1	Tetradecane	1124	24	Corylone	1647
2	Pentadecane	1269	25	cis-muurola-3,5-diene	1658
3	Nonanal	1281	26	β-Damascenone	1668
4	Acetic acid	1293	27	Furaneol	1670
5	Furfural	1307	28	trans-Calamenene	1695
6	3-Methyl-tridecane	1371	29	N-Methylsuccinimide	1708
7	Copaene	1396	30	Butylated Hydroxytoluene	1762
8	5-Methyl-2-furaldehyde	1411	31	Maltol	1765
9	Cyperene	1426	32	1-(1H-pyrrole-2-yl)-ethanone	1768
10	γ-Butyrolactone	1450	33	trans-ß-Ionone	1777
11	4-Hydroxybutyric acid	1451	34	2-Pyrrolecarbaldehyde	1806
12	Benzeneacetaldehyde	1476	35	Pantolactone	1815
13	Pristane	1477	36	5-Methyl tetrahydrofurfuryl alcohol	1836
14	2-Furanmethanol	1492	37	Nerolidol	1876
15	α-Himachalene	1506	38	3,5-dimethyl-2,4(3H,5H)-Furandione	1908
16	5-methyl-2-furanmethanol	1554	39	8α-H-Secoeudesmanolide	1936
17	2(5H)-Furanone	1559	40	γ-Decalactone	1946
18	γ-Gurjunene	1563	41	Rosefuran	1974
19	α-Ionol	1594	42	5-Acetoxymethyl-2-furaldehyde	1975
20	α-Guaiene	1595	43	2,3-Dihydro-3,5-dihydroxy-6-methyl-4h-pyran-4-one	2019
21	α-Muurolene	1604	44	Butyl 2 heptenate	2022
22	α-Humulene	1606	45	4-Methyl-5-thiazolethanol	2069
23	α-Bisabolol	1607	46	5-Hydroxymethylfurfural	2214

[a] Identified via comparison of the mass spectra with the RI. [b] RI: Retention index.

3.4. Sensory Evaluation

To clarify the impact of quality changes on consumer preferences, acceptance, and descriptive analyses were conducted. Roasting for 1 to 2 h resulted in the highest overall preference score (6.25–6.65), followed by roasting for 2.5 h (5.71, 5.75), 3 h (4.65, 5.53), and 0.5 h of roasting resulted in the lowest overall preference score (4.96, 3.84). The acceptance results of different roasting times for unpeeled and peeled potatoes trended similarly (Table 4). The largest difference of overall preference score for peeled and unpeeled sweet potatoes in aroma, flavor, taste, and aftertaste was found after roasting for 0.5 h (4.96 and 3.84, respectively). As the roasting time increased, the overall preference score increased. However, when roasting for 1 h, the aroma of unpeeled roasted potatoes scored significantly higher than that of peeled roasted potatoes (6.51 and 5.75, respectively), which may be related to the higher content of benzeneacetaldehyde created, and the greater content of β-ionone and some sesquiterpenes in roasting unpeeled potatoes contributed sweetness and floral fragrance. After further roasting (2.5 to 3 h), the degradation of monosaccharides caused a reduction in sweetness, an increase in total acidity, and the formation of acetic acid, which significantly reduced the overall preference score. The total acidity of peeled roasted sweet potatoes was higher than unpeeled (0.21 g/100 g and 0.19 g/100 g, DW, respectively), so their overall acceptance score (4.65 and 5.53), flavor score (4.15 and 5.45), and mouthfeel score (5.44 and 6.18) were significantly lower. The overall preference score of the roasted sweet potatoes is affected by the flavor and mouthfeel scores [9]. Descriptive analysis was performed according to Pareto's 80/20 rule, which has been used in many sensory studies [46]. The sensory characteristics of roasted sweet potatoes were further explored by six appearance attributes, six aroma attributes, five flavor attributes, six taste attributes, and three aftertaste attributes (Figure 3). The results showed that 12 samples could be distinguished by PCA as three clusters, the F1 explains about 48.43% of the data, and the F2 explains about 33.65% of the data. Cluster I was the group of samples roasted for 0.5 h. Due to the short roasting time, this cluster had an obvious vanilla aroma, denseness, firmness, chalkiness, and astringent aftertaste. The above-mentioned negative sensory characteristics made it have the lowest overall preference score (aroma, flavor, texture, and aftertaste). Cluster II included unpeeled samples roasted for 1 to 2.5 h and peeled samples roasted for 1 to 2 h. As the group in this cluster had higher yellowness (b* value), the maltose, furfural, 2-furanmethanol, and maltol combined with sesquiterpenoids to form the unique aroma of sweet potato, which enabled consumers to notice the obvious yellow color, fibrous texture, moisture, and sweet potato flavor, sweetness, caramel flavor, and sweet aftertaste in this cluster. Roasted sweet potato with these sensory characteristics can increase consumer preference, which is similar to the sensory attribute results of the yellow-flesh sweet potato mentioned in [10,11]. Cluster III contained unpeeled samples roasted for 3 h and peeled samples roasted for 2.5 to 3 h. This cluster was most affected by caramelization and the Maillard reaction, which causes carbohydrates to crack and polymerize to form caramel and melanin [47,48], increasing the browning index (105.54–108.91), total acidity (0.18 g–0.21 g/100 g, DW), and furans content (Table 3, No. 5, 8, 14, 16, 17, 27, 31, 36, 38, 41, 42, 46). Although furans can exhibit malt and sweet roasting aroma, the significant increase at higher roasting levels produces a burnt aroma [49]. In addition, N-containing compounds (Table 3, No. 29, 32, 34, 45) and acetic acid (Table 3, No. 4) produced a readily apparent burnt smell and sourness, causing quality deterioration and a significant reduction in consumers' overall preference for samples in this cluster, as they noticed the obvious changes of caramel color, caramel aroma, burnt aroma, sour aroma, and burnt flavor. Besides, after roasting 1–2 h at 220 °C, the results of the overall acceptability were around 6.25–6.65 (point 6 indicates like slightly), which corresponds to cluster II in Figure 3. In consumer sensory evaluation, the overall score of cluster II was higher than other clusters (I and III). With increased time of roasting process from 2 h to 3 h, descriptive attributes changed from sweet, sweet potato, and fiber to caramel, sour, and fibrousness. Lower overall acceptability (4.65–5.75) corresponds that over-caramelization and starch liquefying of sweet potatoes [8,50].

Table 4. The average value of consumer acceptance of the sensory quality of sweet potato with different roasting treatments.

Sample	Overall	Visual	Aroma	Flavor	Texture	Aftertaste
Unpeeled-0.5 h	4.96 ± 1.26 [c] ***	5.65 ± 1.38 [a]	5.35 ± 1.08 [b] ***	4.95 ± 1.30 [d] ***	4.98 ± 1.56 [b] ***	5.20 ± 1.15 [cd] ***
Unpeeled-1 h	6.55 ± 1.37 [a]	6.24 ± 1.23 [a]	6.51 ± 1.40 [a] **	6.49 ± 1.43 [ab]	6.47 ± 1.33 [a]	6.71 ± 1.18 [a]
Unpeeled-1.5 h	6.20 ± 1.39 [ab]	5.71 ± 1.47 [a] *	6.27 ± 1.35 [a]	6.31 ± 1.49 [abc]	5.87 ± 1.44 [a] *	5.91 ± 1.55 [abc]
Unpeeled-2 h	6.25 ± 1.46 [ab]	6.25 ± 1.39 [a]	6.67 ± 1.09 [a]	6.56 ± 1.46 [a]	6.47 ± 1.55 [a]	6.25 ± 1.54 [ab]
Unpeeled-2.5 h	5.71 ± 1.61 [bc]	5.87 ± 1.50 [a]	6.56 ± 1.45 [a]	5.65 ± 1.95 [bcd]	6.02 ± 1.67 [a]	5.49 ± 1.59 [bcd]
Unpeeled-3 h	5.53 ± 1.89 [bc] *	5.67 ± 1.60 [a]	6.16 ± 1.55 [a]	5.45 ± 2.09 [cd] **	6.18 ± 1.66 [a] *	4.95 ± 1.95 [d]
Peeled-0.5 h	3.84 ± 1.32 [d] ***	5.18 ± 1.25 [c]	4.47 ± 1.12 [c] ***	3.85 ± 1.38 [c] ***	3.38 ± 1.34 [c] ***	4.18 ± 1.40 [c] ***
Peeled-1 h	6.35 ± 1.27 [ab]	5.91 ± 1.25 [abc]	5.75 ± 1.00 [b] **	6.45 ± 1.26 [a]	6.31 ± 1.36 [a]	6.25 ± 1.28 [a]
Peeled-1.5 h	6.60 ± 1.15 [a]	6.49 ± 1.44 [a] *	6.20 ± 1.46 [ab]	6.47 ± 1.26 [a]	6.53 ± 1.29 [a] *	6.13 ± 1.32 [ab] *
Peeled-2 h	6.65 ± 1.25 [a]	6.51 ± 1.18 [a]	6.87 ± 1.26 [a]	6.67 ± 1.52 [a]	6.53 ± 1.39 [a]	6.31 ± 1.30 [a]
Peeled-2.5 h	5.75 ± 1.65 [b]	6.02 ± 1.35 [ab]	6.51 ± 1.26 [a]	5.45 ± 1.95 [b]	6.24 ± 1.40 [a]	5.31 ± 1.90 [b]
Peeled-3 h	4.65 ± 1.91 [c] *	5.58 ± 1.66 [bc]	5.69 ± 1.94 [b]	4.15 ± 2.01 [c] **	5.44 ± 1.77 [b] *	4.24 ± 1.90 [c] *

1. Each value is expressed as mean ± standard deviation ($n = 60$). 2. Values (a–d) with different letters within the same column ($p < 0.05$). (*) Indicates significant difference in the same roasting time. (* $p < 0.05$, ** $p < 0.01$, *** $p < 0.0001$).

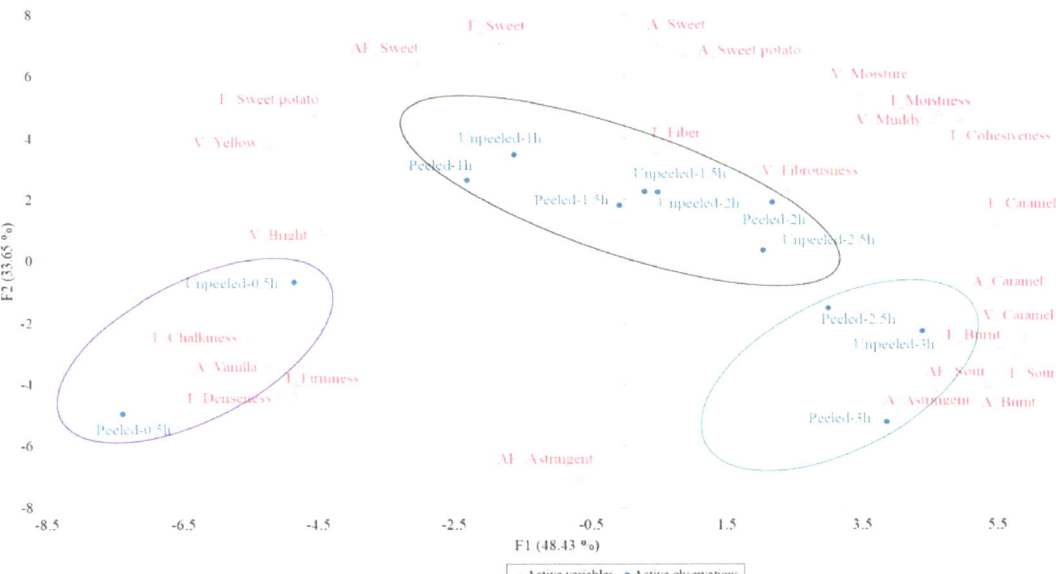

Figure 3. Principle component analysis with (F1 = 48.43% and F2 = 33.65%) variability of all descriptive terms explained for all samples. Abbreviations before attributes: V, visual; A, aroma; F, flavor; T, texture; AF, aftertaste.

4. Conclusions

This study explored the effect of processing methods on the quality of roasted sweet potatoes as measured by consumer preference. This study found that the ideal roasting time has the following effects: starch hydrolysis and thermal cracking reactions (carotenoid degradation, caramelization, the Maillard reaction, and Strecker degradation) change the flesh color from milky white to golden yellow, then to brown, and the browning index had an increasing trend with the roasting time and significant increases in maltose, β-ionone, benzeneacetaldehyde, furfural, maltol, 2-furanmethanol, and sesquiterpenoids, providing fruity, sweet, and caramel-like odors and adding a unique flavor to the roasted sweet potatoes. These results also show that the difference in the composition of volatile compounds due to the degradation of various organic compounds is mainly determined by the roasting time, and the roasting time also has a more significant influence on the overall preference of consumers than whether the sweet potatoes are peeled or not. Comprehensive production cost considerations, quality analysis, and sensory evaluation tests show that the best roasted sweet potato quality is obtained by roasting for 1 to 2 h.

Author Contributions: Conceptualization, L.-Y.L. and P.-Y.C.; methodology, Y.-J.T.; formal analysis, Y.-J.T., L.-Y.L. and P.-Y.C.; resources, M.-H.C.; writing—original draft preparation, Y.-C.C. and P.-Y.C.; writing—review and editing, Y.-C.C. and P.-Y.C.; visualization, K.-M.Y. All authors have read and agreed to the published version of the manuscript.

Funding: This research received no external funding.

Institutional Review Board Statement: Not applicable.

Informed Consent Statement: Not applicable.

Data Availability Statement: The datasets generated for this study are available on request to the corresponding author.

Acknowledgments: This study was appreciated by the council of agriculture under project 110AS-14.1.1-ST-aF.

Conflicts of Interest: The authors declare no conflict of interest.

Appendix A

Table A1. Sensory attributes of sweet potatoes.

	Attribute	Description
Visual	Yellow	Flesh that is yellow in colour.
	Caramel	Appearance associated with brown sugar.
	Fibrousness	Amount of stringy fibers present.
	Moisture	Appearance that is moist.
	Muddy	Appearance that is muddy.
	Bright	Appearance that is bright.
Aroma	Sweet	Aromatic like sugar.
	Caramel	Aromatic associated with brown sugar.
	Sour	Aromatic associated with acid.
	Burnt	An aromatic associated with vegetables that were burnt while cooking.
	Sweet potato	Aromatic associated with cooked sweet potato of TNG57.
	Vanilla	Aromatic notes associated with damp soil, wet foliage or slightly undercooked potatoes. or In-mouth aromatic associated with vanilla and vanillin.
Flavor	Sweet potato	Flavor notes associated with the taste of cooked TNG57.
	Sweet	Tastes like sugar.
	Caramel	Flavor associated with brown sugar.
	Sour	Basic taste stimulated by acid.
	Burnt	The degree of browning or brown spots due to roasting.
Texture	Moistness	The amount of moistness/wetness of the sample in the mouth.
	Cohesiveness	Degree to which sample holds together after chewing.
	Denseness	The solidness/compactness of the sample.
	Firmness	Degree to which the sample retains its shape after lightly squeezing it.
	Chalkiness	Degree to which the mouth feels chalky, like raw potato, very fine particles, often perceived on the roof of the mouth.
	Fiber	The quality of being fibrous.
Aftertaste	Sweet	An aftertaste that leaves a sweetness on the tongue and in the mouth that is pleasant.
	Sour	Aftertaste associated with brown sugar.
	Astringent	Sensation of drying, drawing and/or puckering of any of the mouth surfaces.

References

1. Teow, C.C.; Truong, V.D.; McFeeters, R.F.; Thompson, R.L.; Pecota, K.V.; Yencho, G.C. Antioxidant activities, phenolic and β-carotene contents of sweet potato genotypes with varying flesh colours. *Food Chem.* **2007**, *103*, 829–838. [CrossRef]
2. Blessington, T.; Nzaramba, M.N.; Scheuring, D.C.; Hale, A.L.; Reddivari, L.; Miller, J.C. Cooking methods and storage treatments of potato: Effects on carotenoids, antioxidant activity, and phenolics. *Am. J. Potato Res.* **2010**, *87*, 479–491. [CrossRef]
3. Sablani, S.; Marcotte, M.; Baik, O.; Castaigne, F. Modeling of simultaneous heat and water transport in the baking process. *LWT* **1998**, *31*, 201–209. [CrossRef]
4. Wang, Y.; Kays, S. Contribution of Volatile Compounds to the Characteristic Aroma of BakedJewel'Sweetpotatoes. *J. Am. Soc. Hortic. Sci.* **2000**, *125*, 638–643. [CrossRef]
5. Corrales, C.V.; Lebrun, M.; Vaillant, F.; Madec, M.N.; Lortal, S.; Pérez, A.M.; Fliedel, G. Key odor and physicochemical characteristics of raw and roasted jicaro seeds (*Crescentia alata* KHB). *Food Res. Int.* **2017**, *96*, 113–120. [CrossRef] [PubMed]
6. Staatz, J.; Hollinger, F. *West African Food Systems and Changing Consumer Demands*; FAO: Rome, Italy, 2016.
7. Shi, X.; Dean, L.O.; Davis, J.P.; Sandeep, K.P.; Sanders, T.H. The effects of different dry roast parameters on peanut quality using an industrial belt-type roaster simulator. *Food Chem.* **2018**, *240*, 974–979. [CrossRef] [PubMed]
8. Hou, F.; Mu, T.; Ma, M.; Blecker, C. Sensory evaluation of roasted sweet potatoes influenced by different cultivars: A correlation study with respect to sugars, amino acids, volatile compounds, and colors. *J. Food Process. Preserv.* **2020**, *44*, e14646. [CrossRef]
9. Leksrisompong, P.P.; Whitson, M.E.; Truong, V.D.; Drake, M.A. Sensory attributes and consumer acceptance of sweet potato cultivars with varying flesh colors. *J. Sens. Stud.* **2012**, *27*, 59–69. [CrossRef]
10. Ofori, G.; Oduro, I.; Ellis, W.O.; Dapaah, K.H. Assessment of vitamin A content and sensory attributes of new sweet potato (*Ipomoea batatas*) genotypes in Ghana. *Afr. J. Food Sci.* **2009**, *3*, 184–192.
11. Leighton, C.S.; Schönfeldt, H.C.; Kruger, R. Quantitative descriptive sensory analysis of five different cultivars of sweet potato to determine sensory and textural profiles. *J. Sens. Stud.* **2010**, *25*, 2–18. [CrossRef]

12. Vizzotto, M.; Pereira, E.D.S.; Vinholes, J.R.; Munhoz, P.C.; Ferri, N.M.L.; Castro, L.A.S.D.; Krolow, A.C.R. Physicochemical and antioxidant capacity analysis of colored sweet potato genotypes: In natura and thermally processed. *Cienc. Rural* **2017**, *47*. [CrossRef]
13. Isleroglu, H.; Kemerli, T.; Sakin-Yilmazer, M.; Guven, G.; Ozdestan, O.; Uren, A.; Kaymak-Ertekin, F. Effect of steam baking on acrylamide formation and browning kinetics of cookies. *J. Food Sci.* **2012**, *77*, E257–E263. [CrossRef]
14. Liu, Y.; Sabboh, H.; Kirchhof, G.; Sopade, P. In vitro starch digestion and potassium release in sweet potato from Papua New Guinea. *Int. J. Food Sci. Technol.* **2010**, *45*, 1925–1931. [CrossRef]
15. Chan, C.F.; Chiang, C.M.; Lai, Y.C.; Huang, C.L.; Kao, S.C.; Liao, W.C. Changes in sugar composition during baking and their effects on sensory attributes of baked sweet potatoes. *J. Food Sci. Technol.* **2014**, *51*, 4072–4077. [CrossRef]
16. Picha, D.H. HPLC determination of sugars in raw and baked sweet potatoes. *J. Food Sci.* **1985**, *50*, 1189–1190. [CrossRef]
17. Horwitz, W. *Official Methods of Analysis*; Association of Official Analytical Chemists: Washington, DC, USA, 2020; Volume 222.
18. Liu, S.L.; Jaw, Y.M.; Wang, L.F.; Chuang, G.C.C.; Zhuang, Z.Y.; Chen, Y.S.; Liou, B.K. Evaluation of Sensory Quality for Taiwanese Specialty Teas with Cold Infusion Using CATA and Temporal CATA by Taiwanese Consumers. *Foods* **2021**, *10*, 2344. [CrossRef]
19. Dery, E.K.; Carey, E.E.; Ssali, R.T.; Low, J.W.; Johanningsmeier, S.D.; Oduro, I.; Boakye, A.; Omodamiro, R.M.; Yusuf, H.L. Sensory characteristics and consumer segmentation of fried sweetpotato for expanded markets in Africa. *Int. J. Food Sci. Technol.* **2021**, *56*, 1419–1431. [CrossRef] [PubMed]
20. van Oirschot, Q.E.; Rees, D.; Aked, J. Sensory characteristics of five sweet potato cultivars and their changes during storage under tropical conditions. *Food Qual. Prefer.* **2003**, *14*, 673–680. [CrossRef]
21. Trugo, L.C.; Macrae, R. An investigation of coffee roasting using high performance gel filtration chromatography. *Food Chem.* **1986**, *19*, 1–9. [CrossRef]
22. Clydesdale, F.M. Changes in color and flavor and their effect on sensory perception in the elderly. *Nutr. Rev.* **1994**, *52*, S19. [CrossRef]
23. Chung, H.S.; Kim, D.H.; Youn, K.S.; Lee, J.B.; Moon, K.D. Optimization of roasting conditions according to antioxidant activity and sensory quality of coffee brews. *Food Sci. Biotechnol.* **2013**, *22*, 23–29. [CrossRef]
24. Mccleary, B.V.; Gibson, T.S.; Mugford, D.C. Measurement of total starch in cereal products by amyloglucosidase-α-amylase method: Collaborative study. *J. AOAC Int.* **1997**, *80*, 571–579. [CrossRef]
25. Trancoso-Reyes, N.; Ochoa-Martínez, L.A.; Bello-Pérez, L.A.; Morales-Castro, J.; Estévez-Santiago, R.; Olmedilla-Alonso, B. Effect of pre-treatment on physicochemical and structural properties, and the bioaccessibility of β-carotene in sweet potato flour. *Food Chem.* **2016**, *200*, 199–205. [CrossRef]
26. Lai, Y.C.; Huang, C.L.; Chan, C.F.; Lien, C.Y.; Liao, W.C. Studies of sugar composition and starch morphology of baked sweet potatoes (*Ipomoea batatas* (L.) Lam). *J. Food Sci. Technol.* **2013**, *50*, 1193–1199. [CrossRef] [PubMed]
27. Binner, S.; Jardine, W.G.; Renard, C.M.C.G.; Jarvis, M.C. Cell wall modifications during cooking of potatoes and sweet potatoes. *J. Sci. Food Agric.* **2000**, *80*, 216–218. [CrossRef]
28. Caetano, P.K.; Mariano-nasser, F.A.D.C.; MendonÇa, V.Z.D.; Furlaneto, K.A.; Daiuto, E.R.; Vieites, R.L. Physicochemical and sensory characteristics of sweet potato chips undergoing different cooking methods. *Food Sci. Technol.* **2017**, *38*, 434–440. [CrossRef]
29. Ogliari, R.; Soares, J.M.; Teixeira, F.; Schwarz, K.; da Silva, K.A.; Schiessel, D.L.; Novello, D. Chemical, nutritional and sensory characterization of sweet potato submitted to different cooking methods. *Int. J. Res.-Granthaalayah* **2020**, *8*, 147–156. [CrossRef]
30. Sohail, M.; Khan, R.U.; Afridi, S.R.; Imad, M.; Mehrin, B. Preparation and quality evaluation of sweet potato ready to drink beverage. *ARPN J. Agric. Biol. Sci.* **2013**, *8*, 279–282.
31. Sun, J.B.; Severson, R.F.; Schlotzhauer, W.S.; Kays, S.J. Identifying Critical Volatiles in the Flavor of BakedJewel'Sweetpotatoes [*Ipomoea batatas* (L.) Lam.]. *J. Am. Soc. Hortic. Sci.* **1995**, *120*, 468–474. [CrossRef]
32. Chen, M.X.; Chen, X.S.; Wang, X.G.; Ci, Z.J.; Liu, X.L.; He, T.M.; Zhang, L.J. Comparison of headspace solid-phase microextraction with simultaneous steam distillation extraction for the analysis of the volatile constituents in Chinese apricot. *Agric. Sci. China* **2006**, *5*, 879–884. [CrossRef]
33. Zhou, Y.; Zeng, L.; Liu, X.; Gui, J.; Mei, X.; Fu, X.; Dong, F.; Tang, J.; Zhang, L.; Yang, Z. Formation of (E)-nerolidol in tea (*Camellia sinensis*) leaves exposed to multiple stresses during tea manufacturing. *Food Chem.* **2017**, *231*, 78–86. [CrossRef] [PubMed]
34. Ho, C.T.; Zheng, X.; Li, S. Tea aroma formation. *Food Sci. Hum. Wellness* **2015**, *4*, 9–27. [CrossRef]
35. Ravichandran, R. Carotenoid composition, distribution and degradation to flavour volatiles during black tea manufacture and the effect of carotenoid supplementation on tea quality and aroma. *Food Chem.* **2002**, *78*, 23–28. [CrossRef]
36. Bi, S.; Xu, X.; Luo, D.; Lao, F.; Pang, X.; Shen, Q.; Hu, X.; Wu, J. Characterization of key aroma compounds in raw and roasted peas (*Pisum sativum* L.) by application of instrumental and sensory techniques. *J. Agric. Food Chem.* **2020**, *68*, 2718–2727. [CrossRef] [PubMed]
37. Perez Locas, C.; Yaylayan, V.A. Isotope labeling studies on the formation of 5-(hydroxymethyl)-2-furaldehyde (HMF) from sucrose by pyrolysis-GC/MS. *J. Agric. Food Chem.* **2008**, *56*, 6717–6723. [CrossRef] [PubMed]
38. Liu, J.; Wan, P.; Xie, C.; Chen, D.W. Key aroma-active compounds in brown sugar and their influence on sweetness. *Food Chem.* **2021**, *345*, 128826. [CrossRef]

39. Pu, D.; Zhang, H.; Zhang, Y.; Sun, B.; Ren, F.; Chen, H. Characterization of the key aroma compounds in white bread by aroma extract dilution analysis, quantitation, and sensory evaluation experiments. *J. Food Process. Preserv.* **2019**, *43*, e13933. [CrossRef]
40. Samborska, K.; Bonikowski, R.; Kalemba, D.; Barańska, A.; Jedlińska, A.; Edris, A. Volatile aroma compounds of sugarcane molasses as affected by spray drying at low and high temperature. *LWT* **2021**, *145*, 111288. [CrossRef]
41. Qin, G.; Tao, S.; Cao, Y.; Wu, J.; Zhang, H.; Huang, W.; Zhang, S. Evaluation of the volatile profile of 33 Pyrus ussuriensis cultivars by HS-SPME with GC–MS. *Food Chem.* **2012**, *134*, 2367–2382. [CrossRef] [PubMed]
42. Kang, W.; Li, Y.; Xu, Y.; Jiang, W.; Tao, Y. Characterization of aroma compounds in Chinese bayberry (*Myrica rubra* Sieb. et Zucc.) by gas chromatography mass spectrometry (GC-MS) and olfactometry (GC-O). *J. Food Sci.* **2012**, *77*, C1030–C1035. [CrossRef]
43. Cheng, H.; Qin, Z.H.; Guo, X.F.; Hu, X.S.; Wu, J.H. Geographical origin identification of propolis using GC–MS and electronic nose combined with principal component analysis. *Food Res. Int.* **2013**, *51*, 813–822. [CrossRef]
44. Yuan, F.; Qian, M.C. Aroma potential in early-and late-maturity Pinot noir grapes evaluated by aroma extract dilution analysis. *J. Agric. Food Chem.* **2016**, *64*, 443–450. [CrossRef] [PubMed]
45. Zhou, H.; Luo, D.; Gholamhosseini, H.; Li, Z.; Han, B.; He, J.; Wang, S. Aroma characteristic analysis of Amomi fructus from different habitats using machine olfactory and gas chromatography-mass spectrometry. *Pharmacogn. Mag.* **2019**, *15*, 392.
46. King, S.C.; Meiselman, H.L.; Carr, B.T. Measuring emotions associated with foods in consumer testing. *Food Qual. Prefer.* **2010**, *21*, 1114–1116. [CrossRef]
47. Taş, N.G.; Gökmen, V. Maillard reaction and caramelization during hazelnut roasting: A multiresponse kinetic study. *Food Chem.* **2017**, *221*, 1911–1922.
48. Lund, M.N.; Ray, C.A. Control of Maillard reactions in foods: Strategies and chemical mechanisms. *J. Agric. Food Chem.* **2017**, *65*, 4537–4552. [CrossRef] [PubMed]
49. Guo, S.; Jom, K.N.; Ge, Y. Influence of roasting condition on flavor profile of sunflower seeds: A flavoromics approach. *Sci. Rep.* **2019**, *9*, 1–10. [CrossRef] [PubMed]
50. Komaki, T.; Taji, N. Studies on Enzymatic Liquefaction and Saccharification of Starch: Part VIII. Liquefying Conditions of Corn Starch by Bacterial Alpha-Amylase. *Agric. Biol. Chem.* **1968**, *32*, 860–872. [CrossRef]

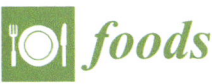

Article

Green Bean, Pea and Mesquite Whole Pod Flours Nutritional and Functional Properties and Their Effect on Sourdough Bread

Angela Mariela González-Montemayor [1], José Fernando Solanilla-Duque [2], Adriana C. Flores-Gallegos [1], Claudia Magdalena López-Badillo [1], Juan Alberto Ascacio-Valdés [1] and Raúl Rodríguez-Herrera [1,*]

[1] Food Research Department, School of Chemistry, Universidad Autónoma de Coahuila, Boulevard Venustiano Carranza and José Cárdenas s/n, Republica Oriente, Saltillo CP 25280, Mexico; angelagonzalez@uadec.edu.mx (A.M.G.-M.); carolinaflores@uadec.edu.mx (A.C.F-G.); cllopezb@uadec.edu.mx (C.M.L.-B.); alberto_ascaciovaldes@uadec.edu.mx (J.A.A.-V.)

[2] Agroindustrial Engineering Department, School of Agrarian Sciences, Universidad del Cauca, Popayán 190002, Colombia; jsolanilla@unicauca.edu.co

* Correspondence: raul.rodriguez@uadec.edu.mx; Tel.: +52-(844)-416-9213

Abstract: In this study, proximal composition, mineral analysis, polyphenolic compounds identification, and antioxidant and functional activities were determined in green bean (GBF), mesquite (MF), and pea (PF) flours. Different mixtures of legume flour and wheat flour for bread elaboration were determined by a simplex-centroid design. After that, the proximal composition, color, specific volume, polyphenol content, antioxidant activities, and functional properties of the different breads were evaluated. While GBF and PF have a higher protein content (41–47%), MF has a significant fiber content (19.9%) as well as a higher polyphenol content (474.77 mg GAE/g) and antioxidant capacities. It was possible to identify Ca, K, and Mg and caffeic and enolic acids in the flours. The legume–wheat mixtures affected the fiber, protein content, and the physical properties of bread. Bread with MF contained more fiber; meanwhile, PF and GBF benefit the protein content. With MF, the specific bread volume only decreased by 7%. These legume flours have the potential to increase the nutritional value of bakery goods.

Keywords: mesquite; legume flour; antioxidant activity; bakery product

1. Introduction

Currently, there is a demand for novel, tasty, and healthy baked goods; bread manufacturing fills the requirements for specific groups that demand products with functional ingredients, that are gluten-free, or that have a high fiber content [1–3]. For the improvement of bread formulations, there is a growing interest in minor cereal, ancient crops, pseudocereals, and legumes, such as oat, rice, corn, sorghum, quinoa, amaranth, buckwheat, chickpea, pea, and soybean, as ingredients for bread making applications [3].

The fortification of wheat flour products with legume flours has been recognized as a viable strategy because legumes are rich in fibers, minerals, phytochemicals, and proteins (compensating the deficiency of the amino acid of the products), and these flours are known for their functionality (water-binding capacity, fat absorption) [4]. Among the legumes used to fortify bread, pea (*Pisum sativum*) is the most investigated.

In bread, there are reports about the inclusion of germinated pea flour [5] and fermented pea flour [6]. The obtained products were of good quality and had high protein and fiber content as well as a higher water absorption capacity along with achieving gluten-free quality products.

Other legumes successfully added into bread are beans (*Phaseolus vulgaris*) and mesquite (*Prosopis* spp.), also known as algarrobo. Regarding beans in an immature form, known as a green bean, no reports of its addition in bakery products are reported. However, white kidney beans [7,8] have been successfully added to bread. Using white

kidney beans, it was possible to obtain bread with a higher protein, fiber, and ash content that also had acceptable sensory (texture and flavor) characteristics and oil and water absorption changes. In mesquite flour, it is documented that it is possible to develop bakery goods such as gluten-free muffins and Panettone bread with increased nutritional values and antioxidant activities [9].

According to our knowledge, specifically, the characteristics of mesquite (*Prosopis glandulosa*) pod flours are limited. It is desirable to compare the effects of these legume flours on bread made with one of the most used legumes, the pea. Owing to the previous antecedents, this study aimed to characterize the obtained flours from mesquite, green bean, and pea whole pods and to incorporate these flours with whole wheat flour into sourdough bread. Sourdough was chosen for its known benefits in improving rheological and sensory qualities and for improving the shelf-life of bread [10].

2. Materials and Methods

2.1. Plant Material

Batches of 12 kg of whole pods of pea (*Pisum sativum*) and green bean (*Phaseolus vulgaris*) were purchased in a local market. The mesquite (*Prosopis glandulosa*) pods were collected in Ramos Arizpe, Coahuila, México (North latitude 25°35′04.4″, West longitude 100°54′50.4″, 1348 masl). All of the samples were rinsed with water and were dried at 50 °C. After, the pods were ground (Moulinex, Écully, France). The flours were sieved to obtain a particle size ranging from 355 and < 75 µm. The pea (PF), green bean (GBF), and mesquite (MF) flours were kept at room temperature in hermetic bags and were covered from light for one week (after this time, the experiments were started).

2.2. Flour Characterization

2.2.1. Proximal Composition

The nutritional analysis of the legume flours was conducted as stated by the following Association of Official Analytical Chemists (AOAC methods) [11]: fat (AOAC 945.16), ash (AOAC 920.181), crude fiber (AOAC 962.09), and total protein (total nitrogen $*$ 6.25) (AOAC 978.02). Then, the carbohydrates were quantified by difference.

2.2.2. Mineral Analysis

For this identification and quantification, 3 g of the different legume flours were placed in the sample cup of an X-Ray Fluorescence (XRF) Spectrometer (Epsilon 1, Malvern Panalytical, Madrid, Spain). The patterns were interpreted with the Omniam software.

2.2.3. Extraction and Determination of Phenolic Content and Profile by RP-HPLC-ESI-MS

For this analysis, the methodologies mentioned by Chen et al. [12] were used. The samples (1 g), which had been previously mixed with 80% methanol (1:10 w/v), were placed in ultrasound equipment (Branson 5510, Marshall Scientific, Hampton, NH, USA at 25 °C for 10 min. Later, to obtain the supernatant, the samples were centrifuged at 4000 g for 10 min. The extraction and centrifugation processes were repeated twice. The supernatants were dried at 40 °C, and the obtained residues were dissolved in methanol and were stored at −80 °C until their use. The phenolic content was determined by mixing 395 µL of distilled water with 5 µL of the sample extract; then, the Folin–Ciocalteu reagent (400 µL) was added. The mix was rested for 5 min, and Na_2CO_3 (0.01 M) was added, and then all of the samples were mixed with water (2.5 mL). Absorbance was determined at 790 nm in a spectrophotometer (Epoch™ microplate, Biotek, Winooski, VT, USA). Gallic acid (GA) was used to prepare the standard curve (0–400 ppm). The phenolic content was expressed as GA equivalents per gram of flour.

The obtained methanolic extracts were used to determine the phenolic profile of the flours using a Varian High Performance Liquid Chromatography (HPLC) system. Reverse phase-high performance liquid chromatography analyses were performed according to the fully described methodology of Hernández-Hernández et al. [13].

2.2.4. Determination of Antioxidant Activity

The methanolic extracts (Section 2.2.3) were also used for these determinations.

The antioxidant activity was evaluated by the 2,2-diphenyl-1-picrylhydrazyl (DPPH), 2,2′-Azino-bis(3-ethylbenzothiazoline-6-sulfonic acid) diammonium salt (ABTS$^\pm$), and ferric reducing antioxidant power (FRAP) methods. Trolox was used as a standard, and the obtained results were expressed as Trolox equivalents (TE) per gram of flour.

The DPPH assay was accomplished according to the methodology described by Molyneux [14] with slight modifications. Briefly, a 60 µM solution was prepared with methanol and the DPPH reagent. Then, 7 µL of each sample with 193 µL of the DPPH methanolic solution was mixed and kept in the dark for 30 min. The absorbance was determined at 517 nm.

For ABTS$^\pm$, according to the modified methodology of Opitz et al. [15], a solution of ABTS$^\pm$ at a concentration of 7 mM was prepared and mixed with $K_2S_2O_8$ at 2.45 mM (1:1 v/v). This ABTS$^\pm$ solution was left to rest for 12 h at 37 °C. Later, the solution was diluted with methanol to reach an absorbance of 0.7 ± 0.02. In the microplate, 5 µL of each sample were added and 95 µL of ABTS$^\pm$ solution. The solutions rested for 1 min before the reading at 734 nm.

For the FRAP assay, the FRAP solution was obtained by mixing TPTZ (2,4,6-Tripyridyl-s-triazine) at 10 mM, $FeCl_3$ (20 mM), and acetate buffer (0.3 M, pH 3.6) in the proportions of 1:1:10 $v/v/v$. Sample solutions (10 µL) were added to the microplate followed by 290 µL of the FRAP solution. Later, the samples were incubated in the dark at 37 °C for 15 min. The absorbance was measured at 593 nm [12].

2.2.5. Functional Activities

The water absorption (WAI) and water solubility (WSI) indexes were calculated following the method reported by Kraithong et al. [16] with modifications. One gram of each flour sample was suspended in 10 mL of distilled water and was mixed for 1 min. Then, the suspensions were stirred and heated in a water bath at 70 °C for 30 min. The next step was centrifugation at 3000 rpm for 10 min. The supernatants were placed into an aluminum container to remove moisture at 105 °C for 12 h. The obtained dry solids were weighted. WAI and WSI were calculated following the equations:

$$\text{WAI (g/g)} = \text{weight of wet sediment/weight of flour sample} \quad (1)$$

$$\text{WSI (\%)} = (\text{weight of dried supernant/weight of flour sample}) \times 100 \quad (2)$$

For the water (WHC) and oil (OHC) holding capacities, 1 g of each flour sample was stirred with 10 mL of distilled water or corn oil (Cristal, AGYDSA, Guadalajara, Jalisco, Mexico). These suspensions were centrifuged at 2200 g for 30 min. The supernatant was recovered and quantified. WHC was expressed as g of held water per g of sample, and the OHC was expressed as g of oil. To determine the organic molecule absorption capacity (OMAC), 3 g of each sample was placed with 10 mL of corn oil for 24 h at 25 °C. Later, the samples were centrifuged at 2000 g for 15 min. OMAC was expressed as the absorbed hydrophobic component and were calculated in g oil/sample g [17].

2.3. Bread Preparation

For bread preparation, legume flours (PF, GBF, and MF), whole wheat flour (WF) (14 g/100 g protein, 2 g/100 g fat, 13 g/100 g fiber, and 54 g/100 g carbohydrates) provided from La Perla, Molinos del Fénix, Saltillo, Coahuila, and salt (natural fluoride iodized salt) from Sal la Fina, Mexico, were used. A type I sourdough supplied by a local bakery (Tres espigas, Saltillo, Mexico) was used as a leavening agent. Water was replaced by aguamiel (sap obtained from agave). This sap is used to obtain pulque, an alcoholic beverage with significant importance in the breadmaking industry and Mexican gastronomy [18]. The aguamiel is rich in carbohydrates (sucrose, glucose, fructose, fructooligosaccharides, and gums) and contains amino acids and phenolic compounds [19]. The primary reason for adding aguamiel is to improve fermentation. This sap was collected from mature *Agave salmiana* plants (8–10 years old) in the town of "Las Mangas" (latitude 25°14′14.9″, longitude 101°10′16″, altitude 1560 masl), which is located near Saltillo, Coahuila, México. This aguamiel (161.5 ± 58.68 g/L total sugars) was pasteurized at 80 °C for 10 min and was kept frozen (−80 °C) until use.

The legume flours (PF, GBF, and MF) and the WF were mixed in the proportions of a simplex-centroid design for treatment mixtures with four different components (Table 1). The proportions of the other ingredients were: 70 g of aguamiel, 2.4 g of salt, and 20 g of sourdough. The first step to make bread treatments was to mix flour, salt, and aguamiel. The obtained doughs were kneaded for 10 min and were left to rest for 1 h. The next step was to add the sourdough and to knead the doughs for another 1 min, and the doughs were left to rest for 1 h and 20 min. Then, the doughs were kept at 4 °C for 24 h. Finally, the samples were baked in a convection oven (HCX Plus 3, San-Son, Naucalpan, Mexico) at 250 °C for 15 min.

Table 1. Treatments for bread elaboration according to a simplex-centroid design with four different components.

Treatment	Flours (g)			
	PF	GBF	MF	WF
1	10	10	0	80
2	0	10	10	80
3	10	0	10	80
4	6.66	6.66	6.66	80
5	20	0	0	80
6	0	20	0	80
7	0	0	20	80
Control	0	0	0	100

PF (pea flour), GBF (green bean flour), MF (mesquite flour), WF (whole-wheat flour).

2.4. Bread Characterization

The bread samples were analyzed for proximal composition with the methods described above. Bread pieces were dried at 130 °C for 1 h in the convection oven (AACC 44-15A) [20].

With the protein, carbohydrate, and fat composition in bread, the caloric value (kcal/100 g) was calculated according to caloric coefficients in the equation [21]:

$$\text{caloric value (kcal/100 g)} = (\text{g protein} \times 4) + (\text{g fat} \times 9) + (\text{g carbohydrates} \times 4) \quad (3)$$

To measure the functional properties of WHC and OHC, the samples were fresh. The loaf volume of the samples was measured (24 h after baking) using the millet seed displacement method (AACC 10-05.01). The specific volume was calculated, dividing the loaf volume by the corresponding loaf weight. The color of the bread crumbs was determined using a Precision Colorimeter NR20XE (3NH, Shenzhen, China; the reported values are from the International Commission on Illumination, for its acronym in French the CIF.Lab system

2.5. Statistical Analyses

The flour experiments were established under a randomized complete block design with three replicates. The data were analyzed using an Analysis of Variance (ANOVA). Differences among the sources of the variations were significant at $p < 0.05$. When it was needed, treatment means were compared using the Tukey multiple range test. The InfoStat/p Software version 2011 p was used for data analysis. A simplex-centroid design for mixtures with four different components: PF, GBF, MF, and WF (Table 1) was used to evaluate the interaction in proximal components (ash, fiber, moisture, protein), color parameters (L*, a*, and b*), loaf bread weight and volume, functional activities (WHC and

OHC), phenol content, and antioxidant activities (by DPPH, ABTS, and FRAP methods). The experimental data were examined with the Scheffe equation:

$$Y = \beta_1 X_1 + \beta_2 X_2 + \beta_3 X_3 + \beta_{12} X_1 X_2 + \beta_{13} X_1 X_3 + \beta_{23} X_2 X_3 + \beta_{123} X_1 X_2 X_3 \quad (4)$$

where Y is the independent variable and where β_1, β_2, β_3, β_{12}, β_{13}, β_{23}, and β_{123} are regression parameters, X_1, X_2, and X_3 are the type of flour in the mixtures. Positive values in binary coefficients indicated synergistic effects, and negative values indicated antagonism. Data were analyzed using the Statgraphic Centurion XVI.I® software. Surface plots and prediction equations were obtained.

3. Results and Discussion

3.1. Proximal Analysis of Flours

The proximal analysis of PF, GBF, and MF (Table 2) showed significant moisture, ash, total fiber, protein, and carbohydrate differences. The moisture varied in a range of 5.97 to 18.71%. The PF moisture was higher than those reported for pea flour (11.22%) [22]. The reported moisture for kidney bean cultivars is between 5.43 to 11.81% [23], comparable to GBF moisture. The *Prosopis chilensis* showed a moisture value of 7.2%, similar to MF [24]. Regarding the fat content, no significant difference was found between the legume flours. The obtained results are according to the statement that legumes contain 1–6% lipids [25], but all of the fat values remained low, around 1%.

Although the statistical analysis showed that the ash content between GBF and MF is not significantly different, it is important to notice the high value (7.06%) of total minerals that GBF contains compared to the other flours. Even though the higher ash content increases the potential of the flour to improve mineral content in the food matrix, an ash content higher than 1% is considered to affect bread, as these molecules interfere with the functional properties of the protein [26].

There is not much information about the nutritional content of green beans. The authors reported ash values that ranged from 3–4.4% in white kidney beans [7,8]. Concerning MF, some of the most studied mesquite species are *P. alba*, *P. nigra*, *P. pallida*, *P. chilensis*, *P. cineraria*, *P. tamarugo*, and *P. juliflora* [9]. The range of mineral content reported in some *Prosopis* species is for *P. alba* 3.09% [27]; meanwhile, for *P. nigra* and *P. pallida*, the ash content is 3.31% and 2.3%, respectively [28,29]. In contrast, dehulled pea flour from different cultivars report ash averages of 2.6 to 3.6%, similar to the ash value PF [30].

Regarding protein content, the higher values were in GBF and PF. These flours contain almost double the total protein compared to MF. Recently, Aquino-Bolaños et al. [31] determined that the protein content in *P. vulgaris* green beans exists in a range of 7 to 12%, much lower than the values obtained in GBF; nonetheless, the protein values in white beans are 36.5–37.1% [7]. This value is close to the one obtained for GBF. The protein content of PF is also higher than expected. A protein content of 21.3–27.2% is reported in dehulled pea flour [30]. However, the flours from the present study were obtained including the whole pod, which may increase the protein content. In the case of PF, Mateos-Aparicio et al. [32] mentioned that the peapod contains 10% protein. Regarding *Prosopis*, the protein value range is also variable between species. In *P. africana* dehulled flour, the protein is in the range of 23 and 25.8% [33], closer to the value obtained in MF; meanwhile, in *P. alba* and *P. nigra*, the protein concentration is about 8% [34].

Despite that, the reported fiber values are higher in the pea pod (about 58%) [32]; in this case, the fiber is much lower in PF and GBF. The fiber values reported for white kidney beans are 15–24% [35]. The MF presented a higher fiber value, approximately two times higher than PF and GBF. In general, most *Prosopis* species offer high fiber content (11 to 31%) [9]. Concerning carbohydrates, GBF and MF had a higher content compared to PF. In red kidney beans, the reported amount of carbohydrates is 58.33% [36], and in common dry beans, Pitura and Arnt [37] reported 60%, which is higher than the value obtained for GBF (32.95%). Similarly, the total carbohydrates reported in different pea landraces are in a range of 38 to 47% [38], which is also higher than PF. The carbohydrates in MF (41.79%) are similar to those reported for *P. pallida* (57.6%) [39] and *P. africana* (46.12%) [40].

The PF and GBF benefits are the high protein content, but GBF has important mineral content. Although the protein content of legumes is one of the foremost studied components, in MF, the fiber content attracts attention.

Table 2. Proximal composition, mineral content, and antioxidant and functional activities of the three legume flours.

Proximal Composition (g/100 g)	PF	GBF	MF
Moisture	18.71 ± 1.35 [a] *	10.86 ± 0.05 [b]	5.97 ± 0.85 [c]
Fat	1.57 ± 0.24 [a]	1.76 ± 0.25 [a]	1.85 ± 0.38 [a]
Ash	3.44 ± 1.25 [b]	7.06 ± 0.19 [a]	5.52 ± 0.33 [a]
Total fiber	9.37 ± 3.43 [b]	6.06 ± 1.95 [b]	19.97 ± 0.11 [a]
Protein	47.5 ± 2.44 [a]	41.31 ± 2.52 [a]	24.71 ± 5.05 [b]
Carbohydrates	19.41 ± 6.09 [b]	32.95 ± 3.20 [a]	41.79 ± 5.43 [a]
Total Polyphenols (mg GA eq/g)	65.83 ± 1.17 [b]	66.34 ± 2.51 [b]	474.77 ± 31.40 [a]
Mineral content (mg/100 g flour)			
Potassium	1839.22 ± 17.04 [c]	4400.12 ± 0.99 [a]	2870.13 ± 21.39 [b]
Calcium	1180.29 ± 35.79 [b]	1880.67 ± 7.48 [a]	1132.86 ± 15.34 [b]
Magnesium	n.d.	n.d.	765.71 ± 39.56 [a]
Phosphorus	128.45 ± 2.43 [b]	223.75 ± 9.98 [a]	243.25 ± 0.80 [a]
Iron	26.34 ± 0.24 [b]	39.17 ± 0.49 [a]	23.13 ± 2.82 [b]
Antioxidant activity (mg TE/g)			
DPPH	21.12 ± 6.06 [b]	10.72 ± 1.25 [b]	204.67 ± 3.79 [a]
ABTS	9.94 ± 7.94 [b]	9.64 ± 2.73 [b]	95.86 ± 0.74 [a]
FRAP	20.01 ± 14.17 [b]	8.46 ± 1.42 [b]	1054.19 ± 64.42 [a]
Functional properties			
WAI (g/g)	4.41 ± 0.11 [b]	7.11 ± 0.13 [a]	2.28 ± 0.12 [c]
WSI (%)	73.66 ± 0.64 [b]	80.61 ± 3.53 [a]	64.87 ± 1.21 [c]
WHC (g water/g sample)	3.80 ± 0.00 [b]	5.77 ± 0.15 [a]	2.07 ± 0.12 [c]
OHC (g oil/g sample)	1.94 ± 0.20 [a]	2.52 ± 0.56 [a]	1.86 ± 0.18 [a]
OMAC (g oil/g sample)	1.60 ± 0.10 [a]	2.03 ± 0.35 [a]	1.66 ± 0.10 [a]

PF (pea flour), GBF (green bean flour), MF (mesquite flour), n.d. (not detected), WHC (water holding capacity), OHC (oil holding capacity), WAI (water absorption index), WSI (water solubility index), OMAC (organic molecule absorption capacity). * Means with a different upper letter ([a,b,c]) in the same line are significantly different at $p < 0.05$ according to the Tukey multiple range test.

3.2. Mineral Content

Through the XRF analysis, at least 47 minerals were detected from the evaluated flour samples. The more abundant minerals are presented in Table 2. In general, the flours mainly contain potassium and calcium. The third most abundant mineral was magnesium, but it was only found in MF. Other essential minerals found in the samples were sulfur, chloride, manganese, copper, and zinc.

Ca, Fe, Zn, K, Na, and Mg have been reported in pea [32]. However, neither Na nor Mg were found in PF. In *P. alba*, *P. juliflora*, *P. Africana*, and *P. pallida* a wide range of minerals are reported, mainly Ca (8–1274 ppm), Fe (5.6–450), Na (5–95 ppm), K (226–460 ppm), and traces of P and Zn [9]. In comparison, MF contains higher amounts of Mg and Fe.

GBF has significantly more Ca, K, and Fe than black bean flour (137.7, 149.12, and 6.5 mg/100 of Ca, K, and Fe) [41].

3.3. Polyphenol Profile and Antioxidant Activity

The RP-HPLC-ESI-MS analysis made it possible to identify 18 different compounds among the three flour samples (Table 3). The 3, 4-DHPEA-EA, and caffeic acid 4-O-glucoside compounds were identified in all of the flour samples. Secoisolariciresinol was only identified in PF and GBF. There are reports of quercetin, kaempferol, p-hydroxybenzoic, vanillic acid, gallic acid, ferulic acid, p-coumaric, and caffeic acid in conventional bean seeds [42]. However, quercetin and caffeic acid were only present in GBF.

Table 3. Phenolic compounds identified in the three legumes flour samples.

Sample	Retention Time (min)	Molecular Mass [M-H]$^{-1}$	Compound	Family
PF	3.727	377.1	3,4-DHPEA-EA	Tyrosols
	4.951	341.0	Caffeic acid 4-O-glucoside	Hydroxycinnamic acids
	13.681	326.1	p-Coumaroyl tyrosine	
	14.802	315.0	Protocatechuic acid 4-O-glucoside	
	16.891	365.0	Secoisolariciresinol (possibility)	Lignans
	19.521	395.1	Unknown	
	29.634	787.0	Patuletin 3-O-glucosyl-(1→6)-[apiosyl(1→2)]-glucoside	Methoxyflavonols
	34.429	933.0	Pedunculagin III	Ellagitannins
GBF	3.709	377.1	3,4-DHPEA-EA	Tyrosols
	4.520	341.0	Caffeic acid 4-O-glucoside	Hydroxycinnamic acids
	15.147	315.0	Protocatechuic acid 4-O-glucoside	
	16.605	365.0	Secoisolariciresinol (possibility)	Lignans
	25.760	378.0	Medioresinol	
	30.332	741.0	Quercetin 3-O-xylosyl-rutinoside	Flavonols
MF	3.667	377.1	3,4-DHPEA-EA	Tyrosols
	4.750	341.1	Caffeic acid 4-O-glucoside	Hydroxycinnamic acids
	15.308	255.0	Pterostilbene	Stilbenes
	19.304	337.1	3-p-Coumaroylquinic acid	Hydroxycinnamic acids
	22.135	275.1	Unknown	
	26.898	593.1	Apigenin 6,8-di-C-glucoside (Vicenin II)	Flavones
	27.844	593.1	Chrysoeriol 7-O-apiosyl-glucoside	Methoxyflavones
	29.999	563.0	Apigenin-6-C-arabinoside-8-C-glucoside (isoschaftoside)	Flavones
	31.224	328.2	Avenanthramide 2f	Methoxycinnamic acids
	35.141	623.1	Isorhamnetin 3-O-glucoside 7-O-rhamnoside	Methoxyflavonols

PF (pea flour), GBF (green bean flour), MF (mesquite flour).

MF was the sample with a variety of other compounds. Many compounds have been identified in different *Prosopis* species pods. In *P. alba* and *P. pallida*, the tentative phenolic compounds of isoschaftoside hexoside, schaftoside hexoside, vicenin II, isoschaftoside, schaftoside, vitexin, and isovitexin were identified [28]. The 1-methoxy-2-propyl acetate, methyldecylamine, hexadecanoic acid, ergosterol acetate, 2,4-dihydroxy-2,5-dimethyl-3(2H)-furan-3-one, and campesterol benzoate compounds were found in the ethanolic extract of *P. juliflora* pods [43]. Recently, Sharifi-Rad et al. [44] characterized the phenolic compounds in the species *P. farcta* through LC-ESI-QTOF-MS/MS. The *P. farcta* has many compounds, ranging from hydroxybenzoic, hydroxycinnamic, hydroxyphenyl acetic acids to flavanols, flavones, isoflavonoids, hydroxycoumarins, tyrosols, lignans, and stilbenes. In addition to vicenin II and isoschaftoside, other different compounds found in MF were pterostilbene and avenanthramide 2f. It is important to highlight that avenanthramide 2f, until now, has only been reported in oats [45].

In *P. sativum* species, the glycosylated flavonol has been described as the principal phenolic compound. Furthermore, other compounds well characterized in *P. sativum* are kaempferol, quercetin, p-coumaric, caffeic, ferulic, and cinnamic acids [46]. The hydroxycinnamic acid of p-coumaroyl tyrosine was found in the PF.

According to Table 2, the highest polyphenol content and antioxidant activity were found in MF. The value of polyphenols content could be related to the antioxidant activity itself. The GBF phenolic compound and antioxidant activity values are similar to those reported by Aquino-Bolaños [31] in green bean landraces. The quantification of total phenolics in green beans reaches 4.9–10.1 mg GA eq/g dw and 23.4 to 45.6 and 14.2 to 44.8 µmol TE/g dw of antiradical activity when using the DPPH and FRAP methods, respectively. Regarding PF, Borges-Martínez et al. [47] studied the variations in the phenolic content and antioxidant activities during pea germination. In the ungerminated pea, the total phenolic content was 584.32 mg GA eq/100 g. The antioxidant activities were 205.3 mg TE/g (DPPH) and 112.1 mg TE/g (FRAP). Both the phenolic content and the antioxidant activities were higher than those obtained in PF.

Brizzolari et al. [48] reported a total phenolic content of 15.3 mg GA eq/kg for mesquite and antioxidant activity of 115 mmol TE/kg (FRAP assay). In *P. alba* and *P. nigra* species, the total phenolic content was reported between 625–1150 mg GA eq/kg, and antioxidant activity was reported between 5.4 and 10.02 µmol TE/100 g sample (by ABTS$^\pm$) [34]. In *P. chilensis* and *P. cineraria*, the polyphenol content ranged from 0.82–2.57 g GA equivalent/100 g and 0.21–13.59 mg GA equivalent/100 g, respectively [49,50]. As these studies mention, most *Prosopis* species are known for their significant polyphenol compounds with high antioxidant activities.

3.4. Functional Activities

The effect of water absorption and retention at different process conditions is determined by the WAI (e.g., viscosity in food) [51]. Kraithong et al. [16] assessed the WAI in rice flour. The WAI of rice flour ranged between 5.44–7.14 g/g, similar to the WAI obtained in this study by GBF (7.11 g/g). The high content of carbohydrates and proteins may contribute to stronger hydrogen bonding. The WSI in GBF was also higher (80.61%), followed by PF with 73.66%; these values indicate an increased number of water-soluble components; nevertheless, high WSI presents adverse effects such as a low ability to preserve food structure. In navy and pinto bean flowers, functional activities of WAI 0.95–1.43 g/g and WSI of 12.20%, respectively [51], have been reported; these differences may be because GBF flour contains more polysaccharides (one of the hydrophilic constituents responsible of water absorption), including the whole pod. The WAI and WSI reported in the mesquite pod flours 2.53 g/g and 36.36% [52], respectively, similar to the WAI obtained in this study (2.28 g/g), but the WSI was higher (64.87%).

Water holding capacity is related to a material's ability, mainly that of proteins, to hold water against gravity; it plays a vital role in releasing the nutritional components of food [53]. Meanwhile, oil holding is associated with the fiber structure [17]. GBF was the sample with the higher WHC (5.77 g water/g sample) (Table 2); despite PF having higher protein content, the nature of the GBF proteins confers this advantage. On the other hand, in raw pinto bean flour, the values of WHC and OHC were 1.7 g water/g sample and 1.4 g oil/g sample [54]. In pea pod fibers, an OHC of 2.85 g oil/g sample and a WHC of 4.64 g water/g sample [55] have been reported. These results are specific for fiber; the interaction between other components and particle sizes affect the matrix and affect these properties [17].

In the case of the OMAC, it is related to the insoluble dietary fiber content; hence, higher OMAC values implied that the samples would have efficient interactions with fat, bile acids, cholesterol, and toxic compounds [56]. The OMAC values ranged between 1.60–2.03 g oil/g sample in the evaluated flours, and no significant differences were found among them.

3.5. Bread Characterization

Table 4 shows the obtained results of the different bread treatments. The fat results are not presented because they were not detected in any sample; this may be because of the low-fat nature of the legume flours and the whole wheat flour. In all of the treatments, the moisture content corresponds to the value of this kind of food between 38–43% [57]. No significant difference was found in ash content, but it is essential to notice that each legume added different minerals types. The bread with MF showed the best fiber parameter, and this was expected, as MF has a higher content than the other flours. Bigne et al. [58] described that the addition of *P. alba* increases the mineral and fiber content of bread.

Another significant difference between the treatments was the carbohydrate content. In this case, the control was higher in carbohydrates, and treatment 1 (with PF and GBF) had the lower content. Between the flours, WF is higher in carbohydrates (54%), and the lower content is in PF. Compared to the other bread with legume flour added, the carbohydrate content is lower. For bread with 30 g of pea flour, Millar et al. [59] reported 50.6% carbohydrate content; in bread with portions of 5 to 15% of *P. pallida* flour, Gonzales-Barron et al. [39] reported a carbohydrate content between 54 to 55%.

Regarding the protein content, the treatment with the addition of GBF and PF had higher content. It is known that the incorporation of legumes has an impact on nutritional properties and technological properties. The effect on technological properties is negative, as the low molecular weight proteins interfere in the gluten structure [26]. Hence, the obtained bread may have a lower volume or higher hardness. Samples with the three flours and the combination of PF and GBF presented lower specific volume values than the control (Figure 1); this can also be attributed to the WSI value since high values affect bread structure preservation. Millar et al. [59] described the addition of yellow pea flour into white bread; compared to the control, substituting 30% of the wheat flour with pea flour decreased the specific bread volume by 19.52%. However, in the present study, the 20% PF (treatment 5) substitution in the dough decreased the bread-specific volume by approximately 11%. In the case of the GBF addition, the specific volume decreased around 27% (treatment 6); this is comparable with the specific volume values obtained by the 15 and 25% substitution of red kidney bean in bread, where the volume decreased 30.32 and 33.47%, respectively [36]. The substitution with MF only reduced the volume by about 7%. The 15, 25, and 35 g/100 g replacement of *P. alba* in bread led to a volume reduction of 5, 7, and 28% [58].

The luminosity of any treatment was not affected in terms of the color parameters, but there are differences in a* and b*. As a* represents the color green to red and as b* represents blue to yellow, the GBF or PF treatments have differences in these parameters because of the greenish color.

Concerning the bread calories, there are no significant differences between treatments, and values are in a range of 217 to 226 kcal/100 g. These results are comparable with the calories in bread with *P. pallida* (355 kcal/100 g) [39] and wholemeal, multi cereal, rye, and oat bread that have values of 242 to 265 kcal/100 g [60].

No major differences were found amid treatments for the polyphenol and antioxidant activities. It has been reported that whole wheat grain cereals are a good source of antioxidants. Moreover, one of the advantages of sourdough is the potentiation of nutritional and functional capacities.

Despite the significant differences in the flour's functional properties, the higher WHC and OHC values correspond to the control bread. These results may be due to protein denaturation during baking or protein degradation during sourdough fermentation [61]. Contrastingly, as the OHC depends on the surface properties, this surface may change in the final product [17]. Moreover, as aguamiel is a carbohydrate source, the sugar molecules bind to water, decrease water activity, and delay the development of the gluten network [62]. The Pearson test presented important correlations between fiber and WHC ($r = -0.72$, $p = 0.0001$), fiber and OHC ($r = -0.50$, $p = 0.0085$), and WHC and OHC ($r = -0.54$, $p = 0.0035$).

Table 4. Proximal composition, antioxidant, and functional activities of sourdough loaves of bread.

	Bread Treatments							
Proximal Composition (g/100 g)	1	2	3	4	5	6	7	Control
Moisture	36.60 ± 1.61 [a*]	35.98 ± 2.05 [a]	34.31 ± 1.05 [a]	35.74 ± 2.05 [a]	34.93 ± 1.42 [a]	36.13 ± 2.46 [a]	33.25 ± 2.91 [a]	38.56 ± 1.60 [a]
Ash	3.29 ± 0.21 [a]	3.95 ± 0.75 [a]	3.33 ± 0.43 [a]	3.24 ± 0.11 [a]	3.43 ± 0.24 [a]	3.62 ± 0.25 [a]	3.81 ± 0.94 [a]	2.85 ± 0.58 [a]
Total fiber	5.18 ± 0.16 [bc]	4.42 ± 0.48 [bc]	5.40 ± 0.29 [abc]	5.63 ± 0.20 [bc]	5.18 ± 0.29 [bc]	4.24 ± 0.47 [c]	6.45 ± 0.90 [a]	2.63 ± 0.24 [d]
Protein	19.77 ± 2.70 [a]	15.35 ± 0.49 [ab]	16.05 ± 2.99 [ab]	17.40 ± 0.42 [ab]	18.02 ± 0.03 [ab]	18.45 ± 0.64 [ab]	14.56 ± 1.53 [ab]	13.13 ± 1.22 [b]
Carbohydrates	34.54 ± 0.61 [b]	40.56 ± 3.93 [ab]	41.88 ± 2.73 [ab]	37.99 ± 2.18 [ab]	37.39 ± 0.06 [ab]	35.94 ± 2.18 [ab]	40.27 ± 0.60 [ab]	43.40 ± 0.82 [a]
Caloric value (kcal/100 g)	217.24 ± 8.37 [a]	223.65 ± 17.71 [a]	231.69 ± 1.03 [a]	221.54 ± 10.38 [a]	221.64 ± 0.35 [a]	217.56 ± 6.18 [a]	219.29 ± 3.72 [a]	226.09 ± 8.17 [a]
Specific volume (cm^3/g)	1.27 ± 0.09 [b]	1.35 ± 0.05 [ab]	1.34 ± 0.15 [ab]	1.26 ± 0.05 [b]	1.47 ± 0.26 [ab]	1.21 ± 0.01 [b]	1.54 ± 0.06 [ab]	1.66 ± 0.15 [a]
Color parameters								
L*	47.28 ± 3.64 [a]	42.03 ± 4.20 [a]	40.65 ± 6.13 [a]	40.88 ± 6.14 [a]	44.97 ± 3.18 [a]	46.37 ± 0.75 [a]	39.24 ± 3.18 [a]	38.03 ± 3.49 [a]
a*	8.27 ± 0.55 [c]	8.94 ± 0.29 [abc]	8.86 ± 0.27 [abc]	8.82 ± 0.39 [abc]	8.52 ± 0.71 [bc]	7.72 ± 0.46 [c]	9.88 ± 0.70 [ab]	10.10 ± 0.50 [a]
b*	21.08 ± 0.61 [a]	19.25 ± 0.55 [ab]	18.51 ± 0.88 [abc]	19.44 ± 1.03 [ab]	20.06 ± 1.08 [a]	20.91 ± 1.39 [a]	16.89 ± 1.06 [bc]	16.48 ± 0.77 [c]
Total Polyphenols (mg GA eq/g)	392.16 ± 91.64 [a]	433.32 ± 98.87 [a]	430.71 ± 57.16 [a]	436.07 ± 34.57 [a]	401.87 ± 52.64 [a]	396.94 ± 85.04 [a]	630.57 ± 266.60 [a]	350.28 ± 59.51 [a]
Antioxidant activity (mg Trolox eq/g)								
DPPH	133.67 ± 62.43 [a]	148.67 ± 65.65 [a]	178.00 ± 18.36 [a]	172.33 ± 12.06 [a]	180.33 ± 6.43 [a]	150.67 ± 22.68 [a]	183.33 ± 15.89 [a]	176.67 ± 9.81 [a]
ABTS	91.15 ± 3.87 [a]	85.46 ± 14.72 [a]	95.13 ± 0.86 [a]	94.64 ± 0.37 [a]	93.50 ± 2.91 [a]	91.07 ± 6.59 [a]	92.24 ± 3.11 [a]	91.96 ± 3.07 [a]
FRAP	920.68 ± 190.08 [a]	923.67 ± 153.24 [a]	992.79 ± 91.13 [a]	995.95 ± 99.85 [a]	961.04 ± 198.43 [a]	908.93 ± 274.54 [a]	995.07 ± 132.92 [a]	809.24 ± 203.44 [a]
Functional properties								
WHC (g water/g sample)	1.03 ± 0.06 [d]	1.63 ± 0.15 [ab]	1.40 ± 0.20 [bc]	1.37 ± 0.12 [abc]	1.10 ± 0.10 [bc]	1.27 ± 0.12 [bc]	1.07 ± 0.12 [bc]	1.87 ± 0.12 [a]
OHC (g oil/g sample)	0.43 ± 0.02 [bc]	0.50 ± 0.05 [a]	0.32 ± 0.04 [c]	0.40 ± 0.01 [abc]	0.36 ± 0.04 [c]	0.33 ± 0.01 [bc]	0.35 ± 0.05 [c]	0.49 ± 0.05 [a]

Sample 1 (10 g PF-10 g GBF-80 g WF), 2 (10 g MF-10 g GBF-80 g WF), 3 (10 g PF-10 g MF-80 g WF), 4 (6.66 g PF-6.66 g GBF-6.66 g MF-80 g WF), 5 (20 g PF-80 g WF), 6 (20 g GBF-80 g WF), 7 (20 g MF-80 g WF), control (100 g WF-aguamiel), PF (pea flour), GBF (green bean flour), MF (mesquite flour), WF (whole-wheat flour), * Means with a different upper letter (a,b,c) in the same line are significantly different at $p < 0.05$ according to the Tukey multiple range test.

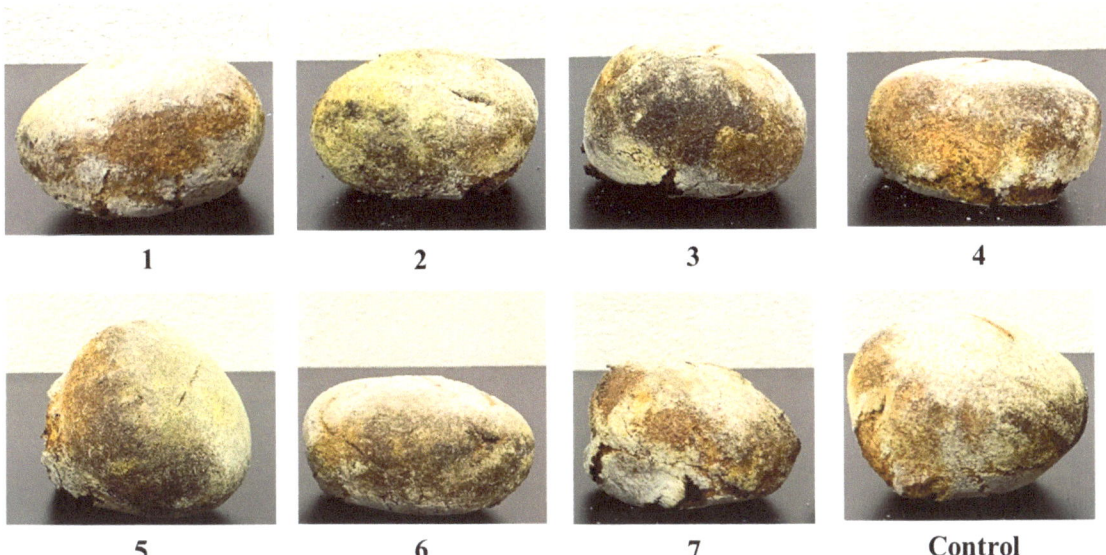

Figure 1. Visual appearance of bread treatments. Picture 1 (10 g PF-10 g GBF-80 g WF), 2 (10 g MF-10 g GBF-80 g WF), 3 (10 g PF-10 g MF-80 g WF), 4 (6.66 g PF-6.66 g GBF-6.66 g MF-80 g WF), 5 (20 g PF-80 g WF), 6 (20 g GBF-80 g WF), 7 (20 g MF-80 g WF), control (100 g WF-aguamiel), PF (pea flour), GBF (green bean flour), MF (mesquite flour), WF (whole-wheat flour).

3.6. Mathematical Model

The presented contour graphics in Figure 2 visually display the effect of the different flours on fiber, protein, carbohydrates, color parameters a* and b*, and specific volume. In the graphics, the color scale presented on the right (ranging from blue to red) goes from lower to higher values. Visually, e.g., for fiber values, a high amount of MF flour is need to increase this parameter, and a higher amount of GBF is needed to decrease fiber. To describe and define these effects, a special cubic model was the best fit for the evaluated variables. The equations of the parameters that had a major influence on the samples were fiber = $2.75 \times WF + 5.35829 \times PF + 4.21429 \times GBF + 6.07029 \times MF$ ($R^2 = 90.98$), protein = $13.13 \times WF + 18.5764 \times PF + 18.6404 \times GBF + 14.0404 \times MF$ ($R^2 = 90.90$), carbohydrates = $38.03 \times WF + 36.9605 \times PF + 35.2725 \times GBF + 44.2485 \times MF$ ($R^2 = 89.61$), a* = $9.9 \times WF + 8.46638 \times PF + 7.85838 \times GBF + 9.82238 \times MF$ ($R^2 = 95.56$), b*= $16.23 \times WF + 20.2126 \times PF + 21.1886 \times GBF + 16.9446 \times MF$ ($R^2 = 98.57$), and specific volume= $1.73 \times WF + 1.38724 \times PF + 1.18324 \times GBF + 1.47524 \times MF$ ($R^2 = 86.51$).

According to the equations, the three legume flours significantly influenced the fiber content, due to its higher value coefficient, the highest impact is due to MF. For the protein value, the significant influence is caused by GBF and PF; meanwhile, MF has a considerable effect on the carbohydrate content.

In a*, there is a synergistic effect because of the similarity in the coefficients, but in b*, the principal effects are those from the PF and GBF. As the legume flours tend to decrease volume, this parameter's positive impact comes from the WF.

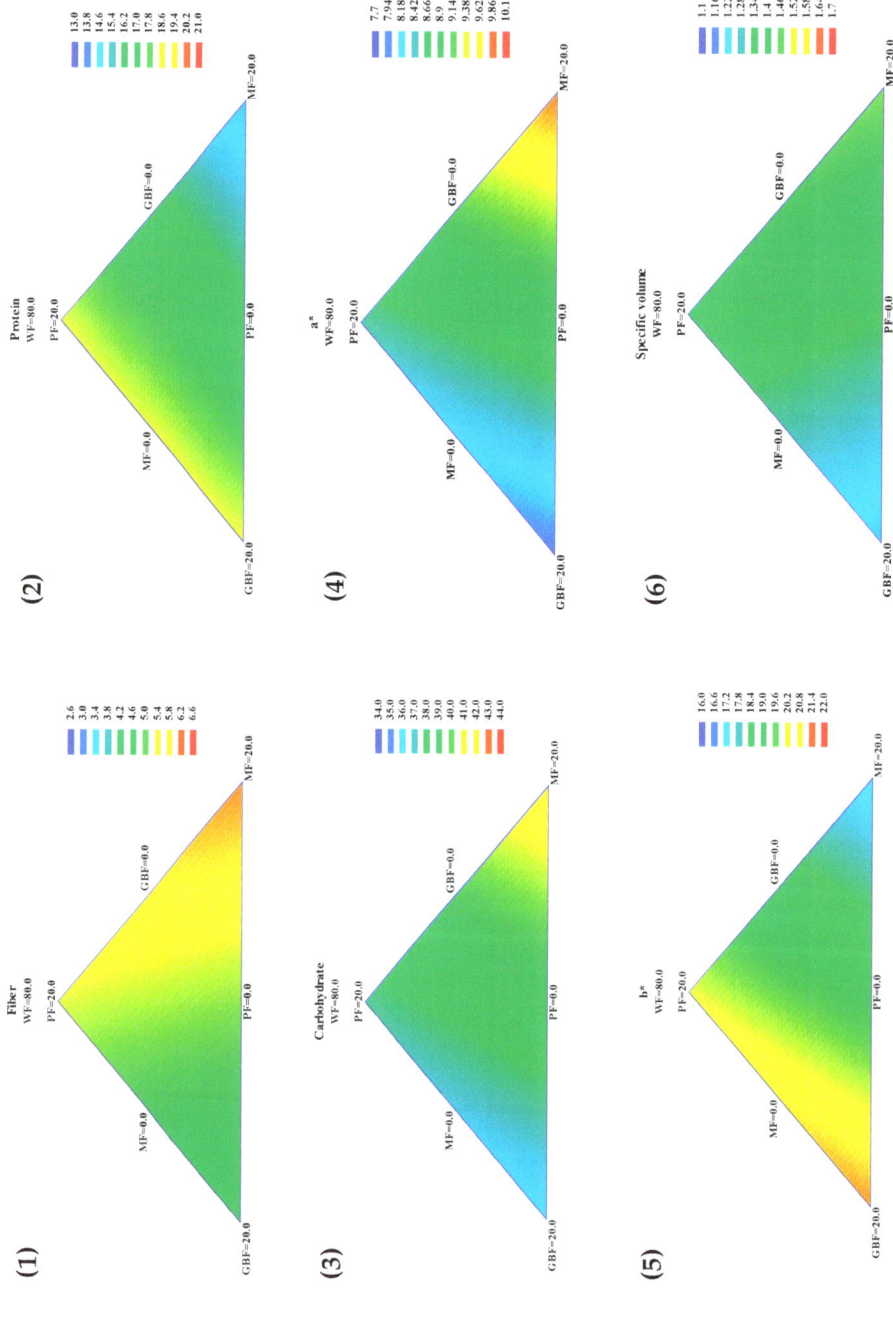

Figure 2. Ternary contour plots of effects of the addition of PF, GBF, MF, and WF on (1) Fiber, (2) Protein, (3) Carbohydrate, color parameters (4) a* and (5) b*, and (6) Specific bread volume.

4. Conclusions

The evaluated legumes presented differences in their proximal composition, mineral content, and antioxidant activities, compared to similarly reported legumes. As the legumes become more important for their nutritional value, their characterization allows whole pods or less-known species to be used.

The pea flour analyzed in this study presented higher protein content compared to other reported pea flours. Green bean flour also showed benefits compared to the red, white, and black beans, making it another option with high protein and a higher mineral content. Additionally, the mesquite flour significantly contributed to the fiber content and significant antioxidant activities. It was possible to obtain bread with a relevant fiber content and with similar color and specific volume than the control. With the obtained mathematical model and more studies of the bread matrix, it is possible to optimize bread potential.

Author Contributions: Conceptualization, J.F.S.-D., A.C.F.-G. and R.R.-H.; data curation, A.M.G.-M.; formal analysis, A.M.G.-M.; funding acquisition, A.C.F.-G. and R.R.-H.; investigation, C.M.L.-B. and J.A.A.-V.; methodology, A.M.G.-M., J.F.S.-D. and A.C.F.-G.; supervision, A.C.F.-G. and R.R.-H.; writing—original draft, A.M.G.-M.; writing—review and editing, A.M.G.-M., J.F.S.-D., A.C.F.-G., C.M.L.-B., J.A.A.-V. and R.R.-H. All authors have read and agreed to the published version of the manuscript.

Funding: This research received no external funding.

Institutional Review Board Statement: Not applicable.

Informed Consent Statement: Not applicable.

Data Availability Statement: The data presented in this study are available on request from the corresponding author. The data are not publicly available due to privacy.

Acknowledgments: This study had financial support from the Universidad Autónoma de Coahuila. González-Montemayor is grateful for receiving funding from the National Council of Science and Technology-Mexico (CONACyT) during her doctoral studies.

Conflicts of Interest: The authors declare no conflict of interest.

References

1. Martins, Z.E.; Pinho, O.; Ferreira, I.M.P.L.V.O. Food industry by-products used as functional ingredients of bakery products. *Trends Food Sci. Technol.* **2017**, *67*, 106–128. [CrossRef]
2. Hager, A.S.; Zannini, E.; Arendt, E.K. Formulating breads for specific dietary requirements. In *Breadmaking: Improving Quality*; Cauvain, S.P., Ed.; Elsevier: Amsterdam, The Netherlands, 2012; pp. 711–735.
3. Collar, C. Bread: Types of Bread. In *Encyclopedia of Food and Health*; Caballero, B., Finglas, P.M., Toldrá, F., Eds.; Elsevier Ltd.: Amsterdam, The Netherlands, 2016; pp. 500–507.
4. Sáez, G.D.; Saavedra, L.; Hebert, E.M.; Zárate, G. Identification and biotechnological characterization of lactic acid bacteria isolated from chickpea sourdough in northwestern Argentina. *LWT* **2018**, *93*, 249–256. [CrossRef]
5. Tuncel, N.B.; Yilmaz, N.; Sener, E. The effect of pea (*Pisum sativum* L.)-originated asparaginase on acrylamide formation in certain bread types. *Int. J. Food Sci. Technol.* **2010**, *45*, 2470–2476. [CrossRef]
6. Bourré, L.; McMillin, K.; Borsuk, Y.; Boyd, L.; Lagassé, S.; Sopiwnyk, E.; Jones, S.; Dick, A.; Malcolmson, L. Effect of adding fermented split yellow pea flour as a partial replacement of wheat flour in bread. *Legum. Sci.* **2019**, *1*, e2. [CrossRef]
7. Ukeyima, M.T.; Dendegh, T.A.; Isusu, S.E. Quality Characteristics of Bread Produced from Wheat and White Kidney Bean Composite Flour. *Eur. J. Nutr. Food Saf.* **2019**, *10*, 263–272. [CrossRef]
8. Hoxha, I.; Xhabiri, G.; Deliu, R. The Impact of Flour from White Bean (*Phaseolus vulgaris*) on Rheological, Qualitative and Nutritional Properties of the Bread. *Open Access Libr. J.* **2020**, *7*, 1–8. [CrossRef]
9. González-Montemayor, A.M.; Flores-Gallegos, A.C.; Contreras-Esquivel, J.C.; Solanilla-Duque, J.F.; Rodríguez-Herrera, R. *Prosopis* spp. functional activities and its applications in bakery products. *Trends Food Sci. Technol.* **2019**, *94*, 12–19. [CrossRef]
10. Galli, V.; Venturi, M.; Pini, N.; Guerrini, S.; Granchi, L.; Vincenzini, M. Liquid and firm sourdough fermentation: Microbial robustness and interactions during consecutive backsloppings. *LWT* **2019**, *105*, 9–15. [CrossRef]
11. *Official Methods of Analysis AOAC Intternational*; AOAC: Rockville, MD, USA, 2000.
12. Chen, D.; Shi, J.; Hu, X.; Du, S. Alpha-amylase treatment increases extractable phenolics and antioxidant capacity of oat (*Avena nuda* L.) flour. *J. Cereal Sci.* **2015**, *65*, 60–66. [CrossRef]

13. Hernández-Hernández, C.; Aguilar, C.N.; Flores-Gallegos, A.C.; Sepúlveda, L.; Rodríguez-Herrera, R.; Morlett-Chávez, J.; Govea-Salas, M.; Ascacio-Valdés, J. Preliminary testing of ultrasound/microwave-assisted extraction (U/M-AE) for the isolation of Geraniin from *Nephelium lappaceum* L. (Mexican Variety) peel. *Processes* **2020**, *8*, 572. [CrossRef]
14. Molyneux, P. The Use of the Stable Free Radical Diphenylpicryl-hydrazyl (DPPH) for Estimating Antioxidant Activity. *Songklanakarin J. Sci. Technol.* **2004**, *26*, 211–219. [CrossRef]
15. Opitz, S.E.W.; Smrke, S.; Goodman, B.A.; Yeretzian, C. Methodology for the measurement of antioxidant capacity of coffee: A validated platform composed of three complementary antioxidant assays. In *Processing and Impact on Antioxidants in Beverages*; Preedy, V., Ed.; Elsevier: Amsterdam, The Netherlands, 2014; pp. 253–264.
16. Kraithong, S.; Lee, S.; Rawdkuen, S. Physicochemical and functional properties of Thai organic rice flour. *J. Cereal Sci.* **2018**, *79*, 259–266. [CrossRef]
17. Escobedo-García, S.; Salas-Tovar, J.A.; Flores-Gallegos, A.C.; Contreras-Esquivel, J.C.; González-Montemayor, A.M. Functionality of *Agave* Bagasse as Supplement for the Development of Prebiotics-Enriched Foods. *Plant. Foods Hum. Nutr.* **2019**, *75*, 96–102. [CrossRef] [PubMed]
18. Lira, A.Q.; Alvarado-Resendiz, M.G.; Simental, S.S.; Martini, J.P.; Reyes-Santamaria, M.I.; Guemes-Vera, N. Use of *Lactobacillus* from Pulque in Sourdough. *Adv. Microbiol.* **2014**, *4*, 969–977. [CrossRef]
19. Villarreal Morales, S.L.; Muñiz Márquez, D.B.; Michel Michel, M.; González Montemayor, A.M.; Escobedo García, S.; Salas Tovar, J.A.; Flores Gallegos, A.C.; Rodríguez Herrera, R. Aguamiel a fresh beverage from *Agave* spp. sap with functional properties. In *Natural Beverages*; Grumezescu, A.M., Holban, A.M., Eds.; Woodhead Publishing: Sawston, UK, 2019; pp. 179–208.
20. AACC International Approved methods of analysis. In *Approved Methods of Analysis*, 11th ed.; AACC International: Saint Paul, MN, USA, 2010.
21. Purić, M.; Rabrenović, B.; Rac, V.; Pezo, L.; Tomašević, I.; Demin, M. Application of defatted apple seed cakes as a by-product for the enrichment of wheat bread. *LWT* **2020**, *130*, 109391. [CrossRef]
22. Saldanha do Carmo, C.; Silventoinen, P.; Nordgård, C.T.; Poudroux, C.; Dessev, T.; Zobel, H.; Holtekjølen, A.K.; Draget, K.I.; Holopainen-Mantila, U.; Knutsen, S.H.; et al. Is dehulling of peas and faba beans necessary prior to dry fractionation for the production of protein-and starch-rich fractions? Impact on physical properties, chemical composition and techno-functional properties. *J. Food Eng.* **2020**, *278*, 109937. [CrossRef]
23. Kan, L.; Nie, S.; Hu, J.; Wang, S.; Cui, S.W.; Li, Y.; Xu, S.; Wu, Y.; Wang, J.; Bai, Z.; et al. Nutrients, phytochemicals and antioxidant activities of 26 kidney bean cultivars. *Food Chem. Toxicol.* **2017**, *108*, 467–477. [CrossRef] [PubMed]
24. Conforti, P.A.; Patrignani, M. Increase in the antioxidant content in biscuits by infusions or *Prosopis chilensis* pod flour. *Open Agric.* **2021**, *6*, 243–253. [CrossRef]
25. Michaels, T.E. Grain Legumes and Their Dietary Impact: Overview. In *Encyclopedia of Food Grains*; Wrigley, C., Corke, H., Seetharaman, K., Faubion, J., Eds.; Academic Press Limited: Cambridge, MA, USA, 2016; Volume 1–4, pp. 265–273.
26. Millar, K.A.; Gallagher, E.; Burke, R.; Mccarthy, S.; Barry-ryan, C. Proximate composition and anti-nutritional factors of fava-bean (*Vicia faba*), green-pea and yellow-pea (*Pisum sativum*) flour. *J. Food Compos. Anal.* **2019**, *82*, 103233. [CrossRef]
27. Sciammaro, L.P.; Ferrero, C.; Puppo, C. Physicochemical and nutritional characterization of sweet snacks formulated with *Prosopis alba* flour. *LWT* **2018**, *93*, 24–31. [CrossRef]
28. Gonzales-Barron, U.; Dijkshoorn, R.; Maloncy, M.; Finimundy, T.; Calhelha, R.C.; Pereira, C.; Stojković, D.; Soković, M.; Ferreira, I.C.F.R.; Barros, L.; et al. Nutritive and bioactive properties of mesquite (*Prosopis pallida*) flour and its technological performance in breadmaking. *Foods* **2020**, *9*, 597. [CrossRef] [PubMed]
29. Romano, N.; Sciammaro, L.; Mobili, P.; Puppo, M.C.; Gomez-Zavaglia, A. Flour from mature *Prosopis nigra* pods as suitable substrate for the synthesis of prebiotic fructo-oligosaccharides and stabilization of dehydrated *Lactobacillus delbrueckii* subsp. bulgaricus. *Food Res. Int.* **2019**, *121*, 561–567. [CrossRef] [PubMed]
30. Arteaga, V.G.; Kraus, S.; Schott, M.; Muranyi, I.; Schweiggert-Weisz, U.; Eisner, P. Screening of twelve pea (*Pisum sativum* L.) cultivars and their isolates focusing on the protein characterization, functionality, and sensory profiles. *Foods* **2021**, *10*, 758. [CrossRef] [PubMed]
31. Aquino-Bolaños, E.N.; Garzón-García, A.K.; Alba-Jiménez, J.E.; Chávez-Servia, J.L.; Vera-Guzmán, A.M.; Carrillo-Rodríguez, J.C.; Santos-Basurto, M.A. Physicochemical Characterization and Functional Potential of *Phaseolus vulgaris* L. and *Phaseolus coccineus* L. Landrace green beans. *Agronomy* **2021**, *11*, 803. [CrossRef]
32. Mateos-Aparicio, I.; Redondo-Cuenca, A.; Villanueva-Suárez, M.J.; Zapata-Revilla, M.A.; Tenorio-Sanz, M.D. Pea pod, broad bean pod and okara, potential sources of functional compounds. *LWT* **2010**, *43*, 1467–1470. [CrossRef]
33. Falade, K.O.; Akeem, S.A. Protein quality of dehulled-defatted African mesquite bean (*Prosopis africana*) flour and protein isolates. *J. Food Meas. Charact.* **2020**, *14*, 3426–3433. [CrossRef]
34. Sciammaro, L.P.; Quintero Ruiz, N.A.; Ferrero, C.; Giacomino, S.; Picariello, G.; Mamone, G.; Puppo, M.C. *Prosopis* spp. powder: Influence of chemical components in water adsorption properties. *Int. J. Food Sci. Technol.* **2021**, *56*, 278–286. [CrossRef]
35. Veber, A.; Zareba, D.; Ziarno, M. Functional fermented beverage prepares from germinated white kidney beans (*Phaseolus vulgaris* L.). In *Milk Substitutes-Selected Aspects*; Ziarno, M., Ed.; IntechOpen: London, UK, 2021; pp. 3–22.
36. Manonmani, D.; Bhol, S.; Bosco, S.J.D. Effect of Red Kidney Bean (*Phaseolus vulgaris* L.) Flour on Bread Quality. *Open Access Libr. J.* **2014**, *3*, 1–6. [CrossRef]

37. Pitura, K.; Arnt, S.D. Characteristics of flavonol glycosides in bean (*Phaseolus vulgaris* L.) seed coats. *Food Chem.* **2019**, *272*, 26–32. [CrossRef]
38. Gebreegziabher, B.G.; Tsegay, B.A. Proximate and mineral composition of Ethiopian pea (*Pisum sativum* var. *abyssinicum* A. Braun) landraces vary across altitudinal ecosystems. *Cogent Food Agric.* **2020**, *6*, 1789421. [CrossRef]
39. Gonzales-Barron, U.; Dijkshoorn, R.; Maloncy, M.; Finimundy, T.; Carocho, M.; Ferreira, I.C.F.R.; Barros, L.; Cadavez, V. Nutritional quality and staling of wheat bread partially replaced with Peruvian mesquite (*Prosopis pallida*) flour. *Food Res. Int.* **2020**, *137*, 109621. [CrossRef]
40. Anhwange, B.; Kyenge, B.; Kukwa, R.; Ishwa, B. Chemical Analysis of *Prosopis africana* (Guill &Perr.) Seeds. *Niger. Ann. Pure Appl. Sci.* **2020**, *3*, 129–140. [CrossRef]
41. Santiago-Ramos, D.; de Dios Figueroa-Cárdenas, J.; Véles-Medina, J.J.; Salazar, R. Physicochemical properties of nixtamalized black bean (*Phaseolus vulgaris* L.) flours. *Food Chem.* **2018**, *240*, 456–462. [CrossRef]
42. Rodríguez Madrera, R.; Campa Negrillo, A.; Suárez Valles, B.; Ferreira Fernández, J.J. Phenolic content and antioxidant activity in seeds of common bean (*Phaseolus vulgaris* L.). *Foods* **2021**, *10*, 864. [CrossRef] [PubMed]
43. Malik, S.K.; Ahmed, M.; Khan, F. Identification of novel anticancer terpenoids from *Prosopis juliflora* (Sw) DC (Leguminosae) pods. *Trop. J. Pharm. Res.* **2018**, *17*, 661–668. [CrossRef]
44. Sharifi-Rad, J.; Zhong, J.; Ayatollahi, S.A.; Kobarfard, F.; Faizi, M.; Khosravi-Dehaghi, N.; Suleria, H.A.R. LC-ESI-QTOF-MS/MS characterization of phenolic compounds from *Prosopis farcta* (Banks & Sol.) J.F.Macbr. And their potential antioxidant activities. *Cell. Mol. Biol.* **2021**, *67*, 189–200. [CrossRef]
45. Schendel, R.R. Phenol content in sprouted grains. In *Sprouted Grains*; Feng, H., Nemzer, B., DeVries, J.W., Eds.; Elsevier Inc.: Amsterdam, The Netherlands, 2019; pp. 247–316.
46. Fahim, J.R.; Attia, E.Z.; Kamel, M.S. The phenolic profile of pea (*Pisum sativum*): A phytochemical and pharmacological overview. *Phytochem. Rev.* **2019**, *18*, 173–198. [CrossRef]
47. Borges-Martínez, E.; Gallardo-Velázquez, T.; Cardador-Martínez, A.; Moguel-Concha, D.; Osorio-Revilla, G.; Ruiz-Ruiz, J.C.; Martínez, C.J. Phenolic compounds profile and antioxidant activity of pea (*Pisum sativum* L.) and black bean (*Phaseolus vulgaris* L.) sprouts. *Food Sci. Technol.* **2021**, *2061*, 1–7. [CrossRef]
48. Brizzolari, A.; Brandolini, A.; Glorio-Paulet, P.; Hidalgo, A. Antioxidant capacity and heat damage of powder products from South American plants with functional properties. *Ital. J. Food Sci.* **2019**, *31*, 731–748. [CrossRef]
49. Schmeda-Hirschmann, G.; Quispe, C.; Soriano, M.D.P.C.; Theodoluz, C.; Jiménez-Aspée, F.; Pérez, M.J.; Cuello, A.S.; Isla, M.I. Chilean *Prosopis* Mesocarp Flour: Phenolic Profiling and Antioxidant Activity. *Molecules* **2015**, *20*, 7017–7033. [CrossRef] [PubMed]
50. Kumar, M.; Govindasamy, P.; Nyola, N.K. In-vitro and in-vivo Anti-Hyperglycemic Potential of *Prosopis cineraria* Pods Extract and Fractions. *J. Biol. Act. Prod. Nat.* **2019**, *9*, 135–140. [CrossRef]
51. Siddiq, M.; Kelkar, S.; Harte, J.B.; Dolan, K.D.; Nyombaire, G. Functional properties of flour from low-temperature extruded navy and pinto beans (*Phaseolus vulgaris* L.). *LWT* **2013**, *50*, 215–219. [CrossRef]
52. De La Rosa, A.P.; Frias-Hernández, J.T.; Olalde-Portugal, V.; González Castañeda, J. Processing, Nutritional Evaluation, and Utilization of Whole Mesquite Flour (*Prosopis laevigata*). *J. Food Sci.* **2006**, *71*, 315–320. [CrossRef]
53. Wu, C.; Ma, W.; Chen, Y.; Navicha, W.B.; Wu, D.; Du, M. The water holding capacity and storage modulus of chemical cross-linked soy protein gels directly related to aggregates size. *LWT* **2019**, *103*, 125–130. [CrossRef]
54. Lin, T.; Fernández-Fraguas, C. Effect of thermal and high-pressure processing on the thermo-rheological and functional properties of common bean (*Phaseolus vulgaris* L.) flours. *LWT* **2020**, *127*, 109325. [CrossRef]
55. Belghith Fendri, L.; Chaari, F.; Maaloul, M.; Kallel, F.; Abdelkafi, L.; Ellouz Chaabouni, S.; Ghribi-Aydi, D. Wheat bread enrichment by pea and broad bean pods fibers: Effect on dough rheology and bread quality. *LWT* **2016**, *73*, 584–591. [CrossRef]
56. Nyam, K.L.; Lau, M.; Tan, C.P. Fibre from pumpkin (*Cucurbita pepo* L.) Seeds and rinds: Physico-chemical properties, antioxidant capacity and application as bakery product ingredients. *Malays. J. Nutr.* **2013**, *19*, 99–110.
57. Rubel, I.A.; Pérez, E.E.; Manrique, G.D.; Genovese, D.B. Fibre enrichment of wheat bread with Jerusalem artichoke inulin: Effect on dough rheology and bread quality. *Food Struct.* **2014**, *3*, 21–29. [CrossRef]
58. Bigne, F.; Puppo, M.C.; Ferrero, C. Fibre enrichment of wheat flour with mesquite (*Prosopis* spp.): Effect on breadmaking performance and staling. *LWT* **2016**, *65*, 1008–1016. [CrossRef]
59. Millar, K.A.; Barry-Ryan, C.; Burke, R.; McCarthy, S.; Gallagher, E. Dough properties and baking characteristics of white bread, as affected by addition of raw, germinated and toasted pea flour. *Innov. Food Sci. Emerg. Technol.* **2019**, *56*, 102189. [CrossRef]
60. Carocho, M.; Morales, P.; Ciudad-Mulero, M.; Fernández-Ruiz, V.; Ferreira, E.; Heleno, S.; Rodrigues, P.; Barros, L.; Ferreira, I.C.F.R. Comparison of different bread types: Chemical and physical parameters. *Food Chem.* **2020**, *310*, 125954. [CrossRef] [PubMed]
61. Coda, R.; Varis, J.; Verni, M.; Rizzello, C.G.; Katina, K. Improvement of the protein quality of wheat bread through faba bean sourdough addition. *LWT* **2017**, *82*, 296–302. [CrossRef]
62. Sahin, A.W.; Zannini, E.; Coffey, A.; Arendt, E.K. Sugar reduction in bakery products: Current strategies and sourdough technology as a potential novel approach. *Food Res. Int.* **2019**, *126*, 108583. [CrossRef] [PubMed]

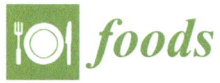 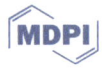

Review

Impact of Non-Thermal Technologies on the Quality of Nuts: A Review

Paola Sánchez-Bravo [1,2], Luis Noguera-Artiaga [2], Vicente M. Gómez-López [3], Ángel A. Carbonell-Barrachina [2], José A. Gabaldón [3] and Antonio J. Pérez-López [4,*]

[1] Laboratory of Fitoquímica y Alimentos Saludables (LabFAS), CEBAS-CSIC, University of Murcia, 25, 30100 Murcia, Spain
[2] Department of AgroFood Technology, Miguel Hernandez University, Carretera de Beniel, km 3.2, 03312 Orihuela, Spain
[3] Catedra Alimentos Para la Salud, Campus de los Jerónimos, Universidad Católica San Antonio de Murcia (UCAM), 30107 Murcia, Spain
[4] Department of Food Technology and Nutrition, Catholic University of San Antonio, Campus de los Jerónimos s/n, 30107 Murcia, Spain
* Correspondence: ajperez@ucam.edu; Tel.: +34-968-278-622

Abstract: Nuts are widely consumed worldwide, mainly due to their characteristic flavor and texture, ease of consumption, and their functional properties. In addition, consumers increasingly demand natural or slightly processed foods with high quality. Consequently, non-thermal treatments are a viable alternative to thermal treatments used to guarantee safety and long shelf life, which produce undesirable changes that affect the sensory quality of nuts. Non-thermal treatments can achieve results similar to those of the traditional (thermal) ones in terms of food safety, while ensuring minimal loss of bioactive compounds and sensory properties, thus obtaining a product as similar as possible to the fresh one. This article focuses on a review of the main non-thermal treatments currently available for nuts (cold plasma, high pressure, irradiation, pulsed electric field, pulsed light, ultrasound and ultraviolet light) in relation to their effects on the quality and safety of nuts. All the treatments studied have shown promise with regard to the inhibition of the main microorganisms affecting nuts (e.g., *Aspergillus*, *Salmonella*, and *E. coli*). Furthermore, by optimizing the treatment, it is possible to maintain the organoleptic and functional properties of these products.

Keywords: almond; cold plasma; high pressure; irradiation; mycotoxin; pistachio; pulsed electric field; pulsed light; ultrasound; ultraviolet light

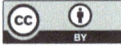

1. Introduction

Nuts are widely consumed worldwide due to their high content of nutrients and bioactive compounds [1]. They can be consumed in different forms and formats, as an appetizer (fresh or toasted), as ingredients (dishes, desserts, ice creams, commercial products, etc.) or as oils [1,2]. Among the great variety of existing dried fruits, the most popular are almonds (*Prunus amigdalis*), hazelnuts (*Corylus avellana*), walnuts (*Juglans regia*) and pistachios (*Pistachia vera*), as well as peanuts (*Arachis hypogea*), which although they are botanically legumes, they are commonly included in the group of dried fruits [2].

Currently, the consumption of nuts is associated with cardioprotective activities (cardiovascular or coronary diseases) and the modulation of other diseases such as cancer [1,3,4]. These activities are mainly due to macronutrients, micronutrients, and other bioactive compounds (proteins, lipid profile, dietary fiber, vitamins, minerals, etc.) that can favorably influence cardiometabolic pathways [2].

However, the consumption of nuts is not risk-free. One of the main risks of consuming nuts is the ingestion of mycotoxin-producing fungi (*Aspergillus flavus*, *Aspergillus parasiticus* and *Aspergillus nonius*, mainly), especially aflatoxins [5]. Aflatoxins cause one of the main risks in agriculture and industry [5,6]. They are carcinogenic, mutagenic, teratogenic, and have immunotoxic properties [7–9]. This fungal contamination not only affects human health but also represents an important economic loss in the food industry [8,10,11].

In addition to fungi, there are other microorganisms that can cause alterations in nuts and affect consumers' health. A clear example is almonds, linked to outbreaks caused by Salmonella in the USA and Canada [12,13]. In addition, similar cases of salmonellosis [14–16] and contamination by *Escherichia coli* [17] have been reported in walnuts.

Currently, most of the processes carried out to control these pathogens are based on heat treatments, and most of the consumed foods are subjected to this type of treatment to ensure their safety and extend their shelf life [18]. In nuts, roasting (in oil or air-oven), pasteurization or blanching are the most used heat treatments [19]. However, although these heat treatments are effective in eliminating the microorganisms present in dried fruits, they entails a loss of sensory and nutritional quality [20,21].

On the other hand, consumers today tend towards natural or minimally processed foods, so there is a need to implement alternative methods to heat treatments for food preservation, improving or at least maintaining the nutritional and sensory quality of the processed products [18]. These new technologies have some advantages over heat treatments, such as the use of low temperatures (20–25 °C), which reduces organoleptic losses in foods due to heat treatments [22].

Therefore, this review aims to establish the advantages and limitations of alternatives to thermal processing (e.g., ultraviolet light, plasma treatments, ultrasound, electrical pulses, etc.) used to obtain safe products while preserving their nutritional and sensory quality.

2. Non-Thermal Treatments

2.1. Ultraviolet Light

UV-C involves the use of light in the spectra range from 200 to 280 nm. Microbial inactivation is caused by the absorption of photons with enough energy to promote a photochemical reaction, resulting in the formation of pyrimidine dimers in the microbial DNA, which impairs cell replication [23].

As mentioned before, UV treatment has increased due to its low cost and easy use in controlling pathogens. However, the inactivation capacity of this technique depends largely on the characteristics of the fruit, such as color or transparency [24], but also the exposure time, microbial species and wavelength [25,26]. In general, the longer the fruit is exposed to UV light and the higher the intensity, the greater the reduction of mycotoxins. In this sense, it has been shown that exposure to ultraviolet-C light in walnuts for 45 min reduced the microbial population of aflatoxin-producing fungi by 4.2 logs, while shorter times (15 and 30 min) reduced contamination by these microorganisms to a lesser extent (1.2 and 3.2 logs, respectively) [27].

In this regard, AFB1 has been shown to be more sensitive to UV radiation at a wavelength of 362 nm due to chemical structural modifications in the terminal furan ring [28]. In peanuts, treatment with ultraviolet radiation (UV-C) at 1080–8370 mJ/cm^2 showed a reduction of 3.1 log CFU/g of *A. flavous* and a reduction of aflatoxin B1 from 14 to 51% [5]. In addition, intensities of 800 µW/cm^2 have proven to be effective in peanuts, where 100% of aflatoxin B1 (AFB1) was inactivated with an exposure of 80 min; lower intensities (200 µW/cm^2) with the same exposure time have presented positive results (approx. 95%) in the inactivation of AFB1 [29]. In pistachios, UV radiation (87.5 µW/cm^2) decreased the AFB1 content by only 22% after 3 h of exposure and after 13 h, 58% inactivation was achieved [30].

Furthermore, it has been established that 15 min of irradiation with UV at 265 nm was sufficient to completely degrade AFB2 and AFG2 and 45 min was sufficient to obtain a degradation percentage of 96.5 and 100% of AFB1 and AFG1, respectively, in peanuts, walnuts and pistachios after 12 weeks of storage [27]. Babaee et al. [31] also showed that UV-C treatments (12 µw/cm) reduce the aflatoxin amount in pistachios, especially AFB2 and AFG2, without reducing total fat content, protein content, total phenolic compounds or carbohydrates. Likewise, in peanuts, an inactivation close to 100% was achieved after 10 h of exposure at 254 nm [32], and as Babaee, et al. reported [31], without affected the physico-chemical and sensory quality of samples.

Aflatoxin inactivation can also be carried out in nut-based products. For example, in peanut oil, UV radiation under an intensity of 800 mW/cm^2 for 30 min produced a degradation of AFB1 [33], and UV treatments at 365 nm during 30 min degraded ~96% of AFB1 [26].

UV light treatments have been shown to be effective in inactivating other microorganisms, such as bacteria (*Salmonella* spp., *Escherichia coli* spp., *Listeria* spp., *Yersinia* spp., *Staphylococcus* spp., etc.) [34–36]. In shelled walnuts, pulsed UV light at 5, 8 and 13 cm (distances from the quartz window) for 1 to 45 s presented a reduction of *Salmonella enteritidi*, with a maximum reduction of 3.18 log cfu/g at 8 cm during 45 s [37]. Likewise, in peanuts and almonds, a reduction of *Salmonella typhimurium* was observed by applying UV-C irradiation of 10 mW/cm^2 for 10–30 min [38].

These results are especially important because UV treatments not only offer an inactivation of pathogenic microorganisms but also do not cause significant changes in the physical and sensory quality of the fruits [5,39].

2.2. Pulsed Electric Field

Pulsed electric field (PEF) treatment consists of the application of repetitive electric field pulses, generally of high intensity (1–40 kV/cm) for a short duration (µs) and a relatively low energy input to a food placed in direct contact with the electrodes. Its main effect on microorganisms is the permeabilization of the cell membranes [40].

PEF is a non-thermal treatment on which much research has been carried out over the last few years, mainly due to its high capacity for being used to extract beneficial components from industry by-products, such as pressing, drying or osmosis itself. It also reduces the detrimental effects arising from conventional heat treatments. This promising PEF technology is an interesting alternative to other classical methods used, such as cooking or microwaving, it has been tested for the separation, stabilization and dehydration of important compounds without affecting their nutritional properties. In addition to improving the extraction processes and energy costs, with this non-thermal technology, it has been seen that stress can be induced in plant cells, thus stimulating the biosynthesis of bioactive components without causing an environmental impact during their extraction [41,42].

The use of this treatment has been applied in food groups such as fruits, vegetables and nuts due to their high nutritional and antioxidant value, linked to their rich composition of proteins, enzymes, phenols, anthocyanins and carotenoids [43–47].

It has been seen that the use of combined treatments, pulsed electric field (PEF) and ultrasound (US) in the evaluation of bioactive compounds in products such as almonds, gave positive results, leading to the highest contents of phenolic compounds and/or flavonoids [48].

There are no data on nut aromas, although the positive effect of this treatment on the extraction of aroma in plants or the preservation of these aromas in food processing, fruits juices and vegetables has been demonstrated. These changes could be possible due to the fact that PEF induces cell permeabilization, facilitating enzyme-substrate reactions after the treatment [49–54].

2.3. Pulsed Light

Pulsed light (PL) is a non-thermal technology initially developed to decontaminate foods by killing microorganisms using pulses of a high-power broad-spectrum light, with the UV-C part being the most lethal [55]. PL can heat samples; however, this is a side effect that should be avoided rather than a pursued effect.

The characterization of PL treatments is usually reported in terms of fluence (J/cm^2), which is the amount of energy imposed on the sample surface divided by the illuminated area of the sample; a more exact definition can be found from Braslavsky [56]. However, this parameter is not always reported, which makes comparison of research findings difficult as has been discussed before [57].

Research about the use of PL in nuts has had three different goals: (i) foodborne pathogen inactivation, (ii) reduction of allergenicity, and (iii) degradation of aflatoxins. Therefore, the potential consequences of PL treatment on the quality of nuts have been studied in the framework of the treatment conditions required to achieve one of these three goals.

In shelled walnuts, the inactivation of *Salmonella* requires 41.2 J/cm^2 to attain a 3.2 log reduction. Under these conditions, no statistical significant changes ($p > 0.05$) in color parameters (L^*, a^* and b^*) nor in lipid oxidation measured by the malondialdehyde (MDA) method were observed [58]. A deeper study about the effect of subjecting shelled walnuts to a fluence of 41.2 J/cm^2 on their quality [59] showed that PL indeed caused quality changes in shelled walnut, but these were mild. PL had no statistically significant ($p > 0.05$) effects on lipid oxidation markers, such as concentration of thiobarbituric acid reactive substances (TBARS) and peroxide value, which is consistent with the absence of rancidity perception reported by a trained sensory panel [58]. Nonetheless, PL significantly ($p < 0.05$) increased the concentration of volatile compounds associated with green/herbaceous odors (e.g., 1-hexanol and hexanal) and decreased compounds related to fruity notes (methyl hexanoate) and citrus odors (D-limonene and nonanal) as determined by gas chromatography/mass spectrometry. A descriptive sensory analysis has shown that the descriptors walnut odor and flavor, nut overall taste and aftertaste received statistically significantly ($p < 0.05$) higher scores; the descriptors sweet and woody odor received lower scores, while 16 other traits such as all those related to color, texture, and rancidity were unaffected. Complementarily, the antioxidant activity and total phenol concentration were not significantly affected ($p > 0.05$) by the PL treatment.

In almond kernels, PL has been successfully applied for reduction of the allergenicity of almond protein extracts [60] but requires an estimate of over 150 J/cm^2, which greatly exceeds the 12 J/cm^2 maximum allowed by the FDA (1996). This fact, together with the high temperature reached (115 °C), the 58.5% water loss and the circumstance that the efficacy of PL is lower in solid matrixes than in liquid ones led to the conclusion that PL was not appropriate for the treatment of almonds due to its low effectiveness and significant negative impact on almond quality. When used to inactivate *Salmonella enteritidis*, Oner [61] reported a 4.1 log reduction and Harguindeguy and Gómez-Camacho [62] reported a 6 log reduction after application of <50 J/cm^2, but no effects on almond quality were studied. Finally, Liu et al. [63] used a 1 min immersion in water as a previous step before subjecting almonds to PL to avoid the detrimental effect of excessive heating on dried almonds observed in their preliminary tests. The dipping of almonds in water followed by a PL treatment for 18 min achieved at least a 5 log reduction of *Salmonella*. The treatment slightly affected almond color, as measured instrumentally, but did not significantly increase the lipid oxidation measured by different methods (peroxide value, total acid number, conjugated diene and TBARS), even after storage at 39 °C for 11 d. Furthermore, no significant effect of the treatment on the appearance and color of almonds was visually observed.

In peanuts, PL has been tested to decrease allergenicity and aflatoxin decontamination. The allergenicity of whole kernels was decreased by PL but required fluences >1600 J/cm^2; the effects of this extreme treatment condition on peanut quality were not reported [64]. PL has also been proven to be able to decrease aflatoxin B1 and B2 concentrations in peanuts with and without skin. No significant ($p < 0.05$) effects were observed when applying >1000 J/cm^2 in the oil quality indicators (free fatty acid, peroxide value and acidity value) but oil color was affected [65]. A study combining the use of citric acid and PL also decreased aflatoxin B1 and B2 concentrations while affecting peanut color; however, no study of oil quality was undertaken in this case [66].

In general, PL causes mild effects on the quality of nut oils. This is striking since the combination of low water activity, the presence of oxygen and UV light favors the oxidation of unsaturated fatty acids, which are abundant in nuts. The detection of changes in oil quality may require a deeper study beyond the classical oil quality indicators because gas chromatography/mass spectrometry and descriptive sensory analysis have revealed changes are not detected by conventional oil oxidation methods. Color is a quality parameter slightly affected in PL-treated nuts. While PL seemed effective for foodborne pathogenic bacteria inactivation, with only mild quality changes, other applications such as allergenicity abatement and aflatoxin degradation require treatment conditions that negatively affect nut quality.

2.4. Ultrasound and High Pressure

Power ultrasound is a part of the sound spectrum ranging from 20 kHz to 1 MHz. Its main inactivation mechanism is acoustic cavitation, which is the formation, growth and implosion of microbubbles within a surrounding medium due to pressure fluctuations induced by ultrasonic waves [40].

For the preservation and quality control of food, this ultrasonic treatment is one of the most investigated, mainly with the objective of reducing the microbial load and inhibiting enzymatic activity, without causing physical–chemical or nutritional changes in food. In addition, this technology usually eliminates microorganisms at levels lower that those reached by thermal treatments and comparable to those reached by current sterilization methods and pasteurization or high pressure [67,68].

It is also used to emulsify oils, sauces and fruit juices and to encapsulate aromas, as this method requires less energy, is economically much more beneficial and improves the efficiency of industrial food processing, including reducing waste and by-products [69–72].

Regarding the effects of this treatment on the nut aromatic profiles, it has not been investigated to date, although research has been carried out in which sensory improvements in parameters such as aroma and flavor in peanuts were observed [73].

A study in which combined pulsed electric field and ultrasound methods were used suggested an improvement in color and a possible stability of volatile compounds in an almond extract [48].

High pressure processing (HPP) is a technology that uses pressures between 100 and 1000 MPa to treat foods submerged in water and packed in a suitable material. The microbial inactivation by HHP is a complex event related to disturbed cell structure organization and metabolism, including, for instance, cell membrane rupture [74].

Most of the research that has been carried out on the application of high pressures has been directed towards the juice industry and other non-alcoholic beverages [75]. For example, in coconut water, a treatment at 593 MPa for 3 min was effective against *E. coli, Salmonella* and *L. monocytogenes* and led to a pleasant sensory profile, similar to that of untreated water [76]. Some recent studies have shown that the application of high pressures (100, 200 and 400 MPa) can even improve the functional properties of pine nut protein [77,78].

On the other hand, the application of HPP has also been analyzed to reduce allergenicity in nuts. Allergic reactions caused by nuts represent 0.5% of the total reactions reported [79]. In this sense, Long et al. [80] showed that applying a treatment of 400, 500 and 600 MPa for 10 min or more in peanuts reduced the immunoreactivity of allergens. Likewise, Hu et al. [81] found that the allergenicity of peanuts decreased with HPP of 60, 90, 120, 150 and 180 MPa. HPP has also been effective in reducing allergens present in soybeans [82,83]; treatments of 300 MPa for 15 min reduced allergens in soybeans and soybean sprouts [83] and in isolated soy protein for baby foods [82].

2.5. Irradiation

γ-rays are high-energy photons produced from radioactive isotopes such as cobalt-60 and cesium-137, with an average total dose equal to or less than 10 kGy. They affect microorganisms and food matrixes by direct disruption of biomolecules such as DNA and by indirect effects due to the interaction between biomolecules and radicals and ions originating from water radiolysis [84]. Irradiation treatments could penetrate through the shell of the nuts and give a homogenous treatment [85].

Directive 1999/3/EC [86] of the European Parliament and of the Council, on the establishment of a community list of foods and food ingredients authorized for treatment with ionizing radiation, establishes a single category of ingredients that can be irradiated throughout the European Union: aromatic herbs, spices and vegetable seasonings (dry). However, Member States were allowed to continue irradiation in other categories authorized before the entry into force of the directive. For this reason, there are currently EU countries where the irradiation of other types of food, such as nuts, still takes place.

The commercial application of irradiation is growing globally, primarily in Asia and in the Americas. However, the trend in the European Union is the opposite, with fewer products being irradiated. In general, irradiation technology is not well understood by the consumer, who tends to have a negative perception of this treatment [87].

One of the problems with nuts is that they can be contaminated by pest damage, mold and yeast, with some of them forming the dangerous aflatoxins (*Aspergillus flavus* and *Aspergillus parasiticus*), which decrease both the quality and shelf life of the nut and are carcinogenic [88–90]. Doses of 20 kGy have proven to be effective in reducing these molds on walnuts (Food Irradiation research technology). In peanuts, doses of 5 kGy and higher significantly decreased (89% approximately) the growth of *A. parasiticus*; however, they did not achieve its complete elimination [91]. In addition, in peanuts, 6 kGy detoxified around 75% of aflatoxin B1 [92].

Microbial pathogens (*Salmonella* and *E. coli*) in nuts are also one of the recent problems associated with these products [12–17]. Irradiation has been shown to be effective against most food pathogens (*Campylobacter jejuni*, *Aeromonas hydrophia*, *Yersinia enterocolitica*, *Salmonella*, *Shigella*, *E. coli*, *Listeria monocytogenes*, and *Staphylococcus aureus*), which have a low tolerance to it, especially in nuts, due to low moisture [85]. Doses between 3 and 5 kGy produce a 4 log cfu/g reduction of *Salmonella* in almonds [93] and reduce, below the detection limit (1 log cfu/g), the concentration of *E. coli*, *Salmonella Thyphimurium* and *L. monocytogenes* in pistachios [94].

Nuts are very susceptible to lipid peroxidation, and therefore, off-flavors and rancidity could be formed during the processing and shelf life [95,96].

The first sensory tests, to determine the formation of off-flavors, in dry fruits such as raw almonds or pistachios, were carried out by O'Mahony et al. [97] and Thomas [98]. No differences were observed in the rancidity parameter, up to irradiated doses of 10 kGy and up to 6 months of storage. Subsequently, Wilson-Kakashita et al. [99] treated walnuts with gamma irradiation doses of up to 20 kGy and did not find any sensory differences in the previously mentioned parameters of off-flavors and rancidity.

Mexis and Kontominas [100] irradiated cashew nuts up to doses of 7 kGy and found that the concentration of volatile compounds, such as alcohols, ketones and aldehydes, increased after being treated, although sensory analysis showed that cashew nuts remained organoleptically acceptable at doses below 3 kGy. Taipina et al. [101] also obtained the same results at irradiation doses of up to 3 kGy in pecan nuts regarding sensory parameters such as aroma and flavor attributes.

With higher irradiation doses up to 7 kGy in pine nut kernels, almonds and hazelnuts, with storage periods of up to 6 months, no sensory differences in flavor were detected [102–104]. Sánchez-Bel et al. [104] reported that irradiation doses up to 7 kGy caused no significant changes in sensory quality.

Recent studies on pistachios have analyzed the evolution of volatile compounds and related sensory parameters, such as taste, at doses of up to 2 kGy; 14 volatile aromatic compounds were found in non-irradiated pistachios. The main compounds at doses lower than 1.5 kGy were terpenes; however, at doses $\geq$ 2 kGy, they were aldehydes, terpenes and alcohols. The amounts of volatile compounds increased in the irradiated product, up to 21; 4 aldehydes and 3 more alcoholic compounds were identified, and these increased with the irradiation doses ($\geq$4 kGy), showing a significant difference ($p < 0.05$). Aldehydes comprised approximately half of the volatile compounds in the sample irradiated at 6 kGy. Aldehyde components, including heptanal, octanal, nonanal and 2-nonenal, and alcohols comprising 1-hexanol, octanol and 1-nonanol were formed during irradiation, as they did not exist previously. Values ranged from 5.95 mg/kg for non-irradiated nuts to 14.97 mg/kg of total volatile compounds for pistachios irradiated at a dose of 6 kGy, for heptanal, with a green sweet taste, and hexanal, an indicator of oxidation and quality of fatty foods, which is one of the main components of irradiated nuts that can be derived from linoleic acid (Frankel, 1983). α-pinene was the most abundant volatile compound in all the samples, as shown by other studies on this dried fruit [105]. The taste of samples was affected ($p < 0.05$) at doses ≥ 2 kGy, obtaining the worst results as the irradiation dose increased to 6 kGy [106].

The authors reported that the oxidation of unsaturated lipids (e.g., unsaturated fatty acids) as a result of irradiation could produce a variety of volatile compounds, including aldehydes, ketones, alcohols and esters, which can significantly affect the organoleptic properties of foods in extremely small quantities [100,107].

2.6. Cold Plasma

Plasma is universally known as the fourth state of matter. It is produced by the ionization of gas particles by adding energy, with the consequent generation of ions, free radicals, molecules in an excited state, and photons [108]. Cold plasma is achieved by generating high electrical discharges at room temperature (or similar), achieving ionic destabilization of the particles [109]. Reactive species such as O, O_3, NO, NO_2, and OH generated by plasma lead to microorganism inactivation and cellular deformation [110]. Applied to food, these electrical discharges destabilize cells, causing membrane damage, protein denaturation, lipid peroxidation, and DNA and/or RNA damage, among others [111]. In addition, it is a technique that does not leave any type of residue and does not raise the temperature of the treated product; thus, it does not greatly affect its original properties [112]. For this reason, cold plasma is being widely investigated for its use as an antimicrobial agent in food, antigerminative, toxin inactivator and biofilm control.

In the case of nuts, the influence of cold plasma as an inactivator of microorganisms has been widely studied in almonds (Table 1). Deng et al. [113] achieved reductions of 5 log cfu/g of *E. coli*, using 30 s treatments with a voltage of 30 kV and 2 kHz. Hertwig et al. [114] also studied the effect on almonds in the case of *Salmonella enteritidis* PT30 and using whole almonds. They studied the application of cold plasma with air at room temperature (20 kV and 15 kHz) and achieved reductions of more than 5 log cfu/g. In addition, in *Salmonella*, Khalili et al. [115] studied the effect of plasma (in addition to *Shigella*), obtaining for both reductions of more than 4 log cfu/g using the gliding arc plasma technique (14 kV, 50 kHz and 4 min of treatment). Shirani et al. [116] studied the effect of plasma on peeled and sliced almonds by applying 17 V and 2.26 A current for different time periods (5, 10, 15, and 20 min). By using 20 min argon cold plasma jet treatment, the total count of almond microorganisms was reduced 2.95 log cfu/g, mold and yeast 1.81 log cfu/g, and *Staphylococcus* aureus 2.72 log cfu/g. Furthermore, almond color, peroxide value and sensory evaluation did not change with this treatment.

In pistachio (Table 1), cold plasma has been studied, mainly for its use in the control of *Aspergillus*. Several authors have shown that this technique is very effective for this microorganism. Makari et al. [117] found that after 3 min of exposure to a power of 130 W, 20 kHz frequency and 15 kV voltage, the spores were undetectable (reduction of 4 log cfu/g). They also reported a reduction in the AFB1 content by up to 60%, without affecting fruit quality. These authors show that the longer the exposure time, the greater the antimicrobial effect achieved. Ghorashi et al. [118] treated whole pistachios using three types of plasma: capacitive coupled plasma (AP-CCP), direct current diode plasma (DC-DP), and inductively coupled plasma (ICP), with the DC-DP being the most effective in the *Aspergillus flavus* reduction rate (5-log reduction; 83%) at 300 W input power, 2 Torr pressure and 20 min irradiation. Tasouji et al. [119] studied the effect of cold plasma, in this case using an Atmospheric Pressure Capacitive Coupled Plasma (AP-CCP) generating device using argon gas, in the reduction of *Aspergillus flavus* in pistachio. These authors obtained a reduction of 4 log fungus reduction (about 67%) by using a power input of 100 W for a 10 min irradiation time, with no alteration on the nut texture. The effect of this technique in pistachios on the decontamination of *Aspergillus brasiliensis* and *E. coli* has also been studied. Pignata et al. [120] used low-pressure gas plasma with three gases: pure argon, pure oxygen and argon-oxygen (50%), with the latter being the most effective. A treatment for 5 min against *Aspergillus brasiliensis* achieved a reduction of 5 logs, and 4 logs in *E. coli*, by applying the treatment for 1 min for decontamination of pistachios [120]. The study demonstrated that a mixture of argon-oxygen-generated plasma was more effective for decontamination than pure oxygen and pure argon. The treatment time of 30 min led to a reduction of 3.5 logs of *Aspergillus brasiliensis* using pure oxygen and pure argon. However, a treatment time of 5 min, 1 min and 15 s led to a reduction of 5.4 logs using an argon and oxygen gas mixture. In *E. coli*, 1 min and 30 s of treatment resulted in 4 log reductions for oxygen and argon, respectively.

This technique has been studied in other nuts, such as peanuts (Table 1). Lin et al. [121] achieved reductions of more than 5 log cfu/g of *Aspergillus flavus* and *Aspergillus niger* using cold plasma with argon (200 W and 5 min of treatment). In addition, the authors specify that microscopically it is observed how this treatment seriously damaged the aflatoxin spores. In walnuts (Table 1), Ahangari et al. [122] observed reductions in the entire content of coliforms and mold through the application of cold plasma (50 W and 20 min). However, in this case, the treatment caused a color change in the samples (darkening).

Cold plasma is an area in which considerable research is being conducted. From what has been shown so far, in the case of nuts, it is a technique that works well as an antimicrobial. It is an inexpensive technique, which has a low environmental impact and which preserves the physical and functional properties of dried fruits. Therefore, it is an emerging technology that deserves to be considered as an alternative in the preservation of nuts. However, research should be focused on obtaining the best combination of processing parameters to achieve the best results.

Table 1. Effect of cold plasma in nuts.

Nut	Processing Conditions Applied	Effects	Reference
Almond	Non-thermal plasma (NTP); 30 s; 30 kV; 2000 H	5-log reduction of *E. coli*.	[113]
	Cold plasma (CP); air; 20 kV; 15 kHz; 15 min	5-log reduction of *Salmonella enteritidis* PT-30	[114]
	NTP; Gliding arc plasma; 14 kV; 50 kHz; 4 min; 6 mm distance	4-log reduction of *Salmonella* and *Shigella*	[115]
	CP; 17 V, 2.26 A; 20 min; 2 cm distance; ambient temperature	3-log reduction of total microorganisms; 1.8-log reduction of molds and yeasts; 2.7-log reduction *Staphylococcus aureu*	[116]
Pistachio	CP; 130 W; 20 kHz; 15 kV; 3 min; ambient temperature	4-log reduction *Aspergillus*; AFB$_1$ reduction of 60%	[117]
	Direct current diode plasma (DC-DP); 300 W; 2 Torr; 20 min	5-log reduction *Aspergillus flavus*	[118]
	Atmospheric pressure capacitive coupled plasma (AP-CCP); argon; 100 W; 10 min; ambient temperature	4-log reduction *Aspergillus flavus*	[119]
	Low pressure cold plasma (LP-CP); O$_2$-Ar, 5 mbar; 20 mm distance; 50 MHz; 400 W; 5 min; ambient temperature	5-log reduction *Aspergillus brasiliensis*; 4-log reduction *E. coli*	[120]
Peanut	CP; Ar; 200 W; 5 min; 1 atm; 4 cm; ambient temperature	5-log reduction *Aspergillus niger* and *Aspergillus flavus*	[121]
Walnut	CP; 500 mTorr; 13.6 MHz; 50 W; 20 min	Total reduction in molds and coliforms	[122]

3. Conclusions and Future Trends

Non-thermal technologies are proving to be efficient in the antimicrobial treatment of nuts. These technologies (cold plasma, high pressure, irradiation, pulsed electric field, pulsed light, ultrasound, and ultraviolet light) have a low environmental impact and a low economic cost; thus, their application can revert directly to the industry and the consumer. Ultraviolet light is effective against mycotoxins, especially those of the aflatoxin group. Pulsed electric field and the application of ultrasound provide good results due to the fact that they cause an increase in the functional properties of nuts. Pulsed light, irradiation and cold plasma have been effective in reducing *Salmonella*, *E. coli* and *Aspergillus*, without affecting the quality of the treated fruit. High-pressure methods are currently in the development phase in nuts because of their great effect on liquid foods. Currently, this technique is being used to study its effect against the inactivation of allergens in food. Non-thermal treatments are proving to be effective for the microbial reduction of nuts; however, to date, tests have been developed with a small amount of product and have not yet been extrapolated to an industrial level for the treatment of large amounts. In the near future, research should focus on the effect against the allergic power that nuts have in a significant part of the population, because some of the non-thermal treatments have achieved promising advances.

Author Contributions: Conceptualization, V.M.G.-L.; methodology, A.J.P.-L.; software, L.N.-A.; validation, P.S.-B., A.J.P.-L. and Á.A.C.-B.; formal analysis, A.J.P.-L.; investigation, V.M.G.-L., L.N.-A., Á.A.C.-B., J.A.G., A.J.P.-L., P.S.-B.; V.M.G.-L., L.N.-A., Á.A.C.-B., J.A.G., A.J.P.-L., P.S.-B.; data curation, V.M.G.-L., L.N.-A., Á.A.C.-B., J.A.G., A.J.P.-L., P.S.-B.; writing—original draft preparation, A.J.P.-L., P.S.-B.; writing—review and editing, Á.A.C.-B., P.S.-B., A.J.P.-L., V.M.G.-L. and L.N.-A.; visualization, A.J.P.-L., P.S.-B.; supervision, Á.A.C.-B.; project administration, P.S.-B.; funding acquisition, J.A.G. All authors have read and agreed to the published version of the manuscript.

Funding: Paola Sánchez-Bravo was funded by the grant for the recall of the Spanish university system for the training of young doctors (Margarita Salas, 04912/2021), funded by the European Union-Next Generation EU and the Ministry of Universities of Spain.

Data Availability Statement: Data is contained within the article.

Conflicts of Interest: The authors declare no conflict of interest.

References

1. Alasalvar, C.; Salvadó, J.-S.; Ros, E. Bioactives and health benefits of nuts and dried fruits. *Food Chem.* **2020**, *314*, 126192. [CrossRef] [PubMed]
2. Ros, E. Health benefits of nut consumption. *Nutrients* **2010**, *2*, 652–682. [CrossRef] [PubMed]
3. Aune, D.; Keum, N.; Giovannucci, E.; Fadnes, L.T.; Boffetta, P.; Greenwood, D.C.; Tonstad, S.; Vatten, L.J.; Riboli, E.; Norat, T. Nut consumption and risk of cardiovascular disease, total cancer, all-cause and cause-specific mortality: A systematic review and dose-response meta-analysis of prospective studies. *BMC Med.* **2016**, *14*, 207. [CrossRef]
4. Becerra-Tomás, N.; Paz-Graniel, I.; Kendall, C.W.C.; Kahleova, H.; Rahelić, D.; Sievenpiper, J.L.; Salas-Salvadó, J. Nut consumption and incidence of cardiovascular diseases and cardiovascular disease mortality: A meta-analysis of prospective cohort studies. *Nutr. Rev.* **2019**, *77*, 691–709. [CrossRef]
5. Udovicki, B.; Stankovic, S.; Tomic, N.; Djekic, I.; Smigic, N.; Trifunovic, B.S.; Milicevic, D.; Rajkovic, A. Evaluation of ultraviolet irradiation effects on *Aspergillus flavus* and aflatoxin b1 in maize and peanut using innovative vibrating decontamination equipment. *Food Control* **2022**, *134*, 108691. [CrossRef]
6. Perrone, G.; Gallo, A.; Logrieco, A.F. Biodiversity of *Aspergillus* section *Flavi* in europe in relation to the management of aflatoxin risk. *Front. Microbiol.* **2014**, *5*, 377. [CrossRef] [PubMed]
7. Roze, L.V.; Hong, S.-Y.; Linz, J.E. Aflatoxin biosynthesis: Current frontiers. *Annu. Rev. Food Sci. Technol.* **2013**, *4*, 293–311. [CrossRef]
8. Wu, Y.; Cheng, J.-H.; Sun, D.-W. Blocking and degradation of aflatoxins by cold plasma treatments: Applications and mechanisms. *Trends Food Sci. Technol.* **2021**, *109*, 647–661. [CrossRef]
9. Yazdanpanah, H. Mycotoxins: Analytical challenges. *Iran. J. Pharm. Sci.* **2011**, *10*, 653–654.
10. Kumar, P.; Mahato, D.K.; Kamle, M.; Mohanta, T.K.; Kang, S.G. Aflatoxins: A global concern for food safety, human health and their management. *Front. Microbiol.* **2017**, *7*, 2170. [CrossRef]

11. Rushing, B.R.; Selim, M.I. Aflatoxin b1: A review on metabolism, toxicity, occurrence in food, occupational exposure, and detoxification methods. *Food Chem. Toxicol.* **2019**, *124*, 81–100. [CrossRef]
12. Hassan-Mohammad, Z.; Murano, E.A.; Moreira, R.G.; Castillo, A. Effect of air- and vacuum-packaged atmospheres on the reduction of *Salmonella* on almonds by electron beam irradiation. *LWT* **2019**, *116*, 108389. [CrossRef]
13. Jeong, S.; Marks, B.P.; Ryser, E.T.; Harte, J.B. The effect of x-ray irradiation on *Salmonella* inactivation and sensory quality of almonds and walnuts as a function of water activity. *Int. J. Food Microbiol.* **2012**, *153*, 365–371. [CrossRef] [PubMed]
14. Blessington, T.; Theofel, C.G.; Mitcham, E.J.; Harris, L.J. Survival of foodborne pathogens on inshell walnuts. *Int. J. Food Microbiol.* **2013**, *166*, 341–348. [CrossRef] [PubMed]
15. Davidson, G.R.; Frelka, J.C.; Yang, M.; Jones, T.M.; Harris, L.J. Prevalence of *Escherichia coli* o157:H7 and *Salmonella* on inshell california walnuts. *J. Food Prot.* **2015**, *78*, 1547–1553. [CrossRef]
16. Zhang, G.; Hu, L.; Melka, D.; Wang, H.; Laasri, A.; Brown, E.W.; Strain, E.; Allard, M.; Bunning, V.K.; Musser, S.M.; et al. Prevalence of *Salmonella* in cashews, hazelnuts, macadamia nuts, pecans, pine nuts, and walnuts in the united states. *J. Food Prot.* **2017**, *80*, 459–466. [CrossRef] [PubMed]
17. Rothschild, M. Canada E. coli Outbreak Tied to Walnuts. Available online: https://www.foodsafetynews.com/2011/04/canada-e-coli-outbreak-tied-to-walnuts/ (accessed on 18 July 2022).
18. Juneja, V.K.; Dwivedi, H.P.; Sofos, J.N. *Microbial Control and Food Preservation: Theory and Practice*; Springer: Berlin/Heidelberg, Germany, 2018.
19. Prakash, A. Non-thermal processing technologies to improve the safety of nuts. In *Improving the Safety and Quality of Nuts*; Woodhead Publishing: Soston, UK, 2013; pp. 35–55.
20. Altemimi, A.; Ali, H.I.; Al-Hilphy, A.R.; Lightfoot, D.A.; Watson, D.G. Electric field applications on dried key lime juice quality with regression modeling. *J. Food Process. Preserv.* **2018**, *42*, e13637. [CrossRef]
21. Picart-Palmade, L.; Cunault, C.; Chevalier-Lucia, D.; Belleville, M.-P.; Marchesseau, S. Potentialities and limits of some non-thermal technologies to improve sustainability of food processing. *Front. Nutr.* **2019**, *5*, 130. [CrossRef]
22. Sonne, A.M.; Grunert, K.G.; Olsen, N.V.; Granli, B.S.; Szabó, E.; Banati, D. Consumers' perceptions of hpp and pef food products. *Br. Food J.* **2012**, *114*, 85–107. [CrossRef]
23. Guerrero, S.N.; Ferrario, M.; Schenk, M.; Fenoglio, D.; Andreone, A. Ultraviolet light. In *Electromagnetic Technologies in Food Science*; Wiley: Hoboken, NJ, USA, 2021; pp. 128–180.
24. Keklik, N.M.; Krishnamurthy, K.; Demirci, A. Microbial decontamination of food by ultraviolet (uv) and pulsed uv light. In *Microbial Decontamination in the Food Industry: Novel Methods and Applications*; Demirci, A., Ngadi, M.O., Eds.; Woodhead Publishing: Soston, UK, 2012; pp. 344–369.
25. Deng, L.-Z.; Tao, Y.; Mujumdar, A.S.; Pan, Z.; Chen, C.; Yang, X.-H.; Liu, Z.-L.; Wang, H.; Xiao, H.-W. Recent advances in non-thermal decontamination techno logies for microorganisms and mycotoxins in low-moisture foods. *Trends Food Sci. Technol.* **2020**, *106*, 104–112. [CrossRef]
26. Mao, J.; He, B.; Zhang, L.; Li, P.; Zhang, Q.; Ding, X.; Zhang, W. A structure identification and toxicity assessment of the degradation products of aflatoxin b1 in peanut oil under uv irradiation. *Toxins* **2016**, *8*, 332. [CrossRef] [PubMed]
27. Jubeen, F.; Bhatti, I.A.; Khan, M.Z.; Zahoor-Ul, H.; Shahid, M. Effect of uvc irradiation on aflatoxins in ground nut (*arachis hypogea*) and tree nuts (*Juglans regia, Prunus duclus and Pistachio vera*). *J. Chem. Soc. Pak.* **2012**, *34*, 1366–1374.
28. Drishya, C.; Yoha, K.S.; Perumal, A.B.; Moses, J.A.; Anandharamakrishnan, C.; Balasubramaniam, V.M. Impact of nonthermal food processing techniques on mycotoxins and their producing fungi. *Int. J. Food Sci. Technol.* **2022**, *57*, 2140–2148. [CrossRef]
29. Chang, M.; Jin, Q.; Liu, Y.; Liu, R.; Wang, X. Efficiency and safety evaluation of photodegradation of aflatoxin b_1 on peanut surface. *Int. J. Food Sci. Technol.* **2013**, *48*, 2474–2479. [CrossRef]
30. Mazaheri, M. Effect of Uv Radiation on Different Concentrations of Aflatoxin b_1 in Pistachio. *Acta Hortic.* **2011**, *963*, 41–46. [CrossRef]
31. Babaee, R.; Karami-Osboo, R.; Mirabolfathy, M. Evaluation of the use of ozone, uv-c and citric acid in reducing aflatoxins in pistachio nut. *J. Food Compost. Anal.* **2022**, *106*, 104276. [CrossRef]
32. Garg, N.; Aggarwal, M.; Javed, S.; Kh, R.K. Studies for optimization of conditions for reducing aflatoxin contamination in peanuts using ultraviolet radiations. *Int. J. Drug Dev. Res.* **2013**, *5*.
33. Diao, E.; Li, X.; Zhang, Z.; Ma, W.; Ji, N.; Dong, H. Ultraviolet irradiation detoxification of aflatoxins. *Trends Food Sci. Technol.* **2015**, *42*, 64–69. [CrossRef]
34. Baysal, A.H. Short-wave ultraviolet light inactivation of pathogens in fruit juices. In *Fruit Juices*; Elsevier: Amsterdam, The Netherlands, 2018; pp. 463–510.
35. Keyser, M.; Müller, I.A.; Cilliers, F.P.; Nel, W.; Gouws, P.A. Ultraviolet radiation as a non-thermal treatment for the inactivation of microorganisms in fruit juice. *Innov. Food Sci. Emerg. Technol.* **2008**, *9*, 348–354. [CrossRef]
36. Unluturk, S.; Atilgan, M.R. Microbial safety and shelf life of uv-c treated freshly squeezed white grape juice. *J. Food Sci.* **2015**, *80*, M1831–M1841. [CrossRef]
37. Izmirlioglu, G.; Demirci, A. Inactivation of salmonella enteritidis on walnuts by pulsed UV treatment. In Proceedings of the ASABE 2018 Annual International Meeting, Detroit, MI, USA, 29 July–1 August 2018.

38. Ruiz-Hernández, K.; Ramírez-Rojas, N.Z.; Meza-Plaza, E.F.; García-Mosqueda, C.; Jauregui-Vázquez, D.; Rojas-Laguna, R.; Sosa-Morales, M.E. Uv-c treatments against *Salmonella typhimurium* atcc 14028 in inoculated peanuts and almonds. *Food Eng. Rev.* **2021**, *13*, 706–712. [CrossRef]
39. Pi, X.; Yang, Y.; Sun, Y.; Wang, X.; Wan, Y.; Fu, G.; Li, X.; Cheng, J. Food irradiation: A promising technology to produce hypoallergenic food with high quality. *Crit. Rev. Food Sci. Nutr.* **2021**, *62*, 1–16. [CrossRef]
40. Gómez-López, V.M.; Pataro, G.; Tiwari, B.; Gozzi, M.; Meireles, M.Á.A.; Wang, S.; Guamis, B.; Pan, Z.; Ramaswamy, H.; Sastry, S.; et al. Guidelines on reporting treatment conditions for emerging technologies in food processing. *Crit. Rev. Food Sci. Nutr.* **2022**, *62*, 5925–5949. [CrossRef]
41. Rábago-Panduro, L.M.; Morales-de la Peña, M.; Martín-Belloso, O.; Welti-Chanes, J. Application of pulsed electric fields pef on pecan nuts *Carya illinoinensis wangenh*. K. Koch: Oil extraction yield and compositional characteristics of the oil and its by-product. *Food Eng. Rev.* **2021**, *13*, 676–685. [CrossRef]
42. Ranjha, M.M.A.N.; Kanwal, R.; Shafique, B.; Arshad, R.N.; Irfan, S.; Kieliszek, M.; Kowalczewski, P.Ł.; Irfan, M.; Khalid, M.Z.; Roobab, U.; et al. A critical review on pulsed electric field: A novel technology for the extraction of phytoconstituents. *Molecules* **2021**, *26*, 4893. [CrossRef]
43. Lin, S.; Liang, R.; Xue, P.; Zhang, S.; Liu, Z.; Dong, X. Antioxidant activity improvement of identified pine nut peptides by pulsed electric field (pef) and the mechanism exploration. *LWT* **2017**, *75*, 366–372. [CrossRef]
44. Niu, D.; Zeng, X.-A.; Ren, E.-F.; Xu, F.-Y.; Li, J.; Wang, M.-S.; Wang, R. Review of the application of pulsed electric fields (pef) technology for food processing in china. *Food Res. Int.* **2020**, *137*, 109715. [CrossRef] [PubMed]
45. Patra, A.; Abdullah, S.; Pradhan, R.C. Review on the extraction of bioactive compounds and characterization of fruit industry by-products. *Bioresour. Bioprocess.* **2022**, *9*, 14. [CrossRef]
46. Saini, A.; Panesar, P.S.; Bera, M.B. Valorization of fruits and vegetables waste through green extraction of bioactive compounds and their nanoemulsions-based delivery system. *Bioresour. Bioprocess.* **2019**, *6*, 26. [CrossRef]
47. Vanga, S.K.; Wang, J.; Jayaram, S.; Raghavan, V. Effects of pulsed electric fields and ultrasound processing on proteins and enzymes: A review. *Processes* **2021**, *9*, 722. [CrossRef]
48. Manzoor, M.F.; Zeng, X.-A.; Rahaman, A.; Siddeeg, A.; Aadil, R.M.; Ahmed, Z.; Li, J.; Niu, D. Combined impact of pulsed electric field and ultrasound on bioactive compounds and ft-ir analysis of almond extract. *J. Food Sci. Technol.* **2019**, *56*, 2355–2364. [CrossRef] [PubMed]
49. Arcena, M.R.; Leong, S.Y.; Then, S.; Hochberg, M.; Sack, M.; Mueller, G.; Sigler, J.; Kebede, B.; Silcock, P.; Oey, I. The effect of pulsed electric fields pre-treatment on the volatile and phenolic profiles of merlot grape musts at different winemaking stages and the sensory characteristics of the finished wines. *Innov. Food Sci. Emerg. Technol.* **2021**, *70*, 102698. [CrossRef]
50. Carpentieri, S.; Režek Jambrak, A.; Ferrari, G.; Pataro, G. Pulsed electric field-assisted extraction of aroma and bioactive compounds from aromatic plants and food by-products. *Front. Nutr.* **2022**, *8*, 792203. [CrossRef]
51. Kanafusa, S.; Maspero, U.; Petersen, M.A.; Gómez Galindo, F. Influence of pulsed electric field-assisted dehydration on the volatile compounds of basil leaves. *Innov. Food Sci. Emerg. Technol.* **2022**, *77*, 102979. [CrossRef]
52. Lee, H.; Choi, S.; Kim, E.; Kim, Y.-N.; Lee, J.; Lee, D.-U. Effects of pulsed electric field and thermal treatments on microbial reduction, volatile composition, and sensory properties of orange juice, and their characterization by a principal component analysis. *Appl. Sci.* **2021**, *11*, 186. [CrossRef]
53. Nandakumar, R.; Eyres, G.T.; Burritt, D.J.; Kebede, B.; Leus, M.; Oey, I. Impact of pulsed electric fields on the volatile compounds produced in whole onions (*Allium cepa* and *Allium fistulosum*). *Foods* **2018**, *7*, 183. [CrossRef]
54. Salehi, F. Physico-chemical properties of fruit and vegetable juices as affected by pulsed electric field: A review. *Int. J. Food Prop.* **2020**, *23*, 1036–1050. [CrossRef]
55. Cudemos, E.; Izquier, A.; Medina-Martínez, M.S.; Gómez-López, V.M. Effects of shading and growth phase on the microbial inactivation by pulsed light. *Czech J. Food Sci.* **2013**, *31*, 189–193. [CrossRef]
56. Braslavsky, S.E. Glossary of terms used in photochemistry, 3rd edition (iupac recommendations 2006). *Pure Appl. Chem.* **2007**, *79*, 293–465. [CrossRef]
57. Gómez-López, V.M.; Bolton, J.R. An approach to standardize methods for fluence determination in bench-scale pulsed light experiments. *Food Bioprocess Technol.* **2016**, *9*, 1040–1048. [CrossRef]
58. Izmirlioglu, G.; Ouyang, B.; Demirci, A. Utilization of pulsed uv light for inactivation of *Salmonella enteritidis* on shelled walnuts. *LWT* **2020**, *134*, 110023. [CrossRef]
59. Gómez-López, V.M.; Noguera-Artiaga, L.; Figueroa-Morales, F.; Girón, F.; Carbonell-Barrachina, Á.A.; Gabaldón, J.A.; Pérez-López, A.J. Effect of pulsed light on quality of shelled walnuts. *Foods* **2022**, *11*, 1186. [CrossRef] [PubMed]
60. Li, Y.; Yang, W.; Chung, S.-Y.; Chen, H.; Ye, M.; Teixeira, A.A.; Gregory, J.F.; Welt, B.A.; Shriver, S. Effect of pulsed ultraviolet light and high hydrostatic pressure on the antigenicity of almond protein extracts. *Food Bioprocess Technol.* **2013**, *6*, 431–440. [CrossRef]
61. Oner, M.E. Inactivation of *Salmonella enteritidis* on almonds by pulsed light treatment. *Acad. Food J. Akad. GIDA* **2017**, *15*, 242–248.
62. Harguindeguy, M.; Gómez-Camacho, C.E. Pulsed light (pl) treatments on almond kernels: *Salmonella enteritidis* inactivation kinetics and infrared thermography insights. *Food Bioprocess Technol.* **2021**, *14*, 2323–2335. [CrossRef]
63. Liu, X.; Fan, X.; Wang, W.; Yao, S.; Chen, H. Wetting raw almonds to enhance pulse light inactivation of *Salmonella* and preserve quality. *Food Control* **2021**, *125*, 107946. [CrossRef]

64. Zhao, X.; Yang, W.; Chung, S.-Y.; Sims, C.A.; Otwell, S.W.; Rababah, T.M. Reduction of ige immunoreactivity of whole peanut (*Arachis hypogaea l.*) after pulsed light illumination. *Food Bioprocess Technol.* **2014**, *7*, 2637–2645. [CrossRef]
65. Abuagela, M.O.; Iqdiam, B.M.; Mostafa, H.; Gu, L.; Smith, M.E.; Sarnoski, P.J. Assessing pulsed light treatment on the reduction of aflatoxins in peanuts with and without skin. *Int. J. Food Sci. Technol.* **2018**, *53*, 2567–2575. [CrossRef]
66. Abuagela, M.O.; Iqdiam, B.M.; Mostafa, H.; Marshall, S.M.; Yagiz, Y.; Marshall, M.R.; Gu, L.; Sarnoski, P. Combined effects of citric acid and pulsed light treatments to degrade b-aflatoxins in peanut. *Food Bioprod. Process.* **2019**, *117*, 396–403. [CrossRef]
67. Zabot, G.L.; Viganó, J.; Silva, E.K. Low-frequency ultrasound coupled with high-pressure technologies: Impact of hybridized techniques on the recovery of phytochemical compounds. *Molecules* **2021**, *26*, 5117. [CrossRef] [PubMed]
68. Zawawi, N.A.F.; Hazmi, N.A.M.; How, M.S.; Kantono, K.; Silva, F.V.M.; Sulaiman, A. Thermal, high pressure, and ultrasound inactivation of various fruit cultivars's polyphenol oxidase: Kinetic inactivation models and estimation of treatment energy requirement. *Appl. Sci.* **2022**, *12*, 1864. [CrossRef]
69. Bhargava, N.; Mor, R.S.; Kumar, K.; Sharanagat, V.S. Advances in application of ultrasound in food processing: A review. *Ultrason. Sonochem.* **2021**, *70*, 105293. [CrossRef]
70. Chavan, P.; Sharma, P.; Sharma, S.R.; Mittal, T.C.; Jaiswal, A.K. Application of high-intensity ultrasound to improve food processing efficiency: A review. *Foods* **2022**, *11*, 122. [CrossRef]
71. Esteban-Lustres, R.; Sanz, V.; Domínguez, H.; Torres, M.D. Ultrasound-assisted extraction of high-value fractions from fruit industrial processing waste. *Foods* **2022**, *11*, 2089. [CrossRef]
72. Taha, A.; Ahmed, E.; Ismaiel, A.; Ashokkumar, M.; Xu, X.; Pan, S.; Hu, H. Ultrasonic emulsification: An overview on the preparation of different emulsifiers-stabilized emulsions. *Trends Food Sci. Technol.* **2020**, *105*, 363–377. [CrossRef]
73. Rudolf, J.L.; Resurreccion, A.V.A. Optimization of trans-resveratrol concentration and sensory properties of peanut kernels by slicing and ultrasound treatment, using response surface methodology. *J. Food Sci.* **2007**, *72*, S450–S462. [CrossRef]
74. Aganovic, K.; Hertel, C.; Vogel, R.F.; Johne, R.; Schlüter, O.; Schwarzenbolz, U.; Jäger, H.; Holzhauser, T.; Bergmair, J.; Roth, A.; et al. Aspects of high hydrostatic pressure food processing: Perspectives on technology and food safety. *Compr. Rev. Food Sci. Food Saf.* **2021**, *20*, 3225–3266. [CrossRef]
75. Pérez-Lamela, C.; Franco, I.; Falqué, E. Impact of high-pressure processing on antioxidant activity during storage of fruits and fruit products: A review. *Molecules* **2021**, *26*, 5265. [CrossRef] [PubMed]
76. Raghubeer, E.V.; Phan, B.N.; Onuoha, E.; Diggins, S.; Aguilar, V.; Swanson, S.; Lee, A. The use of high-pressure processing (HPP) to improve the safety and quality of raw coconut (*Cocos nucifera* L.) water. *Int. J. Food Microbiol.* **2020**, *331*, 108697. [CrossRef] [PubMed]
77. Cao, B.; Fang, L.; Liu, C.; Min, W.; Liu, J. Effects of high hydrostatic pressure on the functional and rheological properties of the protein fraction extracted from pine nuts. *Food Sci. Technol. Int.* **2018**, *24*, 53–66. [CrossRef] [PubMed]
78. Nabi, B.G.; Mukhtar, K.; Arshad, R.N.; Radicetti, E.; Tedeschi, P.; Shahbaz, M.U.; Walayat, N.; Nawaz, A.; Inam-Ur-raheem, M.; Aadil, R.M. High-pressure processing for sustainable food supply. *Sustainability* **2021**, *13*, 13908. [CrossRef]
79. Fleischer, D.M.; Conover-Walker, M.K.; Matsui, E.C.; Wood, R.A. The natural history of tree nut allergy. *J. Allergy Clin. Immunol.* **2005**, *116*, 1087–1093. [CrossRef] [PubMed]
80. Long, F.; Yang, X.; Sun, J.; Zhong, Q.; Wei, J.; Qu, P.; Yue, T. Effects of combined high pressure and thermal treatment on the allergenic potential of peanut in a mouse model of allergy. *Innov. Food Sci. Emerg. Technol.* **2016**, *35*, 133–138. [CrossRef]
81. Hu, C.-Q.; Chen, H.-B.; Gao, J.-Y.; Luo, C.-P.; Ma, X.-J.; Tong, P. High-pressure microfluidisation-induced changes in the antigenicity and conformation of allergen ara h 2 purified from chinese peanut. *J. Sci. Food Agric.* **2011**, *91*, 1304–1309. [CrossRef]
82. Li, H.; Zhu, K.; Zhou, H.; Peng, W. Effects of high hydrostatic pressure treatment on allergenicity and structural properties of soybean protein isolate for infant formula. *Food Chem.* **2012**, *132*, 808–814. [CrossRef]
83. Peñas, E.; Gomez, R.; Frias, J.; Baeza, M.L.; Vidal-Valverde, C. High hydrostatic pressure effects on immunoreactivity and nutritional quality of soybean products. *Food Chem.* **2011**, *125*, 423–429. [CrossRef]
84. Fan, X.; Nicmira, B.A. Gamma Irradiation. In *Electromagnetic Technologies in Food Science*; Wiley: Hoboken, NJ, USA, 2021; pp. 53–73.
85. Sommers, C.H.; Fan, X. *Food Irradiation Research and Technology*; Blackwell Publishing Professional: Ames, IA, USA, 2007; pp. 1–317.
86. European Union. Directive 1999/3/EC of the European Parliament and of the Council of 22 February 1999 on the establishment of a Community list of foods and food ingredients treated with ionising radiation. Consolidated version 22 February 1999. *Off. J. Fur. Communities* **1999**, *13*, 24–25.
87. D'Souza, C.; Apaolaza, V.; Hartmann, P.; Brouwer, A.R.; Nguyen, N. Consumer acceptance of irradiated food and information disclosure—A retail imperative. *J. Retail. Consum. Serv.* **2021**, *63*, 102699. [CrossRef]
88. Diella, G.; Caggiano, G.; Ferrieri, F.; Ventrella, A.; Palma, M.; Napoli, C.; Rutigliano, S.; Lopuzzo, M.; Lovero, G.; Montagna, M.T. Aflatoxin contamination in nuts marketed in italy: Preliminary results. *Ann. Ig.* **2018**, *30*, 401–409.
89. Ebrahimi, A.; Emadi, A.; Arabameri, M.; Jayedi, A.; Abdolshahi, A.; Yancheshmeh, B.S.; Shariatifar, N. The prevalence of aflatoxins in different nut samples: A global systematic review and probabilistic risk assessment. *AIMS Agric. Food* **2022**, *7*, 130–148. [CrossRef]
90. Macri, A.M.; Pop, I.; Simeanu, D.; Toma, D.; Sandu, I.; Pavel, L.L.; Mintas, O.S. The occurrence of aflatoxins in nuts and dry nuts packed in four different plastic packaging from the romanian market. *Microorganisms* **2021**, *9*, 61. [CrossRef] [PubMed]

91. Chiou, R.Y.; Lin, C.M.; Shyu, S.L. Property characterization of peanut kernels subjected to gamma irradiation and its effect on the outgrowth and aflatoxin production by *Aspergillus parasiticus*. *J. Food Sci.* **1990**, *55*, 210–213. [CrossRef]
92. Aziz, N.H.; Moussa, L.A.A.; Far, F.M.E. Reduction of fungi and mycotoxins formation in seeds by gamma-radiation. *J. Food Saf.* **2004**, *24*, 109–127. [CrossRef]
93. Prakash, A. Irradiation of nuts. In *Food Irradiation Research and Technology*, 2nd ed.; Blackwell Publishing Professional: Ames, IA, USA, 2012; pp. 317–336.
94. Song, W.J.; Kim, Y.H.; Kang, D.H. Effect of gamma irradiation on inactivation of *Escherichia coli* O157:H7, *Salmonella* Typhimurium and *Listeria monocytogenes* on pistachios. *Lett. Appl. Microbiol.* **2019**, *68*, 96–102. [CrossRef]
95. Shahidi, F.; John, J.A. 9-oxidative rancidity in nuts. In *Improving the Safety and Quality of Nuts*; Harris, L.J., Ed.; Woodhead Publishing: Soston, UK, 2013; pp. 198–229.
96. Yaacoub, R.; Saliba, R.; Nsouli, B.; Khalaf, G.; Birlouez-Aragon, I. Formation of lipid oxidation and isomerization products during processing of nuts and sesame seeds. *J. Agric. Food. Chem.* **2008**, *56*, 7082–7090. [CrossRef]
97. O'Mahony, M.; Wong, S.Y.; Odbert, N. Initial sensory examination of the effect of postharvest irradiation on almonds. *J. Ind. Irrad. Technol.* **1985**, *3*, 135–140.
98. Thomas, P. Radiation preservation of foods of plant origin. Part vi. Mushrooms, tomatoes, minor fruits and vegetables, dried fruits, and nuts. *Crit. Rev. Food Sci. Nutr.* **1988**, *26*, 313–358. [CrossRef]
99. Wilson-Kakashita, G.; Gerdes, D.L.; Hall, W.R. The effect of gamma irradiation on the quality of english walnuts (*Juglans regia*). *LWT* **1995**, *28*, 17–20. [CrossRef]
100. Mexis, S.F.; Kontominas, M.G. Effect of γ-irradiation on the physicochemical and sensory properties of cashew nuts (*Anacardium occidentale* L.). *LWT* **2009**, *42*, 1501–1507. [CrossRef]
101. Taipina, M.S.; Lamardo, L.C.A.; Rodas, M.A.B.; del Mastro, N.L. The effects of gamma irradiation on the vitamin e content and sensory qualities of pecan nuts (*Carya illinoensis*). *Radiat. Phys. Chem.* **2009**, *78*, 611–613. [CrossRef]
102. Gölge, E.; Ova, G. The effects of food irradiation on quality of pine nut kernels. *Radiat. Phys. Chem.* **2008**, *77*, 365–369. [CrossRef]
103. Koç Güler, S.; Bostan, S.Z.; Çon, A.H. Effects of gamma irradiation on chemical and sensory characteristics of natural hazelnut kernels. *Postharvest Biol. Technol.* **2017**, *123*, 12–21. [CrossRef]
104. Sánchez-Bel, P.; Egea, I.; Romojaro, F.; Martínez-Madrid, M.C. Sensorial and chemical quality of electron beam irradiated almonds (*Prunus amygdalus*). *LWT* **2008**, *41*, 442–449. [CrossRef]
105. Noguera-Artiaga, L.; Salvador, M.D.; Fregapane, G.; Collado-González, J.; Wojdyło, A.; López-Lluch, D.; Carbonell-Barrachina, Á.A. Functional and sensory properties of pistachio nuts as affected by cultivar. *J. Sci. Food Agric.* **2019**, *99*, 6696–6705. [CrossRef] [PubMed]
106. Alinezhad, M.; Hojjati, M.; Barzegar, H.; Shahbazi, S.; Askari, H. Effect of gamma irradiation on the physicochemical properties of pistachio (*Pistacia vera* L.) nuts. *J. Food Meas. Charact.* **2021**, *15*, 199–209. [CrossRef]
107. Frankel, E.N. Volatile lipid oxidation products. *Prog. Lipid Res.* **1983**, *22*, 1–33. [CrossRef]
108. Bourke, P.; Ziuzina, D.; Han, L.; Cullen, P.J.; Gilmore, B.F. Microbiological interactions with cold plasma. *J. Appl. Microbiol.* **2017**, *123*, 308–324. [CrossRef]
109. Misra, N.N.; Schlüter, O.; Cullen, P.J. Chapter 1—plasma in food and agriculture. In *Cold Plasma in Food and Agriculture*; Misra, N.N., Schlüter, O., Cullen, P.J., Eds.; Academic Press: San Diego, CA, USA, 2016; pp. 1–16.
110. Mir, S.A.; Siddiqui, M.W.; Dar, B.N.; Shah, M.A.; Wani, M.H.; Roohinejad, S.; Annor, G.A.; Mallikarjunan, K.; Chin, C.F.; Ali, A. Promising applications of cold plasma for microbial safety, chemical decontamination and quality enhancement in fruits. *J. Appl. Microbiol.* **2020**, *129*, 474–485. [CrossRef]
111. Bora, J.; Khan, T.; Mahnot, N.K. Cold plasma treatment concerning quality and safety of food: A review. *Curr. Res. Nutr. Food Sci.* **2022**, *10*, 427–446. [CrossRef]
112. Pignata, C.; D'Angelo, D.; Fea, E.; Gilli, G. A review on microbiological decontamination of fresh produce with nonthermal plasma. *J. Appl. Microbiol.* **2017**, *122*, 1438–1455. [CrossRef]
113. Deng, S.; Ruan, R.; Mok, C.K.; Huang, G.; Lin, X.; Chen, P. Inactivation of *Escherichia coli* on almonds using nonthermal plasma. *J. Food Sci.* **2007**, *72*, M62–M66. [CrossRef] [PubMed]
114. Hertwig, C.; Leslie, A.; Meneses, N.; Reineke, K.; Rauh, C.; Schlüter, O. Inactivation of *Salmonella enteritidis pt30* on the surface of unpeeled almonds by cold plasma. *Innov. Food Sci. Emerg. Technol.* **2017**, *44*, 242–248. [CrossRef]
115. Khalili, F.; Shokri, B.; Khani, M.-R.; Hasani, M.; Zandi, F.; Aliahmadi, A. A study of the effect of gliding arc non-thermal plasma on almonds decontamination. *AIP Adv.* **2018**, *8*, 105024. [CrossRef]
116. Shirani, K.; Shahidi, F.; Mortazavi, S.A. Investigation of decontamination effect of argon cold plasma on physicochemical and sensory properties of almond slices. *Int. J. Food Microbiol.* **2020**, *335*, 108892. [CrossRef]
117. Makari, M.; Hojjati, M.; Shahbazi, S.; Askari, H. Elimination of *Aspergillus flavus* from pistachio nuts with dielectric barrier discharge (dbd) cold plasma and its impacts on biochemical indices. *J. Food Qual.* **2021**, *2021*, 9968711. [CrossRef]
118. Ghorashi, A.H.; Tasouji, M.A.R.; Kargarian, A. Optimum cold plasma generating device for treatment of *Aspergillus flavus* from nuts surface. *J. Food Sci. Technol.* **2020**, *57*, 3988–3994. [CrossRef]
119. Tasouji, M.A.; Ghorashi, A.H.; Hamedmoosavian, M.T.; Mahmoudi, M.B. Inactivation of pistachio contaminant *Aspergillus flavus* by atmospheric pressure capacitive coupled plasma (ap-ccp). *J. Microbiol. Biotechnol. Food Sci.* **2018**, *8*, 668–671. [CrossRef]

120. Pignata, C.; D'Angelo, D.; Basso, D.; Cavallero, M.C.; Beneventi, S.; Tartaro, D.; Meineri, V.; Gilli, G. Low-temperature, low-pressure gas plasma application on *Aspergillus brasiliensis, Escherichia coli* and pistachios. *J. Appl. Microbiol.* **2014**, *116*, 1137–1148. [CrossRef]
121. Lin, C.-M.; Patel, A.K.; Chiu, Y.-C.; Hou, C.-Y.; Kuo, C.-H.; Dong, C.-D.; Chen, H.-L. The application of novel rotary plasma jets to inhibit the aflatoxin-producing *Aspergillus flavus* and the spoilage fungus, *Aspergillus niger* on peanuts. *Innov. Food Sci. Emerg. Technol.* **2022**, *78*, 102994. [CrossRef]
122. Ahangari, M.; Ramezan, Y.; Khani, M.R. Effect of low pressure cold plasma treatment on microbial decontamination and physicochemical properties of dried walnut kernels (*Juglans regia* L.). *J. Food Process Eng.* **2021**, *44*, e13593. [CrossRef]

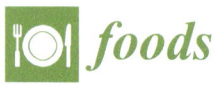

Review

From the Raw Materials to the Bottled Product: Influence of the Entire Production Process on the Organoleptic Profile of Industrial Beers

Ana Belén Díaz [1], Enrique Durán-Guerrero [2,*], Cristina Lasanta [1] and Remedios Castro [2]

[1] Chemical Engineering and Food Technology Department, Faculty of Sciences-IVAGRO, University of Cadiz, Agrifood Campus of International Excellence (CeiA3), Polígono Río San Pedro, s/n, 11510 Puerto Real, Cadiz, Spain

[2] Analytical Chemistry Department, Faculty of Sciences-IVAGRO, University of Cadiz, Agrifood Campus of International Excellence (CeiA3), Polígono Río San Pedro, s/n, 11510 Puerto Real, Cadiz, Spain

* Correspondence: enrique.duranguerrero@uca.es; Tel.: +34-956-016456

Abstract: In the past few years, there has been a growing demand by consumers for more complex beers with distinctive organoleptic profiles. The yeast, raw material (barley or other cereals), hops, and water used add to the major processing stages involved in the brewing process, including malting, mashing, boiling, fermentation, and aging, to significantly determine the sensory profile of the final product. Recent literature on this subject has paid special attention to the impact attributable to the processing conditions and to the fermentation yeast strains used on the aromatic compounds that are found in consumer-ready beers. However, no review papers are available on the specific influence of each of the factors that may affect beer organoleptic characteristics. This review, therefore, focuses on the effect that raw material, as well as the rest of the processes other than alcoholic fermentation, have on the organoleptic profile of beers. Such effect may alter beer aromatic compounds, foaming head, taste, or mouthfeel, among other things. Moreover, the presence of spoilage microorganisms that might lead to consumers' rejection because of their impact on the beers' sensory properties has also been investigated.

Keywords: brewing; maturation; aging; spoilage microorganisms; sensory properties

1. Introduction

Beer is one of the most popular and commonly consumed alcoholic beverages worldwide. However, a remarkable transition has been taking place regarding consumers' preference for traditional 'tasteless' beers, to more complex craft beers, with a growing quota of consumers being interested in new beer styles that exhibit novel sensory characteristics [1]. In addition, a growing consumer segment, comprising people between 21 and 30 years old, seems to be interested in new beer tastes and is willing to pay for these tasty beers, even if more expensive [2]. For this reason, brewers and researchers are investigating the use of alternative raw materials and processing conditions over the different stages of beer brewing so that its organoleptic profile is enhanced [3].

Conventional brewing consists of four main processes: malting, during which enzyme production is activated and endosperm is modified; mashing, during which enzymes hydrolyze starch into fermentable sugars and proteins into aminoacids; boiling, during which resins undergo thermal isomerization and yield bitter taste; fermentation, during which sugars are converted into ethanol [4], and, finally, maturation and bottling (Figure 1). Beer has been traditionally made from malted barley (*Hordeum vulgare*), hops (*Humulus lupulus* L.), water, and yeast. It can also be supplemented with other cereals or sources of sugars known as adjuncts [5,6].

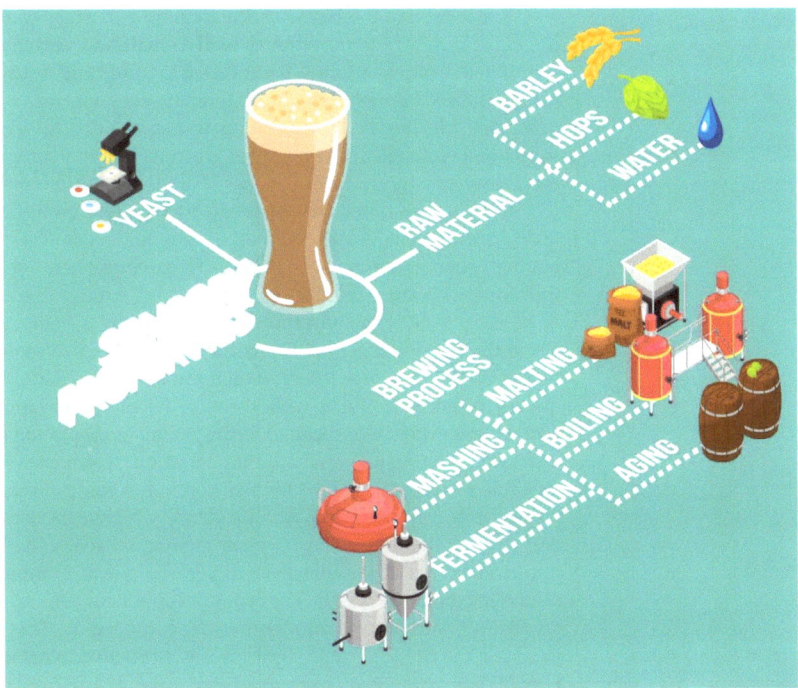

Figure 1. Main factors in the brewing process that have an influence on the sensory properties of beer.

The sensory characteristics of beers play an important role in consumers' acceptance or rejection. As a consequence of this, the number of articles published regarding beer, as well as the number of sensory studies, have increased significantly in the last few years (Figure 2). Beer properties are affected by the variety of barley, yeast, and hops used. Hops provide beers with fruity, spicy, resinous, floral, and wood aromas [7,8].

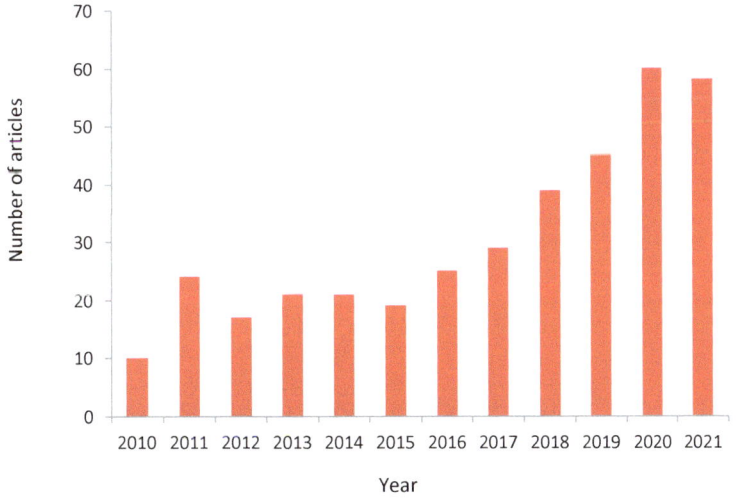

Figure 2. Evolution of the number of works published in Scopus using "beer" and "sensory analysis" as keywords.

Regardless of the Bavarian Purity Law and other country-specific legislations, grain blends and new hop varieties, as well as fruit and vegetables, have been incorporated in recent years into beer brewing in order to modify its sensory profile [9,10]. Such sensory profile is also influenced by the different processing stages involved in the whole brewing practice, including beer maturation and aging. In addition to this, bottle re-fermentation increases beer's effervescence and, given its low oxygen levels due to yeast consumption, the volatile compounds that are associated with off-flavors may be developed [11,12].

It should be noted that between 1000 to 2000 compounds have been found in beers, including alcohols, esters, ketones, aldehydes, organic acids, carboxylic acids, sulfur compounds, phenols, amines, etc. [13,14]. These components are the result of complex reactions that involve a large variety of compounds. Among these, volatile compounds seem to have a key role regarding the aromatic profile of beer, while non-volatile ones, including anthocyanins and phenolic components, affect other sensory attributes such as color, foaming, taste, or mouthfeel, which are also considered as relevant contributors to the quality of beer [15]. It is well known that the abundance of a large number of aroma-active compounds is associated with specific fermentation conditions and to the particular yeast strain being used, which may yield interesting aroma components, such as higher alcohols or esters [16,17]. Other nitrogenous compounds, which may include proteins, polypeptides, amino acids, etc., are also key factors, because they contribute to beer flavor and drinkability, as well as to haze formation, foam stability, and color [18,19]. From a nutritional point of view, beer is rich in carbohydrates, amino acids, vitamins, minerals, and phenolic compounds [20]. The main polyphenols present in beer are flavonoids, tannins, proanthocyanidins, and amino phenolic compounds. These come from the malt and hops used for the brewing and significantly affect the color, flavor, and stability of the final beer [21].

Given beer's considerable concentration of ethanol (0.5–10%), the presence of bitter compounds from hops (~17–55 ppm iso-α-acids), its low pH (3.8–4.7), and its high CO_2 concentration (~0.5% w/w), it represents an inhospitable environment for most microorganisms [22]. However, some spoilage microorganisms, including Gram-positive and Gram-negative bacteria, as well as wild yeasts, are able to grow and cause some undesirable changes in beer's sensory profile. *Lactobacillus* and *Pediococcus* are considered to be the most hazardous bacteria for beer production processes, as they account for around 70% of the microbial spoilage incidents [23].

All these facts considered, it seems rather clear that, in order to produce beer with a variety of sensory profiles that meet current consumers' preferences, brewers may opt for a diversity of raw materials as well as adjuncts, adjust their brewing procedures, or select different yeast strains. The alcoholic fermentation process, being perhaps the most influential factor regarding the sensory characteristics of the final beer, has been investigated in a previous review [24]. Thus, the present review intends to delve into the rest of the potential factors that may affect the organoleptic profile of beers. Such factors have been identified as the main raw materials (barley, water, and hops), as well as the rest of the processes, other than the alcoholic fermentation, involved in beer production—specifically malting, mashing, boiling, maturation, and aging. Any likely effects from a variety of spoilage microorganisms have also been taken into consideration

2. Barley, Malt and Malting

Barley (*Hordeum vulgare* L.) is the most commonly used cereal in beer production, and its endosperm represents the main tissue of the grain, which is mainly composed of starch granules (62.7% of the total grain weight) embedded in a protein matrix [25,26]. Other cereals, such as wheat, rye, oat, triticale, sorghum, maize, etc., can also be used as raw material for beer production [27], as long as we are aware that this procedure may affect the sensory properties of the final beer. It is true that the usage of other cereals may confer beer with new properties and organoleptic features. However, at the same time, the incorporation of new cereals that do not contain the necessary enzymes may involve certain technological issues related to mash lautering, beer filtration, extract recovery, or production forecasting and scaling [28]. As an example, let us mention wheat beer, which is especially consumed in Bavaria and Austria and is characterized by clove-like, banana-like, vanilla, and fresh fruit scents [29,30]. Sorghum beers are described as one of the most subtle beers with regard to their sensory properties and mild taste [31]. Another study where different proportions of sorghum were used concluded that these beers have a lower acetaldehyde and ester content, and a greater proportion of higher alcohols [32]. The same authors described the beers that contained between 30 and 40% oat as better beverages in terms of aroma and taste purity than 100% malted barley beers, which contain lower amounts of lactones and higher alcohols, and a greater proportion of esters [33]. Other studies have concluded that different unmalted cereal adjuncts can replace malted barley at rates of up to 40–60% to produce beers with a sensory profile comparable to that of 100% malted barley beers [21,34].

Different barley genotypes lead to different chemical compositions, i.e., different enzymes and metabolites and, therefore, unequal results are expected from similar malting procedures [35,36]. Beers with higher fruity, floral, and grassy flavors are produced from Golden Promise barley—a classic British spring barley variety with a light malty flavor and beautiful mouthfeel—whereas other beers that are rich in toffee and toasted flavors, while exhibiting lower harshness or astringency, are obtained from Full Pint barley [37]. In this sense, CDC Copeland barley, a two-rowed malting barley, produces neutral flavors and pale colored beers. It has also been reported that, depending on the "terroir" where barley is grown, beers with different flavors can also be obtained [38].

The quality of the barley grain used as raw material is, therefore, another very important factor and it largely depends on agronomic practices, as well as on genetic and environmental variables [39]. Moreover, grain is required to present the adequate plumpness and kernel weight, with a high germination potential ($\geq$95%) and the appropriate protein content. In this regard, barley's protein content should be below 11%, otherwise the proteins that are soluble in wort may confer off-flavors to the final product. Moreover, high protein concentrations traditionally correlate with low carbohydrate levels and lower extract yields. The quality of barley may also be altered by microbial infections, being fungi the most commonly found microorganisms. These can infect barley while in the fields, especially during its wet growing season, while it may infect barley or malt while in storage under moist conditions. Primary gushing is associated with the use of defective malted barley, when harvested under wet conditions, while secondary gushing may be caused by solid particles, which may arise from various sources (dust polluted containers, faulty filtration, haze particles developing in aged beer, etc.), or adsorbed gas residues acting as nuclei for bubble formation. [40]. Primary gushing is derived from the use of malt made from barley spoiled by fungal contamination, especially by certain species of the genus *Fusarium*, which produces hydrophobins, a type of hydrophobic polypeptides that can induce this phenomenon through their interaction with CO_2 molecules [41–44]. *Fusarium* spp. and other fungal pathogens of barley can produce mycotoxins that can survive the brewing process and can, therefore, be found in the final beer [16,44].

Malt contamination with *Aspergillus fumigatus* has been proven to be responsible for a noticeable rancid taste of beer [45]. Fungi growth on malt also has a negative effect on beer foam quality, because of the β-glucanases and xylanases produced that decrease the viscosity of the wort [16]. These and other negative aspects of the fungi that may grow on barley represent a hazard for the organoleptic properties of beer that may lead to consumers' rejection [46]. Barley is also the vehicle for a variety of contaminating microorganisms other than fungi or molds and that may negatively affect the germination of barley prior to malting. *Clostridium* and *Bacillus* bacteria, which are generally associated with the production of butyric acid and sulfides, are amongst these other polluting organisms [47]. An excessive moisture level after completing the kilning or malting roasting process should be avoided if certain barley pollutants are to be prevented. In other words, proper storage and preservation procedures for the barley and the malted barley are crucial factors [16].

Barley is subjected to malting in order to solubilize the proteins and to break down the starch into fermentable sugars. Specific malting procedures also provide beer with characteristic colors and flavors [48]. During the malting process, the grains undergo chemical and structural changes that result in the generation of a number of precursors that will determine the organoleptic properties of the final beer, including its color, aroma, and flavor [49].

The malting process usually involves steeping, germination, and kilning. During the steeping process, cold water (10–15 °C) and oxygen are supplied into hygienic and calibrated kernels in order to maintain moisture levels at approximately 38–45% and promote the germination of the grains. At this stage, the grains' endosperm cell walls and its proteins are broken through the action of certain enzymes, such as protease, amylase, or β-glucanase [50,51]. Different aspect of this process can be improved in several ways, as follows: using standardized seeds to achieve a uniform germination; using plump kernels to achieve maximum malt extract yields; and low protein content to attain higher extract levels and to enhance beer stability [52]. The quality of the malting process can be evaluated through 'fine-grind', which allows measurement of the soluble malt material, including fermentable sugars [53]. Other quality parameters used to evaluate the quality of the malting are kernel size fraction, kernel weight, protein contents, β-glucan, α-amylase activity, viscosity, and soluble nitrogen ratio [54]. Some malt-quality indicators are shown in Table 1 [55].

Table 1. Malt-quality indicators.

Quality Indicator	Recommended Values
Protein content	<10.8%
Kolbach index	38–34%
Extract content	>82%
Extract difference	1.2–1.8%
Viscosity	<1.55 mPa·s
β-glucan in wort	<300 mg/L
Wort color	<3.4 EBC

Germination is ended by drying the grains (moisture content down to 3–4%) through a gradual increment of the temperature from 50 to roughly 85 °C or more (kilning). The kilning process has a crucial impact on beer color and flavor [51], mainly as a result of Maillard reaction, which produces maltoxazine, maltol, isomaltol, and ethyl maltol, among other substances responsible for the caramel, bread, or cotton candy-like flavors in beer [56]. Therefore, through the control of the temperature, Maillard reaction can be adjusted to determine color formation and obtain different types of malt (base, caramel, special, amber, chocolate, or black) [26], which will result in variations of the compounds responsible for wort flavor and for the different organoleptic profiles of the final beers [36,57]. It should also be noted that the melanoidins generated through Maillard reactions may promote the growth of certain undesirable microorganisms. In fact, melanoidins have been used as antimicrobial agents against different pathogenic bacteria strains [58]. Apart from melanoidins, certain malt alkaloids, mainly hordatines, have also been proven to have an influence on beer flavor by increasing its astringency [59,60].

With the aim of reducing the carbon footprint associated with malt production, and given the large energy demand of kilning processes, some recent studies have focused on the usage of undried germinated (green) malt. Even though further studies would be required, the beers that have already been obtained through this methodology presented acceptable specifications with regard to color, pH, alcohol content, and foam stability [61].

Nowadays, brewers can use base malts (e.g., pilsen and pale), specialty malts, and roasted malts in order to produce beers with different flavors [37]. Uniquely flavored and colored beers have been obtained from specialty malts such as Crystal malt (also known as caramel malt), Brown malt, Cara malt, or Black malt, among others [62]. During the roasting operations when using these singular malts, some compounds, such as maltol and isomaltol, can be generated [63], which results in a sweet aroma of the final beer. These malts do not only add color, flavor, and antioxidant activity to wort and beer, but also affect the course of wort fermentation and the production of flavor-active yeast metabolites, such as vicinal diketones or esters [64]. Dark malts may improve foam stability and the mouthfeel of beer, presumably because of the presence of melanoidins [62].

Another aspect to be taken into consideration in relation to malt is that some lactic bacteria can be added in certain cases during the malting and mashing processes, because they compete against natural microflora, thus restricting the growth of certain harmful microorganisms such as fungi or bacteria [65]. Their preservation qualities are associated with the production of some organic acids, such as lactic or acetic acids, together with hydrogen peroxide and bacteriocins [66]. Moreover, bio-acidification increases malt yield and improves malt quality by decreasing its viscosity and shortening the time required for lautering and wort filtration. It has also been demonstrated to improve beer sensory quality and stability [67]. Lactic acid bacteria also produces other organoleptically active compounds besides lactic acid, including organic acids and esters, such as ethyl acetate, aldehydes, higher alcohols, ketones, phenolic, or heterocyclic compounds, and more [68–70].

3. Mashing and Wort

Mashing is an enzymatic process that produces sugars from malt to obtain wort, which is in turn fermented to produce beer. During this stage, the amylases, β-glucanases, and proteases degrade carbohydrates, β-glucans, and proteins, respectively. Their activities are affected by the temperature, pH, and composition of the solution, as well as by the processing time [71]. The action of these enzymes results in a final beer that contains a small amount of residual fermentable sugars (maltose being the most abundant one), a variable amount of dextrins, such as maltodextrin, and a small amount of peptides, which have an influence on the sensory properties and the palate fullness of the final beer.

Water is one of the most important ingredients during this mashing stage, because it represents most of the beer's composition. The chemical composition of water, as well as the presence of pathogenic and/or non-pathogenic microorganisms, also has a considerable influence on the final result, so that it may even spoil beer to the point of rendering it unsuitable for human consumption [72].

The mineral composition of wort and beer, where the principal cations, such as calcium, magnesium, sodium, and potassium, as well as anions, such as sulfate, nitrate, phosphate, chlorides, and silicate, may also determine beer quality. The minor ions are iron, copper, zinc, and manganese [73]. Ions are necessary for the correct course of the fermentation process and for the growth of beneficial microorganisms [74], but also contribute directly to the flavor of beers as non-volatile taste-active compounds [75]. The mineral composition of the wort also depends on the nature of the raw materials [76]. Therefore, this factor must be taken into consideration when using cereals other tan malt.

As an example, Briggs et al. [26] established that the presence of calcium ions in the water used to make beer had a relevant influence on the mashing process and affected final beer flavor. According to Montanari et al. [73], calcium has the capacity to extract fine bittering principles from the hops and to reduce wort color, while sodium contributes to the perceived flavor of the beer by enhancing its sweetness. Other authors [77] have observed that "hard water" (with a high concentrations of salts; pH 8.47 ± 0.08) seemed to be a better extractor of the total carbohydrate content and B vitamins (riboflavin and niacin) than soft water (with a low concentrations of dissolved salts; pH 7.68 ± 0.23), whereas organic acid and iso-α-acid concentrations were not influenced by water pH values. It is a fact that the composition of wort has a great influence on the molecules that result from the fermentation process and, consequently, on the organoleptic profile of final beers. Therefore, as an example, wort sugar content levels and free amino nitrogen and lipids, as well as aeration [78] or temperature [79], are parameters that condition the subsequent production of aromatic esters by the microbiota [80,81]. Sucrose, fructose, glucose, maltose, maltotriose, and some dextrins, with maltose and maltotriose as the most abundant ones, are the main sugars that can be found in wort. Their concentrations depend on the characteristics of the barley and on the malting process [20].

Wort is also moderately rich in amino acids, peptides, and proteins [72]. Some amino acids are required for the healthy growing of yeast. Such amino acids, together with certain small peptides, constitute what is known as Free Amino Nitrogen (FAN). Total FAN is important for the fermentation (via yeast nutrition) and the stability of flavor. A high FAN content may affect beer flavor stability because of the production of vicinal diketones (VDK) such as diacetyl and 2,3-pentanedione, through the differential utilization of amino acids (valine and isoleucine, respectively) by yeast, which may provide beer with a butter- or butterscotch-like flavor or toffee-like flavor, respectively [82].

The releasing of free amino nitrogen and reducing sugars during the mashing stage contributes to a minor set of flavor precursors that can develop during the Maillard reaction, principally during wort boiling [83]. They are transformed during the mashing stage and through the metabolism of the yeasts during the fermentation stage into other new substances that contribute to the organoleptic profile of beer [17,84].

During mashing, a key cascade reaction is also initiated, where the products from lipid oxidation generate hydroperoxides that form active volatile compounds [83].

On the other hand, during this stage, unmalted adjuncts such as rice, wheat, corn, honey, or fruit can be added as an alternative cost-efficient source of extract that enables the production of innovative products that increase the content of bioactive compounds and generate unique flavors and bitterness and improve mouthfeel [5,85,86]. It has been observed that when rice is used in the brewing process, it provides neutral, clean, and dry sensory characteristics, whereas adding corn results in a fuller mouthfeel [87].

More sour, grainy, and sweet corn aroma beers were obtained when 60% torrefied maize was added to the wort [34]. The addition of unmalted barley at up to 50% resulted in beers with a preference rating that was comparable, with regard to odor and taste, to that of all-malt beers [88]. In contrast, when the added unmalted barley reached 90%, it resulted in more astringent beers, while 100% unmalted barley produced final beers with less body and mouthfeel [89].

Certain extracts from medicinal plants can also be added to the wort in order to produce beers with unique sensory characteristics and an increased concentration of various bioactive compounds, such as phenols [90].

4. Hops

Resins and essential oils can be found in the lupulin glands of female hop flowers, which, even when used in small amounts, contribute to bitterness and aroma (sensorially characterized by descriptors such as 'fruity', 'floral', 'spicy', 'herbal', or 'woody') [91,92]. In fact, hops are the main ingredient responsible for the bitterness of beer because of their polyphenols and α-acids contributions [93–95]. Hops contain a complex mixture of volatile compounds (essential oils), among which linalool, geraniol, and 4-methyl-4-sulfanylpentan-2-one are of particular importance [96].

Hop varieties can be classified as aroma hops, dual-purpose hops (aromatic and bitter), and bittering hops (very bitter) [97]. Saaz and the rest of the "noble hops"—Hallertauer Mittelfrüh, Tettnang, and Spalt—belong to the first category and are traditionally used for pilsners and lagers produced in the Bavaria and Bohemia regions. Another Saaz aroma hop, Styrian Goldings, is often preferred for Belgian-style ales. Bitter (high α-acid) or dual-purpose hops such as Citra, Centennial, Cascade, or Amarillo, among others, are typically used for American IPAs [98].

During wort boiling, the humulones (α-acids) that are found in the soft resins of hops are isomerized into isohumulones, which are the main components responsible for the bitterness of beer [99]. It has also been recently observed that the oxidized forms of humulones, humulinones that are present in dry-hopped and hop-forward beers, can also contribute to beer bitterness [100].

During wort boiling, the majority of the volatiles derived from hops are lost through evaporation. Thus, by the late addition of multiple dosages, we can obtain beers with hop aroma but without any extra hop bitterness. So, for a less bitter beer, hops can be added toward the end of the wort boiling stage, or to the whirlpool (late hopping) or to green and bright beer (dry-hopping) [101]. The flavor descriptors that are most often detected in late hopped beers are spicy, noble, herbal, woody, and, to a lesser extent, estery or fruity. Dry-hopping consists of the cold extraction of volatile and non-volatile hop compounds. This technique is widely employed by brewers to increase the aroma and stability of beer flavor [102]. The descriptors that are most frequently found in dry-hopped beers are floral, citrus, or pine [103,104]. Unlike in boiling hopping, dry-hopping does not allow for the thermal isomerization of the α-acids into iso-α-acids, which makes beer more prone to microbial instability [105]. Recent investigations on the microbial contamination hazards associated with dry-hopping techniques have detected spore-forming bacteria such as *Bacillus* spp., as well as Enterobacteriaceae, yeast, and fungi [106].

There is also evidence that the amylolytic enzymes present in hops can biochemically modify dry-hopping beer, which may lead to the degradation of long-chain, unfermentable dextrins into fermentable sugars [107]. This increase in fermentable sugars can, in the presence of yeast, give rise to a slow secondary fermentation, which is referred to as "hop creep" [108]. "Hop creep" represents a problem for brewers, because it modifies the specific density, flavor profile, and alcohol content of beers. Bruner et al. [109] revealed that hop creep resulted in 1.06% (v/v) alcohol increments in dry-hopped lager beers and 0.88% (v/v) in ale ones, over 30 day periods.

Beer aroma can also be modified by adding pure aroma hop extract [110]. Moreover, the addition of hop extracts to unhoped beer has been demonstrated to improve mouthfeel and fullness while increasing the bitter perception of beer [111]. Hop extracts are also commonly added for extra bitterness and to obtain a greater content of aromatic compounds from the different stages of the brewing process [112].

Even though hops have been extensively used since ancient times, they are susceptible to being replaced by other substances that can also provide those molecules responsible for the bitterness of beer, such as artichoke, carqueja, etc. The resulting beers have a similar sensory acceptance to that of commercial beers [113]. While hop oils contribute to beer flavor, the biotransformation of its glycosides [114] not only adds new flavors to the final beer but also plays a significant role in beer flavor stability [115,116].

The type and relative proportions of the molecules provided by the hops (hop bitter acids, phenolic acids, polyphenolic compounds, or volatile compounds) will vary depending on the hop variety. So, once again, genetics plays a relevant role in the process and determines the resulting sensory characteristics, especially with regard to the bitterness and aroma of the final beer [94,95,110,117]. Together with its genetics, the maturity level of hops will also determine the kind of contribution that they make toward a particular flavor or aroma [118,119]. There are also non-volatile compounds in hops, including carboxylic acids, resins, amino acids, carbohydrates, and polyphenols, which are known to have an influence on the taste and mouthfeel characteristics of beer [101,114]. Regarding the polyphenolic fraction, the most important groups of low molecular weight polyphenols present in hops are usually hydroxybenzoic acids, hydroxycinnamic acids, proanthocyanidins, monomeric flavanols, free flavanols, quercetin, kaempferol, and xanthohumol. The composition of polyphenols in beers are, once again, significantly determined by the hop variety used for brewing [120]. Furthermore, their concentration as well as the iso-α-acids content in the wort also varies with the temperature at which the hops are boiled, the boiling time, and the time of hopping [93,121–123]. These iso-α-acids exhibit antimicrobial activity, which means that they can inhibit the growth of some of the contaminating microorganisms that spoil the flavor of beer, acting therefore as preservatives [124]. In fact, the most common microbes responsible for beer spoilage are Gram-positive bacteria, which can actually be inhibited by hops. However, hops do not have the capacity to inhibit the growth of Gram-negative bacteria, such as *Pectinatus frisingensis*, *Pectinatus cerevisiiphilus*, or *Megasphera cerevisiae* [125,126]. Table 2 includes the most frequent microorganisms responsible for beer spoilage.

Table 2. Most common spoilage microorganisms in beer.

	Microorganisms		Compounds Produced	Spoilage Effect	References
Mold	*Aspergillus* sp.	*A. fumigatus*	Mycotoxins	Rancid taste, roughness, stale and moldy flavor	[125,127]
	Fusarium sp.	*F. graminearum* *F. culmorum*	Mycotoxins, hydrophobins, and hydrophobic polypeptides	Gushing	[41,43,46,125]
Yeast	*Brettanomyces* sp.	*B. bruxellensis*	Acetic acid, highly volatile phenolic compounds	Sweat, smoke, and cheese flavors	[128]
		B. anomalus	Tetrahydropyridines	Mousy off-flavor	[129,130]
	Megasphaera sp.	*M. cerevisiae*	Butyric acid, acetic, caproic, isovaleric and valeric acids, acetoin and hydrogen sulphide	Turbidity and off flavors (hydrogen sulphide)	[125]
	Saccharomyces sp.	*S. cerevisiae* var. *diastaticus*	Extracellular glucoamylase	Phenolic off-flavors, overcarbonation, and weakened body	[131,132]
	Wickerhamomyces sp.	*Wickerhamomyces anomalus*	Phenyl ethanol, ethyl propanoate, 2-phenylethyl acetate, and ethyl acetate	Solvent-like aroma	[133]
Bacteria Gram +	*Clostridium* sp.	*C. acetobutylicum*, *C. butyricum*, *C. pasteurianum*, *C. thermosaccharolyticum*	Butyric, propionic, valeric, caproic acids, sulfur compounds	Cheesy, buttery, putrid, and rancid aroma	[16,47,134,135]
	Lactobacillus sp.	*L. brevis*, *L. acetotolerans*, *L. casei*, *L. plantarum* *L. lindneri*	Lactic acid, acetic acid, and diacetyl	Buttery' taste and oily mouthfeel, Turbidity and super-attenuation problems	[136–140]
	Pediococcus sp.	*P. damnosus*	Lactic acid, diacetyl	Sediments, reduced foam stability, sarcina sickness	[125]
Bacteria Gram −	*Acetobacter* sp.	*A. aceti*, *A. hansenii*, *A. liquefaciens*, *A. pasteurianus*	Acetic acid	Ropiness, sour and vinegary flavor	[126,141]
	Gluconobacter sp.	*G. oxydans*	Acetic acid	Cidery note, sour and vinegary flavor	[142]
	Pectinatus sp.	*P. frisingensis*, *P. cerevisiiphilus*	Acetic acid, propionic acid, acetoin, hydrogen sulfide, and methyl mercaptan	Rotten egg, cooked vegetable aromas	[141]

5. Maturation, Storage, and Bottling

Beer is an unstable product whose composition can change during storage and bottling [36] through different types of reaction. Table 3 shows the effects of maturation storage and bottling on the sensory properties of beer.

Table 3. Maturation, storage, and bottling effects that affect the sensory properties of beer.

Stage	Effect	References
Maturation and storage	Extracting wood compounds derived from maturation in oak casks Reducing some off-flavor compounds from previous stages Generally, reducing bitterness and increasing sweetness Increasing volatile compounds Producing microbial compounds that alter beer taste, such as methyl mercaptan, dimethyl sulfoxide, hydrogen sulfide, etc., that promote carbonation, turbidity, superficial films, and excessive viscosity Generating compounds derived from oxidation, including higher alcohols, unsaturated fatty acids, amino acids, and proteins that modify beer flavor	[45,93,126,143–148]
Bottling	Generating sensory-active aldehydes Producing "musty" off-odor derived from cork microbial spoilage or water and other raw materials Increasing the CO_2 derived from the development of contaminants	[47,149–152]
Bottle re-fermentation	Increasing carbonation Promoting effervescence Generating new flavors Reducing oxidation products	[11,17,153]

During the maturation phase, some off-flavor compounds from previous stages may reduce their concentrations and facilitate the production of a more balanced product. The bitterness provided by the hops and by some polyphenols such as gallic acid, flavonoids, and tannins, is also dependent on the specific conditions under which this phase takes place. Generally, during maturation, bitterness decreases and sweetness increases. Nevertheless, the extent to which this phenomenon occurs depends on a number of factors, including the type of beer [93]. In the case of lager beers, certain aromatic changes may take place during storage, together with a linear decrease in bitterness, because of the degradation of isohumulones and/or humulinones, and an increment of sweet aroma, toffee flavor, cardboard taint, and ribes off-flavor [143,144].

Certain compounds such as the furfural extracted from wood, and the esters generated by the esterification reactions that take place between alcohols—mainly ethanol and acids—during beer aging in wood change their concentrations, which increases beer bitterness as greater amounts of tannins are extracted from the wood [93]. Another aspect that should be considered during this particular maturation is that different microorganisms can contribute with different compounds to beer, but their presence will depend on the state and type of wood used for the aging [145]. For example, lambic beer matures in wooden casks, and yeasts such as *Brettanomyces bruxellensis*, *Brettanomyces anomalous*, and *Pichia membranifaciens*; acetic acid bacteria; and the LAB *Pediococcus damnosus* and *Lactobacillus brevis*, among others, play an important role in the process because they contribute to the typical Brett flavor of lambic beer, characterized by spicy and medicinal notes, and also fruity and floral ones. Thus, the ester-synthesizing activity of Brettanomyces contributes to the production of various ethyl esters, such as ethyl caproate or ethyl caprylate, that contribute to floral notes, at concentrations significantly higher than those found in other beers. In addition, the Brettanomyces yeast species that contain a superoxide dismutase enzyme with vinyl phenol reductase activity can form 4-ethylphenol and 4-ethylguaiacol, which are responsible for spicy and medicinal notes. Brettanomyces can also produce isovaleric acid from leucine, and this acid is responsible for sweaty and cheesy flavors, and may also produce mousy off-flavors that are associated with 2-ethyltetrahydropyridine and 2-acetyltetrahydropyridine. The presence of acetic acid and lactic acid bacteria also contributes to the high concentrations of ethyl acetate and ethyl lactate. In addition, acetoin, which is produced by AAB species through the utilization of lactate, may contribute to undesirable buttery notes [146,147].

It is also known that, after bottling, beer flavor is affected by certain chemical reactions that lead to instability, being an indicator of the increment of sensory-active aldehydes, which are generated in the sequence of radical reactions initiated by reactive oxygen species [149,150]. These aldehydes are also produced during mashing and wort boiling, but they decrease during the fermentation stage. It has been demonstrated that hop polyphenols slow down the sensory deterioration of pale lager beer as they suppress the formation of sensory-active aldehydes.

A traditional method to achieve beer carbonation consists of bottle re-fermentation, which is initiated by adding yeast and fermentable carbohydrates. As a result of yeast multiplication, carbonation increases and the concentration of flavor-active compounds is also affected, so that beer aroma and taste are also modified [11]. New flavors are produced as a result of the yeast activity, which incorporates higher alcohols, esters, aldehydes, vicinal diketones, and sulfur compounds that have an influence on beer aroma [17]. So, there are certain yeast strains that produce phenolic flavors resembling clove, smoked meat, or medicinal odors, among others [153]. Furthermore, the increment of carbon dioxide concentrations enhances beer effervescence. An additional effect of bottling is the prevention of oxidative damage, as yeast consumes oxygen.

Another factor to take into account is the presence of contaminants from previous stages that may reach the beer storage phase. During this phase, these contaminants may develop and grow. They can come from the raw materials, such as hops or barley, the latter being considered the main source of potential contamination [125]. In general, these undesirable microorganisms that may be present in the finished beer are not considered pathogenic and, therefore, they do not represent a potential hazard for consumers. However, if they are not eliminated they may still spoil an entire batch of beer [46,145]. The most common way that these contaminating microorganisms alter beer taste is by producing metabolites and other associated by-products, such as methyl mercaptan, dimethyl sulfoxide, or hydrogen sulfide, among others (which will differ depending on the species involved), at concentration levels that would allow a negative impact on the desired characteristics of the target beer. Certain traits in bottled beer, such as misshaped cans due to over-carbonation, turbidity, visible yeast colonies, superficial films, excessive viscosity, or some off-flavors, may act as indicators of a possible contamination [145]. Thus, some bacteria from the *Lactobacilli* genus provide lactic flavor, while others, such as *Pectinatus frisingensis*, *Pectinatus cerevisiiphilus*, or *Megasphaera cerevisiae* can add acetic, manure, rotten egg, or cooked vegetable aromas to beer and make them totally unpalatable for consumers [45,126,145]. The genus *Lactobacilli* is considered to be the most common and best-known bacterial contaminant of beer. Even though only a limited number of species are able to survive the entire brewing process, this type of contamination is more common than one would expect [126]. *Pediococcus* is another important genus of contaminating bacteria, and they produce diacetyl and provide beer with a buttery flavor [126]. *Staphylococcus xylosus* is another contaminating bacterium detected in homebrewed beers (much less common in industrial beers) that makes beer taste like bitter almonds [148]. Not only bacteria but also certain yeasts can be considered as contaminants of beer. These include *Brettanomyces*, *Candida*, *Debaromyces*, *Pichia*, *Hanseniaspora*, *Kluyveromyces*, *Pichia*, and *Torulaspora* [47]. An additional problem derived from contamination is an excessive increment of CO_2 that over pressurizes the packaging and may cause can bursting or bottle caps popping off [151].

There are some microorganisms, such as *Lactobacillus* bacteria (naturally found in barley), that can eliminate certain undesirable microorganisms thanks to the production of antimicrobial compounds that have the capacity to inhibit the growth of other bacteria or fungi [125]. On the other hand, certain compounds from hops (mainly iso-α-acids) can act as preservatives against Gram-positive bacteria [154], but not against *Lactobacillus brevis*— a bacterium whose presence causes turbidity and super-attenuation problems. Other components in beers, such as carbon dioxide or polyphenols, can also act as preservatives and minimize the problems associated with potential contaminations [155].

Beers may also undergo oxidation reactions that can alter their flavor. Higher alcohols, unsaturated fatty acids, amino acids, or proteins generated through Maillard reactions, as well as isohumulones, are some of the compounds involved in such reactions. In this regard, De Francesco et al. [156] found that the addition of some polyphenols-rich extracts to beer before its bottling resulted in more stable beers, while the usage of condensed green tea tannins proved to be ideal for prolonging beer shelf-life.

Finally, and with regard to the bottling stage, it should be mentioned that some high-quality beer brands still use corked bottles. In those cases, the presence of certain compounds derived from the microbiological spoilage of the cork, such as chloroanisoles, bromoanisoles, or chlorophenols, can cause an undesirable "musty" off-odor, even when found at really low concentration levels (ng/L) [157]. Apart from these compounds, geosmin, 2-methylisoborneol, 2-isopropyl-methoxypyrazine, or 2-isobutyl-methoxypyrazine may also be responsible for this type of unpleasant odor. The latter ones may come either from the water or from any of the other raw materials, although they may also come from the brewery itself [152].

As mentioned above, beer contains a large number of natural components that enhance its resistance against undesirable microbiological processes; nevertheless, good brewing practices, from the raw material to the bottled beer, should be followed if high quality products are to be produced. Certain bottling practices, such as purging the bottle with CO_2 prior to bottling, using antioxidants such as sulfur dioxide or ascorbic acid, adding arginine to inhibit the Maillard reaction, preventing oxygen from entering the bottles by means of efficient stoppers, limiting light exposure through the use of brown bottles, etc., are some of the measures to be considered in order to avoid any undesirable chemical and microbiological alteration of bottled beers.

6. Conclusions

The main raw materials for beer production (barley, water, and hops) have a significant impact on the sensory properties of beers. Different barley genotypes have been demonstrated to produce beers with different aroma profile, ranging from fruity and floral aromas to roasted ones. In this respect, some brewers have used specialty malts, which not only add color and flavor, but also have an influence on the course of the fermentation and production of flavor-active yeast metabolites. Protein content in barley is another factor to be monitored, as it can be responsible for the presence of off-flavors in the final product. During the kilning process, on the other hand, germinated barley is subjected to high temperatures that have a considerable impact on the final beer color and flavor as a consequence of the Maillard reactions. These reactions provide beer with certain compounds responsible for the emergence of caramel, bread, or cotton-like flavors. Water, as the major component of beer, may contain certain metal ions that also have a definite influence on beer flavor. The contribution to beer sensory profile from hops largely depends on the hop variety used and on its maturity level. Hops provide volatile compounds and alpha-acids to the wort, the latter ones being isomerized during the boiling stage into isohumulones, which are the main components responsible for beer bitter taste. In order to avoid hop bitterness while providing beer with hop aroma, hops can be added at the end of the boiling stage or after fermentation. This should allow for some of the most common aromatic descriptors, such as floral, citrus, or pine, to be present in the final beer sensorial profile. Alternatively, pure hop extract can be added to improve mouthfeel, fullness, and an increased perception of beer bitterness. Generally, during beer maturation, the aromatic profile of beer changes as bitterness decreases and sweetness increases. Other processes, including aging in wood barrels or bottle refermentation for beer carbonation, have also been demonstrated to change the aroma and flavor of beers. Special attention must be paid to the spoilage microorganisms that may develop during the whole brewing process, because they may definitely affect the sensory properties of beers.

Author Contributions: Conceptualization, C.L. and E.D-G.; writing—original draft preparation, A.B.D., E.D.-G., C.L. and R.C.; writing—review and editing, A.B.D., E.D.-G., C.L.,and R.C.; supervision, E.D.-G.; All authors have read and agreed to the published version of the manuscript.

Funding: This research received no external funding.

Data Availability Statement: Not applicable.

Conflicts of Interest: The authors declare no conflict of interest.

References

1. Betancur, M.I.; Motoki, K.; Spence, C.; Velasco, C. Factors influencing the choice of beer: A review. *Food Res. Int.* **2020**, *137*, 109367. [CrossRef]
2. Einfalt, D. Barley-sorghum craft beer production with Saccharomyces cerevisiae, Torulaspora delbrueckii and Metschnikowia pulcherrima yeast strains. *Eur. Food Res. Technol.* **2021**, *247*, 385–393. [CrossRef]
3. Postigo, V.; García, M.; Cabellos, J.M.; Arroyo, T. Wine Saccharomyces Yeasts for Beer Fermentation. *Fermentation* **2021**, *7*, 290. [CrossRef]
4. van Donkelaar, L.H.G.; Mostert, J.; Zisopoulos, F.K.; Boom, R.M.; van der Goot, A.J. The use of enzymes for beer brewing: Thermodynamic comparison on resource use. *Energy* **2016**, *115*, 519–527. [CrossRef]
5. Humia, B.V.; Santos, K.S.; Schneider, J.K.; Leal, I.L.; de Abreu Barreto, G.; Batista, T.; Machado, B.A.S.; Druzian, J.I.; Krause, L.C.; da Costa Mendonça, M.; et al. Physicochemical and sensory profile of Beauregard sweet potato beer. *Food Chem.* **2020**, *312*, 126087. [CrossRef]
6. Salanță, L.C.; Coldea, T.E.; Ignat, M.V.; Pop, C.R.; Tofană, M.; Mudura, E.; Borșa, A.; Pasqualone, A.; Anjos, O.; Zhao, H. Functionality of Special Beer Processes and Potential Health Benefits. *Processes* **2020**, *8*, 1613. [CrossRef]
7. Machado, J.C.; Faria, M.A.; Ferreira, I.M.P.L.V.O. Hops: New Perspectives for an Old Beer Ingredient. In *Natural Beverages*; Elsevier: Amsterdam, The Netherlands, 2019; pp. 267–301.
8. Martins, C.; Brandão, T.; Almeida, A.; Rocha, S.M. Unveiling the lager beer volatile terpenic compounds. *Food Res. Int.* **2018**, *114*, 199–207. [CrossRef]
9. Donadini, G.; Porretta, S. Uncovering patterns of consumers' interest for beer: A case study with craft beers. *Food Res. Int.* **2017**, *91*, 183–198. [CrossRef]
10. Li, F.; Shi, Y.; Boswell, M.; Rozelle, S. Craft beer in China. In *Economic Perspectives on Craft Beer*; Garavaglia, C., Swinnen, J., Eds.; Palgrave Macmillan: Cham, Switzerland, 2017.
11. Derdelinckx, G.; Neven, H.; Demeyer, I.; Delvaux, F. Belgian special beers: Refermented beers, white and wheat beers, amber and dark beers, spiced and hoppy beers. *Belgian J. Brew. Biotechnol.* **1995**, *20*, 67–73.
12. Nizet, S.; Gros, J.; Peeters, F.; Chaumont, S.; Robiette, R.; Collin, S. First evidence of the production of odorant polyfunctional thiols by bottle refermentation. *J. Am. Soc. Brew. Chem.* **2013**, *71*, 15–22. [CrossRef]
13. Liu, M.; Zeng, Z.; Xiong, B. Preparation of novel solid-phase microextraction fibers by sol–gel technology for headspace solid-phase microextraction-gas chromatographic analysis of aroma compounds in beer. *J. Chromatogr. A* **2005**, *1065*, 287–299. [CrossRef]
14. Cortacero-Ramírez, S.; Hernáinz-Bermúdez De Castro, M.; Segura-Carretero, A.; Cruces-Blanco, C.; Fernández-Gutiérrez, A. Analysis of beer components by capillary electrophoretic methods. *TrAC Trends Anal. Chem.* **2003**, *22*, 440–455. [CrossRef]
15. Romero-Medina, A.; Estarrón-Espinosa, M.; Verde-Calvo, J.R.; Lelièvre-Desmas, M.; Escalona-Buendía, H.B. Renewing Traditions: A Sensory and Chemical Characterisation of Mexican Pigmented Corn Beers. *Foods* **2020**, *9*, 886. [CrossRef]
16. Bokulich, N.A.; Bamforth, C.W. The Microbiology of Malting and Brewing. *Microbiol. Mol. Biol. Rev.* **2013**, *77*, 157–172. [CrossRef]
17. Pires, E.J.; Teixeira, J.A.; Brányik, T.; Vicente, A.A. Yeast: The soul of beer's aroma—A review of flavour-active esters and higher alcohols produced by the brewing yeast. *Appl. Microbiol. Biotechnol.* **2014**, *98*, 1937–1949. [CrossRef]
18. Fontana, M.; Buiatti, S. Amino Acids in Beer. In *Beer in Health and Disease Prevention*; Academic Press: Cambridge, MA, USA, 2009; pp. 273–284. [CrossRef]
19. Poveda, J.M. Biogenic amines and free amino acids in craft beers from the Spanish market: A statistical approach. *Food Control* **2019**, *96*, 227–233. [CrossRef]
20. He, Y.; Dong, J.; Yin, H.; Zhao, Y.; Chen, R.; Wan, X.; Chen, P.; Hou, X.; Liu, J.; Chen, L. Wort composition and its impact on the flavour-active higher alcohol and ester formation of beer—A review. *J. Inst. Brew.* **2014**, *120*, 157–163. [CrossRef]
21. Deng, Y.; Lim, J.; Lee, G.H.; Hanh Nguyen, T.T.; Xiao, Y.; Piao, M.; Kim, D. Brewing rutin-enriched lager beer with buckwheat malt as adjuncts. *J. Microbiol. Biotechnol.* **2019**, *29*, 877–886. [CrossRef]
22. Olaniran, A.O.; Hiralal, L.; Mokoena, M.P.; Pillay, B. Flavour-active volatile compounds in beer: Production, regulation and control. *J. Inst. Brew.* **2017**, *123*, 13–23. [CrossRef]
23. Garcia-Garcia, J.H.; Galán-Wong, L.J.; Pereyra-Alférez, B.; Damas-Buenrostro, L.C.; Pérez, E.; Carlos Cabada, J. Distribution of lactobacillus and pediococcus in a brewery environment. *J. Am. Soc. Brew. Chem.* **2017**, *75*, 312–317. [CrossRef]
24. Romero-Rodríguez, R.; Durán-Guerrero, E.; Castro, R.; Díaz, A.B.; Lasanta, C. Evaluation of the influence of the microorganisms involved in the production of beers on their sensory characteristics. *Food Bioprod. Process.* **2022**, *135*, 33–47. [CrossRef]

25. Briggs, D. *Malts and Malting*; Springer Science & Business Media: Berlin/Heidelberg, Germany, 1998.
26. Briggs, D.E.; Boulton, C.A.; Brookes, P.A.; Stevens, R. *Brewing: Science and Practice*; CRC Press: Cambridge, UK, 2004.
27. Gąsior, J.; Kawa-Rygielska, J.; Kucharska, A. Carbohydrates profile, polyphenols content and antioxidative properties of beer worts produced with different dark malts varieties or roasted barley grains. *Molecules* **2020**, *25*, 3882. [CrossRef] [PubMed]
28. Phiarais, B.P.N.; Mauch, A.; Schehl, B.D.; Zarnkow, M.; Gastl, M.; Herrmann, M.; Zannini, E.; Arendt, E.K. Processing of a Top Fermented Beer Brewed from 100% Buckwheat Malt with Sensory and Analytical Characterisation. *J. Inst. Brew.* **2010**, *116*, 265–274. [CrossRef]
29. Langos, D.; Granvogl, M.; Schieberle, P. Characterization of the key aroma compounds in two Bavarian wheat beers by means of the sensomics approach. *J. Agric. Food Chem.* **2013**, *61*, 11303–11311. [CrossRef]
30. Yin, H.; Dong, J.; Yu, J.; Chang, Z.; Qian, Z.; Liu, M.; Huang, S.; Hu, X.; Liu, X.; Deng, Y.; et al. A preliminary study about the influence of high hydrostatic pressure processing on the physicochemical and sensorial properties of a cloudy wheat beer. *J. Inst. Brew.* **2016**, *122*, 462–467. [CrossRef]
31. Coulibaly, W.H.; Florent N'guessan, K.; Coulibaly, I.; Cot, M.; Rigou, P.; Djè, K.M. Influence of Freeze-Dried Yeast Starter Cultures on Volatile Compounds of Tchapalo, a Traditional Sorghum Beer from Côte d'Ivoire. *Beverages* **2016**, *2*, 35. [CrossRef]
32. Schnitzenbaumer, B.; Karl, C.A.; Jacob, F.; Arendt, E.K. Impact of Unmalted White Nigerian and Red Italian Sorghum (*Sorghum bicolor*) on the Quality of Worts and Beers Applying Optimized Enzyme Levels. *J. Am. Soc. Brew. Chem.* **2013**, *71*, 258–266. [CrossRef]
33. Schnitzenbaumer, B.; Kerpes, R.; Titze, J.; Jacob, F.; Arendt, E.K. Impact of Various Levels of Unmalted Oats (*Avena sativa* L.) on the Quality and Processability of Mashes, Worts, and Beers. *J. Am. Soc. Brew. Chem.* **2012**, *70*, 142–149. [CrossRef]
34. Yorke, J.; Cook, D.; Ford, R. Brewing with Unmalted Cereal Adjuncts: Sensory and Analytical Impacts on Beer Quality. *Beverages* **2021**, *7*, 4. [CrossRef]
35. Bettenhausen, H.M.; Benson, A.; Fisk, S.; Herb, D.; Hernandez, J.; Lim, J.; Queisser, S.H.; Shellhammer, T.H.; Vega, V.; Yao, L.; et al. Variation in Sensory Attributes and Volatile Compounds in Beers Brewed from Genetically Distinct Malts: An Integrated Sensory and Non-Targeted Metabolomics Approach. *J. Am. Soc. Brew. Chem.* **2020**, *78*, 136–152. [CrossRef]
36. Bettenhausen, H.M.; Barr, L.; Broeckling, C.D.; Chaparro, J.M.; Holbrook, C.; Sedin, D.; Heuberger, A.L. Influence of malt source on beer chemistry, flavor, and flavor stability. *Food Res. Int.* **2018**, *113*, 487–504. [CrossRef]
37. Herb, D.; Filichkin, T.; Fisk, S.; Helgerson, L.; Hayes, P.; Meints, B.; Jennings, R.; Monsour, R.; Tynan, S.; Vinkemeier, K.; et al. Effects of barley (*Hordeum vulgare* L.) variety and growing environment on beer flavor. *J. Am. Soc. Brew. Chem.* **2017**, *75*, 345–353. [CrossRef]
38. Kyraleou, M.; Herb, D.; O'reilly, G.; Conway, N.; Bryan, T.; Kilcawley, K.N. The impact of terroir on the flavour of single malt whisk(E)y new make spirit. *Foods* **2021**, *10*, 443. [CrossRef]
39. McMillan, T.; Tidemann, B.D.; O'Donovan, J.T.; Izydorczyk, M.S. Effects of plant growth regulator application on the malting quality of barley. *J. Sci. Food Agric.* **2020**, *100*, 2082–2089. [CrossRef]
40. Casey, G.P. Primary Versus Secondary Gushing and Assay Procedures Used to Assess Malt/Beer Gushing Potential. *MBAA Tech. Q.* **1996**, *33*, 229–235.
41. Sarlin, T. *Detection and Characterisation of Fusarium hydrophobins Inducing Gushing in Beer*; Aalto University School of Chemical Technology: Espoo, Finland, 2012.
42. Deckers, S.M.; Vissers, L.; Khalesi, M.; Shokribousjein, Z.; Verachtert, H.; Gebruers, K.; Pirlot, X.; Rock, J.M.; Ilberg, V.; Titze, J.; et al. Thermodynamic view of primary gushing. *J. Am. Soc. Brew. Chem.* **2013**, *71*, 149–152. [CrossRef]
43. Deckers, S.M.; Venken, T.; Khalesi, M.; Gebruers, K.; Baggerman, G.; Lorgouilloux, Y.; Shokribousjein, Z.; Lberg, V.; Schönberger, C.; Titze, J.; et al. Combined Modeling and Biophysical Characterisation of CO_2 Interaction with Class II Hydrophobins: New Insight into the Mechanism Underpinning Primary Gushing Sylvie. *J. Am. Soc. Brew. Chem.* **2012**, *70*, 257–261. [CrossRef]
44. Pascari, X.; Marin, S.; Ramos, A.J.; Sanchis, V. Relevant Fusarium Mycotoxins in Malt and Beer. *Foods* **2022**, *11*, 246. [CrossRef]
45. Kyselová, L.; Brányik, T. *Quality Improvement and Fermentation Control in Beer*; Elsevier Ltd.: Amsterdam, The Netherlands, 2015; ISBN 9781782420248.
46. Hill, A.E. Microbiological stability of beer. In *Handbook of Alcoholic Beverages: Beer, a Quality Perspective*; Bamforth, C.W., Russell, I., Stewart, G., Eds.; Academic Press: Cambridge, MA, USA; Elsevier: New York, NY, USA, 2009; pp. 163–183. ISBN 9780126692013.
47. Back, W. Color atlas and handbook of beverage biology. In *Color Atlas and Handbook of Beverage Biology*; Fachverlag Hans Carl: Numberg, Germany, 2005.
48. Gupta, M.; Abu-Ghannam, N.; Gallaghar, E. Barley for brewing: Characteristic changes during malting, brewing and applications of its by-products. *Compr. Rev. Food Sci. Food Saf.* **2010**, *9*, 318–328. [CrossRef]
49. Chandra, G.S.; Proudlove, M.O.; Baxter, E.D. The structure of barley endosperm—An important determinant of malt modification. *J. Sci. Food Agric.* **1999**, *79*, 37–46. [CrossRef]
50. Iimure, T.; Sato, K. Beer proteomics analysis for beer quality control and malting barley breeding. *Food Res. Int.* **2013**, *54*, 1013–1020. [CrossRef]
51. Justé, A.; Malfliet, S.; Lenaerts, M.; De Cooman, L.; Aerts, G.; Willems, K.A.; Lievens, B. Microflora during malting of barley: Overview and impact on malt quality. *Brew. Sci.* **2011**, *64*, 22–31.

52. Mather, D.E.; Tinker, N.A.; LaBerge, D.E.; Edney, M.; Jones, B.L.; Rossnagel, B.G.; Legge, W.G.; Briggs, K.G.; Irvine, R.B.; Falk, D.E.; et al. Regions of the genome that affect grain and malt quality in a North American two-row Barley Cross. *Crop Sci.* **1997**, *37*, 544–554. [CrossRef]
53. Heuberger, A.L.; Broeckling, C.D.; Kirkpatrick, K.R.; Prenni, J.E. Application of nontargeted metabolite profiling to discover novel markers of quality traits in an advanced population of malting barley. *Plant Biotechnol. J.* **2014**, *12*, 147–160. [CrossRef]
54. Fox, G.P.; Panozzo, J.F.; Li, C.D.; Lance, R.C.M.; Inkerman, P.A.; Henry, R.J. Molecular basis of barley quality. *Aust. J. Agric. Res.* **2003**, *54*, 1081–1101. [CrossRef]
55. Kunze, W. *Technology Brewing and Malting*; VLB: Berlin, Germany, 2010.
56. Coghe, S.; Martens, E.; D'Hollander, H.; Dirinck, P.J.; Delvaux, F.R. Sensory and Instrumental Flavour Analysis of Wort Brewed with Dark Specialty Malts. *J. Inst. Brew.* **2004**, *110*, 94–103. [CrossRef]
57. Dack, R.E.; Black, G.W.; Koutsidis, G.; Usher, S.J. The effect of Maillard reaction products and yeast strain on the synthesis of key higher alcohols and esters in beer fermentations. *Food Chem.* **2017**, *232*, 595–601. [CrossRef]
58. Rufián-Henares, J.A.; Morales, F.J. Antimicrobial activity of melanoidins. *J. Food Qual.* **2007**, *30*, 160–168. [CrossRef]
59. Inui, T.; Tsuchiya, F.; Ishimaru, M.; Oka, K.; Komura, H. Different Beers with Different Hops. Relevant Compounds for Their Aroma Characteristics. *J. Agric. Food Chem.* **2013**, *61*, 4758–4764. [CrossRef] [PubMed]
60. Kageyama, N.; Inui, T.; Fukami, H.; Komura, H. The science of beer elucidation of chemical structures of components responsible for beer aftertaste. *J. Am. Soc. Brew. Chem.* **2018**, *69*, 255–259. [CrossRef]
61. Dugulin, C.A.; Acuña Muñoz, L.M.; Buyse, J.; De Rouck, G.; Bolat, I.; Cook, D.J. Brewing with 100% green malt-process development and key quality indicators. *J. Inst. Brew.* **2020**, *126*, 343–353. [CrossRef]
62. Hornsey, I.S. *Brewing*; Royal Society of Chemistry: London, UK, 2013.
63. Yahya, H.; Linforth, R.S.T.; Cook, D.J. Flavour generation during commercial barley and malt roasting operations: A time course study. *Food Chem.* **2014**, *145*, 378–387. [CrossRef]
64. Coghe, S.; D'Hollander, H.; Verachtert, H.; Delvaux, F.R. Impact of dark specialty malts on extract composition and wort fermentation. *J. Inst. Brew.* **2005**, *111*, 51–60. [CrossRef]
65. Perretti, G.; Floridi, S.; Turchetti, B.; Marconi, O.; Fantozzi, P. Quality Control of Malt: Turbidity Problems of Standard Worts Given by the Presence of Microbial Cells. *J. Inst. Brew.* **2011**, *117*, 212–216. [CrossRef]
66. Lowe, D.P.; Arendt, E.K. The use and effects of lactic acid bacteria in malting and brewing with their relationships to antifungal activity, mycotoxins and gushing: A review. *J. Inst. Brew* **2004**, *110*, 163–180. [CrossRef]
67. Kim, D.Y.; Kim, J.; Kim, J.H.; Kim, W.J. Malt and wort bio-acidification by *Pediococcus acidilactici* HW01 as starter culture. *Food Control* **2021**, *120*, 107560. [CrossRef]
68. Rozada-Sánchez, R.; Sattur, A.P.; Thomas, K.; Pandiella, S.S. Evaluation of *Bifidobacterium* spp. for the production of a potentially probiotic malt-based beverage. *Process Biochem.* **2008**, *43*, 848–854. [CrossRef]
69. Salmeron, I.; Fuciños, P.; Charalampopoulos, D.; Pandiella, S.S. Volatile compounds produced by the probiotic strain *Lactobacillus plantarum* NCIMB 8826 in cereal-based substrates. *Food Chem.* **2009**, *117*, 265–271. [CrossRef]
70. Salmerón, I.; Loeza-Serrano, S.; Pérez-Vega, S.; Pandiella, S.S. Headspace Gas Chromatography (HS-GC) Analysis of Imperative Flavor Compounds in Lactobacilli-fermented Barley and Malt Substrates. *Food Sci. Biotechnol* **2015**, *24*, 1363–1371. [CrossRef]
71. Rübsam, H.; Gastl, M.; Becker, T. Determination of the influence of starch sources and mashing procedures on the range of the molecular weight distribution of beer using field-flow fractionation. *J. Inst. Brew.* **2013**, *119*, 139–148. [CrossRef]
72. Anderson, H.E.; Santos, I.C.; Hildenbrand, Z.L.; Schug, K.A. A review of the analytical methods used for beer ingredient and finished product analysis and quality control. *Anal. Chim. Acta* **2019**, *1085*, 1–20. [CrossRef]
73. Montanari, L.; Mayer, H.; Marconi, O.; Fantozzi, P. Minerals in Beer. In *Beer in Health and Disease Prevention*; Elsevier: Amsterdam, The Netherlands, 2009; pp. 359–365.
74. Sterczyńska, M.; Stachnik, M.; Poreda, A.; Pużyńska, K.; Piepiórka-Stepuk, J.; Fiutak, G.; Jakubowski, M. Ionic composition of beer worts produced with selected unmalted grains. *LWT* **2021**, *137*, 110348. [CrossRef]
75. Schoenberger, C.; Krottenthaler, M.; Back, W. Sensory and Analytical Characterization of Nonvolatile Taste-Active Compounds in Bottom-Fermented Beers. *MBAA Tech. Q.* **2002**, *39*, 210–217.
76. Poreda, A.; Bijak, M.; Zdaniewicz, M.; Jakubowski, M.; Makarewicz, M. Effect of wheat malt on the concentration of metal ions in wort and brewhouse by-products. *J. Inst. Brew.* **2015**, *121*, 224–230. [CrossRef]
77. Punčochářová, L.; Pořízka, J.; Diviš, P.; Štursa, V. Study of the influence of brewing water on selected analytes in beer. *Potravin. Slovak J. Food Sci.* **2019**, *13*, 507–514. [CrossRef]
78. Webersinke, F.; Klein, H.; Flieher, M.; Urban, A.; Jäger, H.; Forster, C. Control of Fermentation By-Products and Aroma Features of Beer Produced with Scottish Ale Yeast by Variation of Fermentation Temperature and Wort Aeration Rate. *J. Am. Soc. Brew. Chem.* **2018**, *76*, 147–155. [CrossRef]
79. Kucharczyk, K.; Tuszyński, T. The effect of temperature on fermentation and beer volatiles at an industrial scale. *J. Inst. Brew.* **2018**, *124*, 230–235. [CrossRef]
80. Verstrepen, K.J.; Derdelinckx, G.; Dufour, J.; Winderickx, J.; Thevelein, J.M.; Pretorius, I.S.; Delvaux, F.R.; Box, P.O.; Osmond, G.; Sa, A. Flavor active esters adding fruitiness to beer. *J. Biosci. Bioeng.* **2003**, *96*, 110–118. [CrossRef]
81. Loviso, C.L.; Libkind, D. Synthesis and regulation of flavor compounds derived from brewing yeast: Esters. *Rev. Argent. Microbiol.* **2018**, *50*, 436–446. [CrossRef]

82. Krogerus, K.; Gibson, B.R. 25 th Anniversary Review: Diacetyl and its control during brewery fermentation. *J. Inst. Brew.* **2013**, *119*, 86–97. [CrossRef]
83. Hughes, P. Beer flavor. In *Beer, A quality Perspective. Handbook of Alcoholic Beverages*; Academic Press: Cambridge, MA, USA; Elsevier: Amsterdam, The Netherlands, 2009; pp. 61–83.
84. Ferreira, I.; Guido, L. Impact of Wort Amino Acids on Beer Flavour: A Review. *Fermentation* **2018**, *4*, 23. [CrossRef]
85. Kok, Y.J.; Ye, L.; Muller, J.; Ow, D.S.-W.; Bi, X. Brewing with malted barley or raw barley: What makes the difference in the processes? *Appl. Microbiol. Biotechnol.* **2019**, *103*, 1059–1067. [CrossRef]
86. Mehra, R.; Kumar, H.; Kumar, N.; Kaushik, R. Red rice conjugated with barley and rhododendron extracts for new variant of beer. *J. Food Sci. Technol.* **2020**, *57*, 4152–4159. [CrossRef]
87. Bogdan, P.; Kordialik-Bogacka, E. Alternatives to malt in brewing. *Trends Food Sci. Technol.* **2017**, *65*, 1–9. [CrossRef]
88. Kunz, T.; Müller, C.; Mato-Gonzales, D.; Methner, F.-J. The influence of unmalted barley on the oxidative stability of wort and beer. *J. Inst. Brew.* **2012**, *118*, 32–39. [CrossRef]
89. Steiner, E.; Auer, A.; Becker, T.; Gastl, M. Comparison of beer quality attributes between beers brewed with 100% barley malt and 100% barley raw material †. *J. Sci. Food Agric.* **2012**, *92*, 803–812. [CrossRef]
90. Ducruet, J.; Rébénaque, P.; Diserens, S.; Kosińska-Cagnazzo, A.; Héritier, I.; Andlauer, W. Amber ale beer enriched with goji berries—The effect on bioactive compound content and sensorial properties. *Food Chem.* **2017**, *226*, 109–118. [CrossRef]
91. Baiano, A. Craft beer: An overview. *Compr. Rev. Food Sci. Food Saf.* **2020**, *20*, 1829–1856. [CrossRef]
92. De Keukeleire, D. Fundamentals of beer and hop chemistry. *Quim. Nova* **2000**, *23*, 108–112. [CrossRef]
93. Luo, Y.; Kong, L.; Xue, R.; Wang, W.; Xia, X. Bitterness in alcoholic beverages: The profiles of perception, constituents, and contributors. *Trends Food Sci. Technol.* **2020**, *96*, 222–232. [CrossRef]
94. Oladokun, O.; Tarrega, A.; James, S.; Cowley, T.; Dehrmann, F.; Smart, K.; Cook, D.; Hort, J. Modification of perceived beer bitterness intensity, character and temporal profile by hop aroma extract. *Food Res. Int.* **2016**, *86*, 104–111. [CrossRef]
95. Oladokun, O.; Tarrega, A.; James, S.; Smart, K.; Hort, J.; Cook, D.; Lafontaine, S.R.; Shellhammer, T.H.; Ceola, D.; Huelsmann, R.D.; et al. The impact of hop bitter acid and polyphenol profiles on the perceived bitterness of beer. *Food Chem.* **2016**, *205*, 212–220. [CrossRef]
96. Almaguer, C.; Schönberger, C.; Gastl, M.; Arendt, E.K.; Becker, T. Humulus lupulus—A story that begs to be told. A review. *J. Inst. Brew.* **2014**, *120*, 289–314. [CrossRef]
97. Krofta, K. Comparison of quality parameters of Czech and foreign hop varieties. *Plant Soil Environ.* **2003**, *49*, 261–268. [CrossRef]
98. Buarque, B.S.; Davies, R.B.; Hynes, R.M.; Kogler, D.F. *Hops, Skip & a Jump: The Regional Uniqueness of Beer Styles*; UCD Centre for Economic Research Working Paper Series; WP2020/31; Geary Institute; University College Dublin: Dublin, Ireland, 2020.
99. Verzele, M.; De Keukeleire, D. Chemistry and Analysis of Hop and Beer Bitter Acids. In *Developments in Food Science*; Verzele, M., De Keukeleire, D., Eds.; Elsevier: Amsterdam, The Netherlands, 1991; Volume 27, ISBN 0444881654.
100. Hahn, C.D.; Lafontaine, S.R.; Pereira, C.B.; Shellhammer, T.H. Evaluation of Nonvolatile Chemistry Affecting Sensory Bitterness Intensity of Highly Hopped Beers. *J. Agric. Food Chem.* **2018**, *66*, 3505–3513. [CrossRef]
101. Rettberg, N.; Biendl, M.; Garbe, L.A. Hop aroma and hoppy beer flavor: Chemical backgrounds and analytical tools—A review. *J. Am. Soc. Brew. Chem.* **2018**, *76*, 1–20. [CrossRef]
102. Lafontaine, S.R.; Shellhammer, T.H. Investigating the Factors Impacting Aroma, Flavor, and Stability in Dry-Hopped Beers. *MBAA Tech. Q.* **2019**, *56*, 13–23.
103. Eyres, G.T.; Dufour, J.P. Hop Essential Oil: Analysis, Chemical Composition and Odor Characteristics. In *Beer in Health and Disease Prevention*; Academic Press: Cambridge, MA, USA; Elsevier: Amsterdam, The Netherlands, 2009; pp. 239–254.
104. Castro, R.; Díaz, A.B.; Durán-Guerrero, E.; Lasanta, C. Influence of different fermentation conditions on the analytical and sensory properties of craft beers: Hopping, fermentation temperature and yeast strain. *J. Food Compos. Anal.* **2022**, *106*, 104278. [CrossRef]
105. Caballero, I.; Blanco, C.A.; Porras, M. Iso-α-acids, bitterness and loss of beer quality during storage. *Trends Food Sci. Technol.* **2012**, *26*, 21–30. [CrossRef]
106. Jelínek, L.; Müllerova, J.; Karavín, M.; Dostalek, P. The secret of dry hopped beers—Review. *Kvas. Prum.* **2018**, *64*, 287–296. [CrossRef]
107. Kirkpatrick, K.R.; Shellhammer, T.H. A Cultivar-Based Screening of Hops for Dextrin Degrading Enzymatic Potential. *J. Am. Soc. Brew. Chem.* **2018**, *76*, 247–256. [CrossRef]
108. Stokholm, A.; Shellhammer, T.H. *Hop Creep–Technical Brief*; Brewers Association: Boulder, CO, USA, 2020.
109. Bruner, J.; Williams, J.; Fox, G. Further Exploration of Hop Creep Variability with *Humulus lupulus* Cultivars and Proposed Method for Determination of Secondary Fermentation. *MBAA Tech. Q.* **2020**, *57*, 169–176. [CrossRef]
110. Oladokun, O.; James, S.; Cowley, T.; Dehrmann, F.; Smart, K.; Hort, J.; Cook, D. Perceived bitterness character of beer in relation to hop variety and the impact of hop aroma. *Food Chem.* **2017**, *230*, 215–224. [CrossRef] [PubMed]
111. Van Opstaele, F.; Goiris, K.; De Rouck, G.; Aerts, G.; De Cooman, L. Production of novel varietal hop aromas by supercritical fluid extraction of hop pellets—Part 2: Preparation of single variety floral, citrus, and spicy hop oil essences by density programmed supercritical fluid extraction. *J. Supercrit. Fluids* **2012**, *71*, 147–161. [CrossRef]
112. Sanz, V.; Torres, M.D.; López Vilariño, J.M.; Domínguez, H. What is new on the hop extraction? *Trends Food Sci. Technol.* **2019**, *93*, 12–22. [CrossRef]

113. Schuina, G.L.; Quelhas, J.O.F.; de Castilhos, M.B.M.; de Carvalho, G.B.M.; Del Bianchi, V.L. Alternative production of craft lager beers using artichoke (*Cynara scolymus* L.) as a hops substitute. *Food Sci. Technol.* **2020**, *40*, 157–161. [CrossRef]
114. Ting, P.L.; Ryder, D.S. The bitter, twisted truth of the hop: 50 years of hop chemistry. *J. Am. Soc. Brew. Chem.* **2017**, *75*, 161–180. [CrossRef]
115. Aron, P.M.; Shellhammer, T.H. A discussion of polyphenols in beer physical and flavour stability. *J. Inst. Brew.* **2010**, *116*, 369–380. [CrossRef]
116. Ting, P.L.; Lusk, L.; Refling, J.; Kay, S.; Ryder, D. Identification of antiradical hop compounds. *J. Am. Soc. Brew. Chem.* **2008**, *66*, 116–126. [CrossRef]
117. Machado, J.C.; Lehnhardt, F.; Martins, Z.E.; Kollmannsberger, H.; Gastl, M.; Becker, T.; Ferreira, I.M.P.L.V.O. Prediction of Fruity-Citrus Intensity of Beers Dry Hopped with Mandarina Bavaria Based on the Content of Selected Volatile Compounds. *J. Agric. Food Chem.* **2020**, *68*, 2155–2163. [CrossRef]
118. Lafontaine, S.; Varnum, S.; Roland, A.; Delpech, S.; Dagan, L.; Vollmer, D.; Kishimoto, T.; Shellhammer, T. Impact of harvest maturity on the aroma characteristics and chemistry of Cascade hops used for dry-hopping. *Food Chem.* **2019**, *278*, 228–239. [CrossRef]
119. Schnaitter, M.; Wimmer, A.; Kollmannsberger, H.; Gastl, M.; Becker, T. Influence of hop harvest date of the 'Mandarina Bavaria' hop variety on the sensory evaluation of dry-hopped top-fermented beer. *J. Inst. Brew.* **2016**, *122*, 661–669. [CrossRef]
120. Biendl, M.; Engelhard, B.; Forster, A.; Gahr, A.; Lutz, A.; Mitter, W.; Schmidt, R.; Schönberger, C. *Hops: Their Cultivation, Composition and Usage*; Fachverlag Hans Carl: Nuremberg, Germany, 2014.
121. Forster, A.; Gahr, A. On the Fate of Certain Hop Substances during Dry Hopping. *Brew. Sci.* **2013**, *66*, 93–103.
122. Richter, T.M.; Silcock, P.; Algarra, A.; Eyres, G.T.; Capozzi, V.; Bremer, P.J.; Biasioli, F. Evaluation of PTR-ToF-MS as a tool to track the behavior of hop-derived compounds during the fermentation of beer. *Food Res. Int.* **2018**, *111*, 582–589. [CrossRef]
123. Machado, J.C.; Faria, M.A.; Melo, A.; Martins, Z.E.; Ferreira, I.M.P.L.V.O. Modeling of α-acids and xanthohumol extraction in dry-hopped beers. *Food Chem.* **2019**, *278*, 216–222. [CrossRef]
124. Dysvik, A.; La Rosa, S.L.; De Rouck, G.; Rukke, E.-O.; Westereng, B.; Wicklund, T. Microbial Dynamics in Traditional and Modern Sour Beer Production. *Appl. Environ. Microbiol.* **2020**, *86*. [CrossRef]
125. Vaughan, A.; O'Sullivan, T.; Van Sinderen, D. Enhancing the microbiological stability of malt and beer—A review. *J. Inst. Brew.* **2005**, *111*, 355–371. [CrossRef]
126. Sakamoto, K.; Konings, W.N. Beer spoilage bacteria and hop resistance. *Int. J. Food Microbiol.* **2003**, *89*, 105–124. [CrossRef]
127. Morgavi, D.P.; Boudra, H.; Jouany, J.P.; Michalet-Doreau, T.F.B. Effect and stability of gliotoxin, an *Aspergillus fumigatus* toxin, on in vitro rumen fermentation. *Food Addit. Contam.* **2004**, *21*, 871–878. [CrossRef]
128. Suiker, I.M.; Wösten, H.A. Spoilage yeasts in beer and beer products. *Curr. Opin. Food Sci.* **2022**, *44*, 100815. [CrossRef]
129. Michel, M.; Meier-Dörnberg, T.; Jacob, F.; Methner, F.; Wagner, R.S.; Hutzler, M. Review: Pure non-Saccharomyces starter cultures for beer fermentation with a focus on secondary metabolites and practical applications. *J. Inst. Brew.* **2016**, *122*, 569–587. [CrossRef]
130. Kheir, J.; Salameh, D.; Strehaiano, P.; Brandam, C.; Lteif, R. Impact of volatile phenols and their precursors on wine quality and control measures of Brettanomyces/Dekkera yeasts. *Eur. Food Res. Technol.* **2013**, *237*, 655–671. [CrossRef]
131. Priest, F.; Campbell, I. *Brewing Microbiology*; Priest, F., Campbell, I., Eds.; Springer: New York, NY, USA, 2003.
132. Hutzler, M.; Riedl, R.; Koob, J.; Jacob, F. Fermentation and spoilage yeasts and their relevance for the beverage industry. *Brew. Sci.* **2012**, *65*, 33–52.
133. Basso, R.F.; Alcarde, A.R.; Portugal, C.B. Could non-Saccharomyces yeasts contribute on innovative brewing fermentations? *Food Res. Int.* **2016**, *86*, 112–120. [CrossRef]
134. Stewart, G. Butyric Acid. In *The Oxford Companion to Beer*; Oliver, G., Ed.; Oxford University Press: Oxford, UK, 2012.
135. Brožová, M.; Kubizniaková, P.; Matoulková, D. Brewing microbiology-bacteria of the genus Clostridium. *Kvas. Prum.* **2018**, *64*, 242–247. [CrossRef]
136. Chou, C.H.; Liu, C.W.; Yang, D.J.; Wu, Y.H.S.; Chen, Y.C. Amino acid, mineral, and polyphenolic profiles of black vinegar, and its lipid lowering and antioxidant effects in vivo. *Food Chem.* **2015**, *168*, 63–69. [CrossRef]
137. Liu, J.; Li, L.; Peters, B.M.; Li, B.; Deng, Y.; Xu, Z.; Shirtliff, M.E. Draft genome sequence and annotation of *Lactobacillus acetotolerans* BM-LA14527, a beer-spoilage bacteria. *FEMS Microbiol. Lett.* **2016**, *363*, fnw201. [CrossRef]
138. Liu, J.; Li, L.; Li, B.; Peters, B.M.; Deng, Y.; Xu, Z.; Shirtliff, M.E. First study on the formation and resuscitation of viable but nonculturable state and beer spoilage capability of *Lactobacillus lindneri*. *Microb. Pathog.* **2017**, *107*, 219–224. [CrossRef]
139. Liu, J.; Li, L.; Peters, B.M.; Li, B.; Chen, L.; Deng, Y.; Xu, Z.; Shirtliff, M.E. The viable but nonculturable state induction and genomic analyses of *Lactobacillus casei* BM-LC14617, a beer-spoilage bacterium. *Microbiologyopen* **2017**, *6*, e00506. [CrossRef]
140. Liu, J.; Li, L.; Li, B.; Peters, B.M.; Deng, Y.; Xu, Z.; Shirtliff, M.E. Study on spoilage capability and VBNC state formation and recovery of *Lactobacillus plantarum*. *Microb. Pathog.* **2017**, *110*, 257–261. [CrossRef]
141. Paradh, A.D. Gram-negative spoilage bacteria in brewing. In *Brewing Microbiology*; Elsevier: Amsterdam, The Netherlands, 2015; Volume 5, pp. 175–194. ISBN 9781782423317.
142. Bradfield, M.F.A.; Mohagheghi, A.; Salvachúa, D.; Smith, H.; Black, B.A.; Dowe, N.; Beckham, G.T.; Nicol, W. Continuous succinic acid production by *Actinobacillus succinogenes* on xylose-enriched hydrolysate. *Biotechnol. Biofuels* **2015**, *8*, 181. [CrossRef] [PubMed]

143. Lermusieau, G.; Noël, S.; Liégeois, C.; Collin, S. Nonoxidative mechanism for development of trans-2-nonenal in beer. *J. Am. Soc. Brew. Chem.* **1999**, *57*, 29–33. [CrossRef]
144. Ferreira, C.S.; Bodart, E.; Collin, S. Why craft brewers should be advised to use bottle refermentation to improve late-hopped beer stability. *Beverages* **2019**, *5*, 39. [CrossRef]
145. Spedding, G.; Aiken, T. Sensory analysis as a tool for beer quality assessment with an emphasis on its use for microbial control in the brewery. In *Brewing Microbiology. Managing Microbes, Ensuring Quality and Valorising Waste*; Elsevier: Amsterdam, The Netherlands, 2015; pp. 375–404.
146. Bongaerts, D.; De Roos, J.; De Vuyst, L. Technological and Environmental Features Determine the Uniqueness of the Lambic Beer Microbiota and Production Process. *Appl. Environ. Microbiol.* **2021**, *87*, e00612-21. [CrossRef]
147. De Roos, J.; Verce, M.; Weckx, S.; De Vuyst, L. Temporal Shotgun Metagenomics Revealed the Potential Metabolic Capabilities of Specific Microorganisms during Lambic Beer Production. *Front. Microbiol.* **2020**, *11*, 1692. [CrossRef]
148. Yu, Z.; Luo, Q.; Xiao, L.; Sun, Y.; Li, R.; Sun, Z.; Li, X. Beer-spoilage characteristics of Staphylococcus xylosus newly isolated from craft beer and its potential to influence beer quality. *Food Sci. Nutr.* **2019**, *7*, 3950–3957. [CrossRef]
149. Nobis, A.; Kwasnicki, M.; Lehnhardt, F.; Hellwig, M.; Henle, T.; Becker, T.; Gastl, M. A Comprehensive Evaluation of Flavor Instability of Beer (Part 2): The Influence of De Novo Formation of Aging Aldehydes. *Foods* **2021**, *10*, 2668. [CrossRef]
150. Mikyška, A.; Jurková, M.; Horák, T.; Slabý, M. Study of the influence of hop polyphenols on the sensory stability of lager beer. *Eur. Food Res. Technol.* **2022**, *248*, 533–542. [CrossRef]
151. de Oliveira Gomes, F.; Guimaraes, B.P.; Ceola, D.; Ghesti, G.F. Advances in dry hopping for industrial brewing: A review. *Food Sci. Technol.* **2021**, 2061. [CrossRef]
152. McGarrity, M.J.; McRoberts, C.; Fitzpatrick, M. Identification, Cause, and Prevention of Musty Off-Flavors in Beer. *MBAA Tech. Q.* **2003**, *40*, 44–47.
153. Štulíková, K.; Novák, J.; Vlček, J.; Šavel, J.; Košin, P.; Dostálek, P. Bottle Conditioning: Technology and Mechanisms Applied in Refermented Beers. *Beverages* **2020**, *6*, 56. [CrossRef]
154. Sakamoto, K.; Van Veen, H.W.; Saito, H.; Kobayashi, H.; Konings, W.N. Membrane-bound ATPase contributes to hop resistance of *Lactobacillus brevis*. *Appl. Environ. Microbiol.* **2002**, *68*, 5374–5378. [CrossRef]
155. Hammond, J.; Brennan, M.; Price, A. The control of microbial spoilage of beer. *J. Inst. Brew.* **1999**, *105*, 113–120. [CrossRef]
156. de Francesco, G.; Bravi, E.; Sanarica, E.; Marconi, O.; Cappelletti, F.; Perretti, G. Effect of Addition of Different Phenolic-Rich Extracts on Beer Flavour Stability. *Foods* **2020**, *9*, 1638. [CrossRef]
157. Chatonnet, P.; Bonnet, S.; Boutou, S.; Labadie, M.D. Identification and Responsibility of 2,4,6-Tribromoanisole in Musty, Corked Odors in Wine. *J. Agric. Food Chem.* **2004**, *52*, 1255–1262. [CrossRef]

MDPI AG
Grosspeteranlage 5
4052 Basel
Switzerland
Tel.: +41 61 683 77 34

Foods Editorial Office
E-mail: foods@mdpi.com
www.mdpi.com/journal/foods

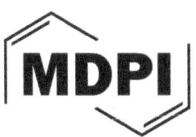

Disclaimer/Publisher's Note: The title and front matter of this reprint are at the discretion of the Guest Editors. The publisher is not responsible for their content or any associated concerns. The statements, opinions and data contained in all individual articles are solely those of the individual Editors and contributors and not of MDPI. MDPI disclaims responsibility for any injury to people or property resulting from any ideas, methods, instructions or products referred to in the content.

www.ingramcontent.com/pod-product-compliance
Lightning Source LLC
LaVergne TN
LVHW072335090526
838202LV00019B/2421